Global Applications of Indian Psychology:

Therapeutic and Strategic Models

Anuradha Sathiyaseelan
Christ University, India

Sathiyaseelan Balasundaram
Christ University, India

IGI Global
PUBLISHER of TIMELY KNOWLEDGE

A volume in the Advances in Psychology, Mental Health, and Behavioral Studies (APMHBS) Book Series

Published in the United States of America by
IGI Global
Information Science Reference (an imprint of IGI Global)
701 E. Chocolate Avenue
Hershey PA, USA 17033
Tel: 717-533-8845
Fax: 717-533-8661
E-mail: cust@igi-global.com
Web site: http://www.igi-global.com

Library of Congress Cataloging-in-Publication Data

Names: Sathiyaseelan, Anuradha, 1971- editor. | Balasundaram, Sathiyaseelan, 1968- editor.
Title: Global applications of Indian psychology : therapeutic and strategic models / edited by Anuradha Sathiyaseelan, Sathiyaseelan Balasundaram.
Description: Hershey, PA : Information Science Reference, [2024] | Includes bibliographical references and index. | Summary: "The book provides an interdisciplinary lens in viewing Indian Psychology and its application with multiple disciplines"-- Provided by publisher.
Identifiers: LCCN 2023038675 (print) | LCCN 2023038676 (ebook) | ISBN 9781668497784 (hardcover) | ISBN 9781668497791 (ebook)
Subjects: LCSH: Psychology--Religious aspects--Hinduism. | Psychology--India. | Psychology, Applied. | Hinduism--Psychology.
Classification: LCC BL1215.P87 G56 2024 (print) | LCC BL1215.P87 (ebook) | DDC 155.8/954--dc23/eng/20231031
LC record available at https://lccn.loc.gov/2023038675
LC ebook record available at https://lccn.loc.gov/2023038676

This book is published in the IGI Global book series Advances in Psychology, Mental Health, and Behavioral Studies (APMHBS) (ISSN: 2475-6660; eISSN: 2475-6679)

British Cataloguing in Publication Data
A Cataloguing in Publication record for this book is available from the British Library.

All work contributed to this book is new, previously-unpublished material. The views expressed in this book are those of the authors, but not necessarily of the publisher.

For electronic access to this publication, please contact: eresources@igi-global.com.

Advances in Psychology, Mental Health, and Behavioral Studies (APMHBS) Book Series

Harish C. Chandan
Argosy University, USA
Bryan Christiansen
Southern New Hampshire University, USA

ISSN:2475-6660
EISSN:2475-6679

Mission

The complexity of the human mind has puzzled researchers and physicians for centuries. While widely studied, the brain still remains largely misunderstood.

The **Advances in Psychology, Mental Health, and Behavioral Studies (APMHBS)** book series presents comprehensive research publications focusing on topics relating to the human psyche, cognition, psychiatric care, mental and developmental disorders, as well as human behavior and interaction. Featuring diverse and innovative research, publications within APMHBS are ideally designed for use by mental health professionals, academicians, researchers, and upper-level students.

Coverage

- Human Behavior
- Emotional Health
- Cognition
- Counseling & Therapy
- Treatment & Care
- Developmental Disorders
- Personality Disorders
- Eating Disorders
- Trauma & Stress
- Anxiety

IGI Global is currently accepting manuscripts for publication within this series. To submit a proposal for a volume in this series, please contact our Acquisition Editors at Acquisitions@igi-global.com or visit: http://www.igi-global.com/publish/.

The Advances in Psychology, Mental Health, and Behavioral Studies (APMHBS) Book Series (ISSN 2475-6660) is published by IGI Global, 701 E. Chocolate Avenue, Hershey, PA 17033-1240, USA, www.igi-global.com. This series is composed of titles available for purchase individually; each title is edited to be contextually exclusive from any other title within the series. For pricing and ordering information please visit http://www.igi-global.com/book-series/advances-psychology-mental-health-behavioral/110200. Postmaster: Send all address changes to above address.

Titles in this Series

For a list of additional titles in this series, please visit: www.igi-global.com/book-series

Stabilization Approaches That Empower Clients Through Mental Health Crises
Isabel Logan (Southern Connecticut State University, USA) and Cheryl A. Green (Yale New Haven Health-Bridgeport Hospital, USA & Abilene Christian University, USA)
Medical Information Science Reference • copyright 2023 • 202pp • H/C (ISBN: 9781799882282) • US $360.00 (our price)

Modern Perspectives and Current Trends in Asian Education, Psychology, and Sociology
Pannee Suanpang (Suan Dusit University, Thailand)
Information Science Reference • copyright 2023 • 295pp • H/C (ISBN: 9781668473757) • US $240.00 (our price)

Developmental Language Disorders in Childhood and Adolescence
Dimitra V. Katsarou (University of the Aegean, Greece)
Information Science Reference • copyright 2023 • 436pp • H/C (ISBN: 9798369306444) • US $230.00 (our price)

Changing the Stigma of Mental Health Among African Americans Moving From Denial to Acceptance
LaVelle Hendricks (Texas A&M University, Commerce, USA) and Dimitra Smith (Texas A&M University, Commerce, USA)
Information Science Reference • copyright 2023 • 367pp • H/C (ISBN: 9781668489185) • US $240.00 (our price)

Facilitating Social Justice, Service Delivery, and Advocacy Through Multicultural Counseling Competencies
Keith B. Wilson (University of Kentucky, USA) and Si-Yi Chao (University of Kentucky, USA)
Information Science Reference • copyright 2023 • 369pp • H/C (ISBN: 9781668461556) • US $215.00 (our price)

Combining Exercise and Psychotherapy to Treat Mental Health
Lara Carneiro (United Arab Emirates University, UAE) and Felipe Schuch (Universidade Federal de Santa Maria, Brazil)
Medical Information Science Reference • copyright 2024 • 300pp • H/C (ISBN: 9781668460405) • US $325.00 (our price)

Exploring the Benefit of Creative Arts Therapies for Children, Adolescents, and Adults
Nava R. Silton (Marymount Manhattan College, USA)
Information Science Reference • copyright 2023 • 293pp • H/C (ISBN: 9781668478561) • US $215.00 (our price)

Perspectives and Considerations on Navigating the Mental Healthcare System
Susan Van Alstyne (Centenary University, USA)

IGI Global
PUBLISHER of TIMELY KNOWLEDGE

701 East Chocolate Avenue, Hershey, PA 17033, USA
Tel: 717-533-8845 x100 • Fax: 717-533-8661
E-Mail: cust@igi-global.com • www.igi-global.com

The book is dedicated to the ancient sages, scholars, and practitioners whose timeless wisdom and profound insights continue to inspire and guide us. It is an homage to the rich traditions of Indian psychology and philosophy that have contributed to the understanding of the human mind, consciousness, and behavior. We are grateful to those who have preserved and transmitted this valuable knowledge throughout the ages. They have contributed to the global exploration of Indian psychology by providing a unique perspective that enriches the field of contemporary psychology. We dedicate this book to all those who seek knowledge, promote diversity of thought, and strive to improve the well-being of others.

Table of Contents

Detailed Table of Contents

theoretical lens based on 'practical rationality,' which can substantiate the use of qualitative methods for collecting data on mindfulness and help develop a higher orientation of experience among individuals. The authors concluded that mindfulness is an individual-level process that workplace factors and systems can influence. In addition, the purpose of initiating mindfulness should not be towards more 'hedonic' reasons like stress management. Instead, the purpose should be more 'eudemonic.'

Indian psychology is characterized by its diverse and rich traditions that have evolved over several centuries. This chapter tries to fulfill four objectives: 1) To provide a brief overview of the concept of self in Bhagavad Gita; 2) to give a brief overview of the two frameworks for moksha given in the Bhagavad Gita with the help of empirical evidence of current research; 3) to propose a conceptual model using Triguna Framework and Trimarg Framework; and 4) to provide the implications of the proposed model. The chapter begins with an explanation of the Indian philosophical understanding of self from the lens of Bhagavad Gita. In the second section, an effort has been made to compare and contrast the two frameworks given in Bhagavad Gita for Moksha. The last section introduces a conceptual model to enhance sattva guna and reduce the rajas and tamas gunas to attain atmabodha that can have positive psychological implications in modern times.

Spiritual leadership is a holistic leadership approach through which organizational members can experience their connection with their spiritual realities. With the help of spiritual leadership, employees can find the inner motivation to show the necessary altruism to serve for the common good and vision. Thus, they find the opportunity to experience meaning in their workplace. This study has focused on spiritual leadership and its possible effects on person-organization fit and turnover intentions among Turkish academicians. Moreover, in this study, the mediator effect of person-organization fit in the relationship between spiritual leadership and turnover intentions has been examined. The research model has been investigated among academicians from various Turkish universities. In the related field research, 190 usable surveys were obtained, and the research data has been examined in SPSS 20. Results showed spiritual leadership has a negative effect on turnover intentions and person-organization fit acts as a mediator in this relationship.

In the new millennium, therapies of Indian psychology have gained renewed interest as a distinct and holistic approach to understanding the mind and human behavior. The essence of psychotherapy existed in India since time immemorial submerged in social structures, religion, ancient scriptures, mystics,

Foreword

॥ यस्तु सर्वाणि भूतान्यात्मन्येवानुपश्यति। सर्वभूतेषु चात्मानं ततो न विजुगुप्सते ॥

"There is but one Self, and that is present in all beings; he who sees all beings in the Self, and the Self in all beings, he never turns away in hatred."

- Isa Upanishad, Verse 6

With these timeless words, we embark on a scholarly journey through the captivating pages of *Global Applications of Indian Psychology: Therapeutic and Strategic Models*. This ancient wisdom encapsulates the very essence of interconnectedness and unity, echoing a universal truth that resonates with the very heart of our academic exploration.In a global context, interconnectedness can be applied to foster a sense of global citizenship and solidarity. It encourages people to recognize that they are part of a larger whole, connected to all living beings and the planet. This philosophy can inspire efforts in global cooperation, environmental sustainability, and cross-cultural understanding.

At Christ (Deemed to be University), we have always been committed to upholding the torch of interdisciplinary education, seamlessly bridging the spiritual and the empirical, the traditional and the contemporary. This book stands as a testament to our enduring commitment to unveil the hidden treasures of Indian psychology and facilitate their dissemination across the world.

Within the pages of this compendium, distinguished authors embark on a captivating voyage through the intricate realms of yoga, meditation, Ayurveda, and other ancient practices. These practices have gained international recognition for their benefits in promoting mental and physical well-being. These practices are now used globally as tools for stress management, health improvement, and mental health support.They unveil the therapeutic and strategic relevance of these age-old traditions in today's complex world. Each contribution is a unique prism, refracting the brilliance of Indian psychology into various fields, from enhancing mental health to fostering visionary leadership, from reimagining education to facilitating conflict resolution.

Moreover, interdisciplinary education, as emphasized in this book, is crucial in the global context. It allows individuals to draw from various fields and traditions, including spiritual and empirical knowledge, to address complex global challenges. The fusion of traditional wisdom and contemporary knowledge can lead to innovative solutions for issues like climate change, healthcare, and social justice.

The synergy of scholarly creativity and academic rigor in this compendium invites us to transcend the boundaries of conventional knowledge. The wisdom encapsulated within these pages promises not only to deepen our understanding of the human psyche but also to redefine our approach to the pressing challenges of our age. Applying Indian psychology in a global forum encourages individuals and scholars to think outside the box and explore innovative approaches to complex problems. This mindset is essential in addressing global challenges where conventional solutions may fall short. It promotes creativity, critical thinking, and adaptability on a global scale.

Global Applications of Indian Psychology: Therapeutic and Strategic Models is more than just a book; it is a captivating intellectual odyssey. We wholeheartedly encourage the readers to immerse themselves in the profound wisdom of these pages, where they will discover the enduring principles of Indian psychology and how they can reshape their worldview and personal growth.

In the spirit of academic enlightenment, creative inquiry, and global synergy, I extend my heartfelt welcome as we embark on this transformative journey through the profound realms of Indian psychology. May this book catalyze wisdom and unity, embodying the undying spirit of the Isa Upanishad, emphasizing the universality of the wisdom found in Indian psychology, and encouraging a sense of unity and shared purpose among people of diverse backgrounds.

In closing, as we embark on this transformative journey through the profound realms of Indian psychology, let us remember that the wisdom contained within these pages is not bound by borders or confined by time. It is a treasure trove of knowledge and insights that have the power to transcend cultural, geographical, and temporal constraints. We encourage the readers to embrace this intellectual odyssey and allow it to be a source of inspiration and guidance in their personal and professional lives. May the enduring principles of Indian psychology continue to light the path toward a more harmonious, interconnected, and enlightened world for all. With great anticipation and gratitude for their participation, we invite them to join us in exploring the rich tapestry of Indian psychology's global applications.

With great anticipation and intellectual enthusiasm,

Fr Joseph CC
Christ University, India

Preface

In contemporary psychological research and practice, *Global Applications of Indian Psychology: Therapeutic and Strategic Models* represents a profound exploration of the therapeutic and strategic models derived from Indian traditions. The book provides an overview of the application of Indian psychological principles in a global context, addressing various aspects of personal development, strategic decision-making, and well-being. There is no doubt that the Indian philosophy of psychology, which is deeply rooted in ancient texts and theories such as Yoga, Ayurveda, Vedanta, and Buddhist psychology, offers a unique perspective with regard to understanding the human mind, consciousness, and behavior. Throughout this text, readers will gain a thorough understanding of these age-old traditions and their relevance and applicability to modern life. The book presents a scientific examination of the principles and practices of Indian psychology in a global context. As a bridge between traditional Indian knowledge systems and the contemporary academic and scientific discourse, this book offers a unique perspective. By combining ancient wisdom with modern scientific methodologies, the book aims to provide readers with an in-depth exploration of the therapeutic and strategic applications of Indian psychology.

With the scientific community increasingly recognizing the value of integrating diverse perspectives in psychology, the purpose of this book is to contribute to the ongoing discussion by highlighting the unique insights and methodologies that Indian psychology brings to the table. In adopting a global perspective, we address the urgent need to explore alternative models for psychological well-being and strategic decision-making. In order to become familiar with the dynamics of Indian Psychological principles in our daily lives, the book encompasses scholars, researchers, practitioners, and students from several related fields in addition to psychology. This book can be used by both experienced professionals and students who are just embarking on their academic journeys. It provides insights and practical applications that cater to a wide range of interests and levels of expertise. The book demonstrates the ever-evolving landscape of psychology and the importance of embracing a variety of perspectives as part of the pursuit of knowledge.

Chapter 1, "Indian Psychology: Challenges, Strategies, and Prospects in Education," introduces the reader to the challenges and opportunities in the field of Indian psychology. It highlights the erosion of India's rich psychological heritage due to westernization and globalization. The chapter points out the biases within society and the educational system that have hindered the recognition and dissemination of Indian psychology. It emphasizes the need for rigorous research to substantiate the contributions of Indian psychology in understanding human cognition, behavior, and consciousness. The chapter advocates for dispelling misconceptions and fostering awareness to promote Indian psychology as a respected field. Collaboration and increased research are suggested as ways for Indian psychology to claim its rightful place within the global academic community.

Chapter 2, "An Overview of Mindfulness Based on Practical Rationality," describes the concept of mindfulness, emphasizing the need for a deeper understanding beyond quantitative methods. It connects mindfulness with various theories, such as trait activation theory and broad and build theory, providing a theoretical lens based on "practical rationality." The chapter suggests the use of qualitative methods for collecting data on mindfulness to enhance the individual's experience. It advocates a shift from "hedonic" reasons to "eudemonic" ones for practicing mindfulness. By offering a novel perspective on mindfulness, the chapter contributes to more effective and holistic applications of mindfulness in various contexts.

Chapter 3, "Atman's Awakening: Bhagavad Gita's Path to Moksha Through Karma Yoga and Atma-bodha," explores the rich tradition of Indian psychology by focusing on the Bhagavad Gita. It aims to provide a brief overview of the concept of self in the Bhagavad Gita, two frameworks for moksha, and a proposed conceptual model using empirical evidence. The chapter connects ancient wisdom with modern research to highlight the enduring relevance of Indian psychology. By discussing the implications of the proposed model, it contributes to a deeper understanding of mental well-being and consciousness, using the Bhagavad Gita as a foundational text.

Chapter 4, "Effect of Spiritual Leadership on Intention to Quit: Mediator Effect of Person-Organization Fit," explores the holistic approach of spiritual leadership in the context of Turkish academicians. It explores how spiritual leadership can positively impact turnover intentions and the mediating role of person-organization fit. The research model is examined among academicians from various Turkish universities. By demonstrating the negative effect of spiritual leadership on turnover intentions and the significance of person-organization fit as a mediator, the chapter provides insights into the practical implications of spiritual leadership in the workplace. It underscores the importance of finding inner motivation and meaning in work, ultimately contributing to a more profound understanding of leadership in a spiritual context.

Chapter 5, "Existence of Therapeutic Techniques in Indian Psychology," reflects on the renewed interest in therapeutic techniques rooted in Indian psychology. It acknowledges the existence of psychotherapeutic elements in India for centuries, submerged in various traditions. The popularity of Indian psychology in the West, driven by practices like mindfulness and meditation, is highlighted. The chapter emphasizes that Indian psychology is not a substitute for modern evidence-based approaches to mental health care but offers a unique perspective on understanding mental well-being. By bridging ancient traditions with contemporary practices, it contributes to a holistic understanding of mental health.

Chapter 6, "From Ancient Wisdom to Modern Science: Indian Psychology for the Modern Age," explores the traditional significance of psychology, yoga, and Ayurveda in India and their continued relevance in contemporary times. It discusses the global recognition of these disciplines for their holistic approach to well-being. The chapter helps understand psychological problems and remedies through the practices of yoga and Ayurveda. It aims to provide valuable insights for students, corporate professionals, scholars, and researchers, promoting the integration of Indian wisdom in modern life.

Chapter 7, "Holistic Approach as a Strategy for Special Education in India," addresses the challenges of special education in India, emphasizing the need for a holistic approach that considers regional adaptations and multidisciplinary methods. It traces the roots of Indian philosophical perspectives in education and offers a framework for effective assessment. The chapter has important implications for improving education and assessment practices, especially for individuals with hidden disabilities like learning disabilities.

Chapter 8, "Interconnections of Yogic Practices With Mental Health," explores the holistic impact of various yogic practices on mental health, including pranayama, pratyahara, and others. It contextualizes these practices within the biopsychosocial model, highlighting their potential to enhance well-being. The cost-effectiveness and absence of side effects compared to pharmacological treatments make yoga an attractive adjunctive therapeutic agent. The chapter promotes the use of yoga as a complementary form of treatment to improve biopsychosocial well-being, provided that properly trained professionals are involved.

Chapter 9, "Mahabharata Immersion: The Praxis of Antaranga Sadhana – A Pathway to Personal Transformation," describes the Mahabharata Immersion (MI) process, a unique approach to personal transformation and introspection. It focuses on the introspective practices that lead to meditative witnessing of inner processes. Participants in MI write reflective journals on their experiences, which form the basis for understanding inner transformation and self-reflection. The chapter offers a comprehensive understanding of the MI process and its potential to facilitate personal growth and self-awareness.

Chapter 10, "Management Practices on Execution Effectiveness of Strategies Based on Thirukkural," focuses on management skills based on the principles found in Thirukkural, particularly the chapters on execution focus and mode of execution. It emphasizes the importance of execution in constructing effective strategies and sustaining team motivation. The chapter provides valuable insights for management professionals seeking guidance from ancient wisdom to improve their strategic execution.

Chapter 11, "Mindfulness-Based Interventions: Applications in Western and Indian Psychology," provides a comprehensive examination of Mindfulness-Based Interventions (MBIs) in both Western and Indian psychology. It discusses the efficacy of MBIs and their applications in diverse cultural contexts. By emphasizing cultural sensitivity and inclusiveness, it offers insights for psychological practice and future research, demonstrating the potential of MBIs to improve well-being and reduce psychological distress.

Chapter 12, "Spiritual Intelligence and Srimad Bhagavad Gita," explores the teachings of Srimad Bhagavad Gita and offers a unique perspective on human behavior and suffering. It analyzes Chapter 2, focusing on dualistic realism and the concept of "Sthitaprajnasamadhistsa" or "state of Steady Intelligence." The chapter sheds light on the potential for individuals to attain a state of permanent happiness and provides an alternative viewpoint to understand human experiences.

Chapter 13, "The Concept of Mindfulness: Perspectives From Major Religions Practiced in India," examines mindfulness through the lens of various religions practiced in India. It provides a framework for individuals to integrate mindfulness principles from their religious scriptures into their daily lives, addressing psychological issues. The chapter has significance for religious practitioners, managers, therapists, and researchers in the field of Indian psychology, offering a multi-religious perspective on mindfulness.

Chapter 14, "The Power of Words: Daily Life Practices Incorporating Teachings From Indian Psychology," explores the transformative potential of language, drawing from Indian philosophies like Sabda Sakti and the concept of "Shabda Brahman." It delves into the therapeutic impact of positive language and its influence on cognitive processes, self-perception, and relationships. The chapter highlights the interconnectedness of language and psychology, offering insights for daily practices and well-being.

Chapter 15, "Therapeutic Potential of Ayurvedic Practices for Mental Health of Geriatric Population: A Personalized Ayurvedic Protocol," addresses the growing issue of mental disorders among the elderly and presents a personalized model based on Ayurvedic principles. It offers a practical framework for maintaining the mental health of the geriatric population through dietary and lifestyle modifications, Rasayana drugs, and Panchakarma procedures. The chapter has implications for healthcare professionals and policymakers seeking effective approaches to address mental health challenges in aging populations.

The book *Global Applications of Indian Psychology: Therapeutic and Strategic Models* provides a unique perspective on understanding the human mind, consciousness, and behavior. Bringing together ancient Indian wisdom and modern scientific methodologies, it has the potential to enhance the landscape of contemporary psychology. The book addresses the urgent need to integrate diverse perspectives and alternative models to improve psychological well-being and make strategic decisions. There is an emphasis on the valuable insights and methodologies that Indian psychology brings to the global discourse on psychology. Readers will gain a comprehensive understanding of Indian psychological traditions, their relevance, and their applicability to modern life through the chapters presented in this book. With the scientific community increasingly recognising the importance of diverse viewpoints, this book stands as a testament to the ongoing discussions in the field of psychology. It provides a forum for scholars, researchers, practitioners, and students in various related fields to explore the therapeutic and strategic applications of Indian psychology. By examining these applications in detail, the book contributes to the expansion of psychological knowledge.

In addition to providing insights and practical applications tailored to a wide range of interests and expertise levels, this book serves as a valuable resource for both professionals and students embarking on their academic journeys. This book highlights the ever-evolving nature of psychology and the significance of embracing multiple perspectives in the pursuit of knowledge. As a whole, the book is poised to contribute to the field, providing a holistic and culturally enriched approach to understanding human behavior and well-being. As part of the growing body of literature that recognizes the importance of traditional knowledge systems in the modern world, it encourages a deeper exploration and integration of these valuable insights into psychological practice and research.

Anuradha Sathiyaseelan
Christ University, India

Sathiyaseelan Balasundaram
Christ University, India

Acknowledgment

We express our heartfelt gratitude to all those who have contributed to the realization of this book, "Global Applications of Indian Psychology: Therapeutic and Strategic Model." This project has been a collective endeavor, and we are deeply appreciative of the support, insights, and dedication that have made it possible. We are immensely thankful to our colleagues, researchers, and scholars from diverse fields who have shared their expertise, perspectives, and knowledge to enrich the content of this book. Your contributions have added depth and breadth to our understanding of Indian psychology.

We would also like to acknowledge and thankful to Dr Rama Raju (Emeritus Professor and Retired HoD – Jyoti Nivas Collage, India), Dr. Soumya RR (Assistant Professor – Christ University, India), Dr. Maryanne Pais (Assistant Professor and HoD – St. Joseph's College of Commerce, India), Ms Roseline Gomes (Assistant Professor and Head – Jyoti Nivas College, India), Dr. Anita Mary Vadivel (Assistant Professor – Vidyashilp University, India), Dr Rekha Ahuja (Assistant Professor and HoD- St. Joseph's evening College, India), Dr. Satheesh Varma (Assistant Professor – Chinmaya Vishwa Vidyapeeth, India), Dr. Maxim Pereira (Associate Professor – Sampurna Montfort College, India), Dr. Maya Rathnasabapathy (Professor and Head – VIT- Chennai, India), Dr. Deviga Subramani (Assistant Professor – Christ University, India), Dr. Sreeja Gangadharan (Assistant Professor – Christ University, India), Dr Vijay M (Assistant Professor – Christ University, India), and Ms. Malvika Parakh (Junior Research Fellow – Christ University, India) for critically reviewing different book chapters.

We would like to acknowledge the continuous support from Dr Fr Jose CC, the Vice Chancellor of CHRIST (Deemed to be University), India, for providing the conducive environment and resources that facilitated the creation of this book. To our families and friends, who have stood by us with unwavering support and encouragement throughout this journey, we offer our heartfelt thanks. Their understanding and patience have been instrumental in the ability to undertake this project. Finally, to the readers and scholars who seek knowledge and inspiration from the pages of this book, we extend our warmest appreciation. The quest for understanding and the commitment to the exploration of diverse perspectives in psychology drive our shared pursuit of wisdom and well-being.

Chapter 1
Indian Psychology: Challenges, Strategies, and Prospects in Education

Anuradha Sathiyaseelan
https://orcid.org/0000-0001-6771-9413
Christ University, India

Sathiyaseelan Balasundaram
Christ University, India

Bishal Patangia
https://orcid.org/0000-0002-7693-3275
Christ University, India

R. R. Soumya
https://orcid.org/0000-0003-3808-8725
Christ University, India

ABSTRACT

Knowledge dissemination has been a hallmark of Indian tradition for millennia, particularly in the area of human biology and behavior. Westernization and globalization, however, have caused a gradual erosion of this rich heritage, resulting in waning interest among the populace. As a discipline, Indian Psychology faces a number of formidable challenges. The number of preconceived biases within society, the Westernized educational system, and the shortage of faculty with expertise in Indian psychology hinder the recognition and dissemination of the field. A dearth of research studies directly related to Indian psychology is also hindering its development and recognition. Emphasis was given on the importance of thorough research to substantiate its contributions to the understanding of human cognition, behavior, and consciousness. Promoting Indian psychology as an important and respected field requires dispelling misconceptions and fostering awareness. Through collaboration and increased research, Indian psychology can rightfully claim its place within the global academic community.

DOI: 10.4018/978-1-6684-9778-4.ch001

1. INTRODUCTION TO INDIAN PSYCHOLOGY

Psychology is a derivative of philosophy, and is now an amalgamation of numerous other disciplines. It is predominantly a western concept now. Not just because of its origins, but because of where the records lie or who writes them. Indian psychology means the ideas and approaches can be derived from the Indian culture and philosophies thousands of years back in India (Sharma, 2021). Ancient Indian scriptures have descriptions of cognition, perception, thinking, consciousness, and self-actualization. The Vedas and the Upanishads, dated back to 600 BC, have mentioned the above concepts with steps to achieve them (Sedlmeier & Srinivas, 2016).

Unfortunately, these scriptures have not been used to disseminate knowledge. Instead, it was handed down from the Guru (teacher) to the Sishya (disciple) by word of mouth, specifically to specific communities.. Hence most of the knowledge was lost (Sivananda, 1999). For any scientific discipline, what is remembered is what is taken down. Much history remains unknown to us because no documentation was maintained. What is left out is now understood by only a few people because (1) the language it is written in – Sanskrit, most of us are not trained in this language, and (2) modernization led us to the western world and its knowledge. More preference is given to western education by both students and their parents (Malviya, 2021). On the one hand, we can be proud that modernization and globalization are suitable for broader knowledge. Still, on the other hand, we should not discourage the knowledge of our ancestors and lose it (Mason & De la Torre, 2000).

The philosophies given by our ancestors have their roots in consciousness as well as yoga. Indian literature states how mental status has been examined thoroughly (Avasthi et al., 2013). It takes on a life-affirming worldview. It emphasizes spirituality and is therefore not restricted to individuals of Indian descent but can transcend across borders, encompassing all of humanity. 'Yoga' does not refer to the philosophical school or its subsets (such as *raja yoga* or *hatha yoga*). It refers to a conscious effort to be one with the Divine (Rao, 1979). The life-affirming spirituality entails one that is a force used to accept human nature and transcend reality for the Divine to manifest itself. This consciousness-based approach to psychology can make a significant contribution to psychology globally (Cornelissen, 2013). Its principles are being increasingly studied all across the world. The link between emotions, feelings and physiological reactions has been studied well and documented in the Ayurveda. In the past half-century, due to the efforts of the Indian Government and actions of the practitioners western world has accepted Ayurveda and its practices. More people are coming to India seeking Ayurveda treatment (Jaiswal & Williams, 2016).

After 1960 when humanistic psychology emerged in the western world, psychology readers started to pay more attention to the theories, methods, and approaches proposed and practiced by the Indians thousands of years back (CLAY, 2002). One idea had a significant role in linking modern Psychology to Indian traditions and early Indian philosophies – Maslow's theory about self-actualization and transcendental self-actualization. In his book, Abraham Maslow mentions the derivations of hierarchical need from the Pancha kosha concept (Heylighen, 1992). Pancha kosha is the basic five sheaths of human existence (Müller, 1879). Indian psychology became highly relevant after this. Some branches of Psychology that borrow at length from Indian writings are Parapsychology, Psychology of Religion and Transpersonal Psychology, Psychology of Mysticism, and Psychology of Consciousness. Psychology literature is now infused with terms such as Jain Psychology, Oriental Psychology, Yoga Psychology, and Buddhist Psychology, amongst others. These are indeed significant achievements for streams of Psychology that are not western. Publications in the field of Indian Psychology are indeed increasing, with more than 40 books having been published in the field. Attempts are undoubtedly being made to integrate Indian Psychology with modern Western Psychology (MATHEW, 2001). After all, psychology is constantly evolving, and new approaches to existing concepts are being taken up.

Euro-American norms for the last century have dominated the learning and teachings of Indian Psychology. In 1916, when Calcutta University set up the first Department of Psychology, it introduced its content and theories, which were considered universal, even though imported from the West. At the commencement of the century, psychologists in India focused on bringing up theories of sensation and perception from the classics. Once cognition began to be studied by Western psychologists, Indian psychologists too started examining it. Publications emerged, with Jadunath Sinha authoring a book on cognition in 1958. Moreover, in 1981, he published a book on Emotions and the Will, after modern Psychology began emphasizing emotions.

2. TEACHING AND LEARNING INDIAN PSYCHOLOGY

Teaching psychology in India can be challenging without the burden of highlighting Indian Psychology. Psychology is still associated with a lot of stigma and taboo. Students, who take it up, often enter the academic field holding many stereotypes and biases – some of which are not abolished even after formally studying the subject. When one thinks about psychology as a discipline, one does not usually think of Indian Psychology as a branch. Using the availability heuristic, we often associate Psychology with western scripts. It takes more time and effort to bring to surface records about Indian Psychology as opposed to other domains within the field. As such, this would also increase the challenges of teaching Indian Psychology. However, modern Western Psychology has been increasingly interested in Indian, Eastern, and Asian psychology, making them more known to the general population.

While the western notions of Psychology and Philosophy accentuate matter as the foundation, Indian Philosophy, on the other hand, stresses consciousness. This concept could be better integrated into the academic syllabi for students, thereby introducing them to Indian Psychology. Till now, the Western materialistic paradigm is what has dictated the teaching style and content practically all across the world. The mind is seen primarily as an instrument of cognition that divides, analyses, and synthesizes phenomena around us. However, with this view, the subtler layers of consciousness are often overlooked (Huppes, 2011). Another problem with teaching psychology in India is that one cannot easily access documents authored by Indian Psychologists. Today, research paper after paper has been published about a variety of topics within Psychology – but most of them by western authors. A student will not associate any Indian elements with Psychology if they are rarely exposed to any Indian psychological research. We almost only find Euro-American papers, and even amongst the Asian authors, Indians are hard to find!

When it comes to Indian Psychology, even those research papers published on the topic are not authored by too many Indians. Western researchers seem to be taking up more interest in Indian Psychology. Nevertheless, this does not mean there are no valuable researches authored by Indian researchers that provide insight into Indian Psychology (Dalal & Misra, 2010; Dalal, 2011; Manickam, 2008). Perhaps a bias exists in not seeing Indian Psychology as 'developed' enough, and they must fight against the misperception. Not enough coverage is given to the many accomplishments of Indian psychologists. Furthermore, thus, they, unfortunately, remain hidden in the shadows. Sometimes Indian Psychology is also viewed as religious babble. This is untrue. As mentioned earlier, even yoga is seen as a medium through which to get a better understanding of one's consciousness. It is not religious but is more spiritual. This perspective has its merits and may be able to connect with many individuals on a level that cognitive and behavioral approaches cannot.

Psychology has also been seen as external. The behaviorist paradigm has reigned supreme. The cognitive-behavioral approach is the most accurate or helpful today. Indian Psychology tends to look within. This is why consciousness is given so much emphasis. It is time to raise awareness about Indian Psychology and bust the myths that currently act as obstacles to its further progress. For this discipline to develop and grow, Indian Psychology should be viewed as equally important and relevant as other sub-fields within Psychology. Indians themselves should make more endeavors to bring focus to this discipline by conducting more research and publishing it. Indian Psychology will not be able to be taught well if the mindset the students come with is not favorable. For the Indian ethos that Indian Psychology contains to permeate into today's minds, they must find Indian Psychology to hold some value and meaning to them. This value, which indeed exists, must be made evident and public.

A student will not associate any Indian elements with Psychology if they are rarely exposed to any Indian psychological research. The educational board must consciously incorporate more Indian psychology topics into the curriculum of undergraduate and postgraduate psychology programs. At the same time, professors and students should try to liven up the classroom experience by bringing in instances closer to home. It is essential to be acquainted with a variety of viewpoints to achieve a better understanding of how a concept is being perceived. As learners of Psychology, it is necessary to remain open-minded. However, the subject of Indian Psychology emerged among students in recent years with significantly poor backgrounds due to a lack of enough information. As mentioned earlier, poor research finds and collaboration in Indian Psychology limits the knowledge, which is a significant challenge for students to be motivated enough to explore Indian Psychology. Further, very few universities in the country have any specific subject, such as Indian Psychology. As teaching itself is a challenge, studying Indian Psychology has become more complicated and needs more steps to be taken, making it easy for the student to identify and explore Indian Psychology. International students are more interested in how Indian tradition displays psychology than students in India. Various research papers are published authored by western investigators with fewer or no Indian investigators (Paranjpe, 2011). However, in the academic year 2019-20, a significant rise in international students enrolled in Indian universities for undergraduate and postgraduate (Aishe, 2021). An increase in the rate of international student enrollment in Indian colleges could significantly act as a way to deliver and collaborate with native researchers on the in-depth investigation of the psychological phenomenon with the integration of indigenous concepts of Indian Psychology.

Teaching-learning is a process. We cannot teach or learn anything in a day. Creating an environment with many opportunities will make this process efficient and likable. Indian Psychology must not be seen as inept or backward. Many of its core tenets are centuries old. Today, they must be adapted and engaged with modern findings. The seed for such an initiative is evident from the Government's initiatives on international Yoga day. Such initiatives promote and help in motivating academicians to explore more in the field of Indian Psychology.

3. CULTURAL BIAS IN PSYCHOLOGY

Addressing cultural bias in mainstream psychology is vital for creating an inclusive and representative field that accurately captures diverse human experiences (Pedersen, 2003). Cultural bias, characterized by favoring certain cultural groups over others, can result in incomplete or inaccurate understandings of behavior (Sayegh et al., 2023). This bias manifests in assumptions about cultural norms, values, and behaviors, along with the underrepresentation of certain cultural groups in research (Sayegh et al., 2023). One approach to tackle this bias is by enhancing cultural awareness, sensitivity, and humility in training and service delivery, challenging biases in assessment methods (Sayegh et al., 2023). Another strategy involves integrating diversity, equity, inclusion, and justice (DEIJ) issues in psychological assessment to reduce inequities caused by cultural bias (Sayegh et al., 2023). Recognizing the intersectionality of cultural bias with other forms of bias, such as gender and disability, is essential for a comprehensive understanding of human behavior (Olkin & Pledger, 2003; Pickar, 2008).

To effectively combat cultural bias, there is a need to promote diversity research in psychology, encouraging the inclusion of ethnic minority perspectives in research and increasing the representation of diverse researchers (Miranda & Gutter, 2002). Challenging cognitive biases that contribute to cultural bias is crucial, and reflective practice and supervision can aid psychologists in critically examining their biases (Schaffer & Rodolfa, 2020). Addressing cultural bias necessitates a multifaceted approach, including cultural awareness, DEIJ integration, diversity research promotion, and reflective practice, to foster inclusivity and accuracy in understanding human behavior.

The cultural bias present in mainstream psychology significantly influences the teaching and learning of Indian psychology, which encompasses unique cultural perspectives, values, and practices (Juntunen et al., 2001). Cultural bias, rooted in Western norms and values, may create a clash of cultures and cultural discontinuity for Indian students, implying that they should minimize their cultural identity to conform to mainstream expectations (Juntunen et al., 2001). This can lead to alienation and hinder the full engagement with and understanding of Indian psychology.

Furthermore, bias in curriculum content and teaching methodologies can perpetuate Western-centric views and marginalize Indian psychology, contributing to a limited understanding of its unique contributions (Gupta, 2015). The underrepresentation of Indian researchers in psychology further reinforces Western perspectives, hindering the development of culturally relevant theories.

To address these issues, cultural sensitivity should be promoted in teaching Indian psychology by integrating Indian philosophical and cultural perspectives into the curriculum (Gupta, 2015). Recognizing and valuing the unique contributions of Indian psychology can foster a more comprehensive understanding of human behavior grounded in cultural context. Increasing the representation of Indian researchers in psychology is also crucial, achieved through supporting Indian students in pursuing higher education and research, and fostering collaboration with Western psychologists (Juntunen et al., 2001).

Therefore, addressing cultural bias in mainstream psychology is essential for creating an inclusive field. This bias significantly impacts the teaching and learning of Indian psychology, emphasizing the need for cultural sensitivity, inclusivity, and increased representation of Indian perspectives.

4. COLONIAL INFLUENCE IN TEACHING INDIAN PSYCHOLOGY

Historical Context and Theoretical Underpinnings

There are persistent and indelible imprints of colonialism throughout the educational landscape of Indian psychology. This influence is deeply rooted in the historical crucible of British colonial rule, during which the contours of knowledge dissemination, particularly in the field of psychology, were profoundly altered (Sharma, 2006). This historical juncture is characterized by the entrenched privilege accorded to Western psychological theories and models within the academic edifice-a phenomenon that has persisted and grown in the post-colonial era (Daniels et al., 2011).

As a result of the development of Western psychological paradigms during colonial rule, a trajectory of sustained Western epistemological dominance was set in motion. This dominance, similar to an intellectual hegemony, has left an enduring legacy on the educational infrastructure of post-colonial India. Psychological education was designed from the ground up with Western frameworks taking precedence, creating a knowledge hierarchy that is now intrinsic to the disciplinary fabric of Indian psychology (Jabin et al., 2022).

The ascendancy of Western psychological theories is not merely an isolated occurrence, but rather a sign of a broader phenomenon, which is epistemological colonization. As a consequence of this process, indigenous and cultural perspectives, rooted in the deep historical and philosophical foundations of the Indian subcontinent, are being pushed to the margins of academic discourse. As a result of the overt privileging of Western paradigms, marginalization is not an accident, but rather the result of a complex interaction of power dynamics that perpetuates a knowledge hierarchy favoring Western epistemological frameworks (Hwang, 2004).

Indigenous epistemologies are marginalized within the educational milieu not simply as a consequence of intellectual predilections, but as a result of a more intricate and insidious narrative of the production and dissemination of knowledge. The deliberate relegation of indigenous and cultural perspectives underscores a structural bias ingrained within the educational apparatus, in which Western paradigms are upheld as normative, universal, and, by extension, more 'scientific'. Systemic biases produce epistemic subalternity in which indigenous ways of knowing are subjugated and positioned as an ancillary part of the purported universality of Western epistemologies (McCarty et al., 2005).

As a consequence, colonial influence remains a foundational bedrock for Indian psychology education, both in terms of curriculum and ethos. It is necessary to examine carefully and to undertake concerted efforts on behalf of decolonization if we are to perpetuate this knowledge hierarchy, which is often unacknowledged (Phiri et al., 2023). To foster a more inclusive and equitable pedagogical landscape within Indian psychology, it is imperative for educators to develop a nuanced understanding of the historical trajectory and mechanisms of colonial influence.

Pedagogical Modalities: Replication of Western Methodologies

Beyond the theoretical contours, the colonial legacy is evident in the methodological frameworks adopted for the dissemination of knowledge in Indian psychology education. Replication of Western pedagogical methodologies, rooted in didactic lectures, seminars, and examination-centric assessments, serves as a poignant example of the colonial legacy permeating the education system.

The traditional Western teaching methods of unidirectional transmission of knowledge from instructor to student have been seamlessly incorporated into the pedagogical landscape of Indian psychology. The integration of these two approaches, while ostensibly pragmatic, appears to be at odds with the intrinsic nature of Indian psychology, which is often characterized by an experiential and holistic approach. The didactic nature of these pedagogical methodologies tends to overlook the contextual richness of indigenous psychological phenomena, rendering them susceptible to oversimplification and misrepresentation (Avasthi et al., 2013).

While lecture-centric formats are pragmatic within certain educational paradigms, they inadvertently perpetuate a unidirectional flow of information. Consequently, it inhibits the development of critical perspectives among students and hinders their ability to engage in a nuanced exploration of culturally specific manifestations of psychological phenomena (Miller et al., 2013). In addition, the lack of space for interactive learning and experiential engagement limits the students' ability to develop a comprehensive understanding that transcends the confines of theoretical frameworks (Grassini, 2023).

In addition to merely disseminating information, the didactic approach has profound implications for identity and cultural narratives. Pedagogical modalities with inherent unidimensionality exacerbate students' estrangement from their cultural narratives. The rigid confines of a lecture-based paradigm prevent a nuanced understanding of Indian psychology that is deeply rooted in experiential and contextually embedded dimensions. This distances students from the rich and diverse cultural tapestry that should ideally aid their understanding of psychological phenomena within the context of India (Hoshmand, 2007; Wilson, 2007).

It is clear that the replication of Western pedagogical methodologies represents more than a pragmatic educational strategy; it reveals a profound disjunction between epistemology and culture. Inconsistencies between these methodologies' didactic approach and Indian psychology's inherently experiential and holistic nature point to a misalignment that impedes the development of a comprehensive understanding of indigenous psychological phenomena. To address this incongruity, it is necessary to reevaluate pedagogical practices in a way that embraces experiential learning and fosters an interactive engagement with Indian psychology's multifaceted dimensions. A transformative reorientation may lead to a decolonization of Indian psychology education, ushered in by a pedagogical ethos that is more culturally sensitive and inclusive.

Marginalization of Indigenous Perspectives: A Pedagogical Gap

Indigenous and cultural perspectives are profoundly marginalized and neglected in the teaching of Indian psychology as a result of colonial influence. Consequently, this phenomenon permeates both instructional practices and curriculum design, cementing a pervasive bias that underlines the enduring legacy of colonialism (Paranjpe, 2002).

In Indian psychology textbooks, Western psychological paradigms are accorded preeminence, positioning them as the only and most credible source of scientific information. As a result of this discursive landscape, indigenous and cultural perspectives often occupy the margins, are isolated in separate sections, or are entirely omitted from the narrative as a whole. A tacit hierarchy is perpetuated by such pedagogical partitioning that implicitly attribute normativity and universal applicability to Western psychological frameworks, thereby implicitly diminishing the perceived validity of indigenous epistemologies (Chaudhary et al., 2022).

Discourse separation constitutes a pernicious form of epistemic hegemony, in which the dominant Western paradigms are put on a pedestal, while alternative perspectives are marginalized. The educational materials perpetuate this hierarchy, which reinforces the primacy of Western conceptualizations, while marginalizing indigenous and cultural approaches to understanding psychological phenomena (Adams et al., 2018).

Additionally, the temporal dimension of the educational trajectory exacerbates the colonial legacy. In academic trajectories, indigenous and cultural perspectives are typically not introduced until the graduate level, which results in a significant delay in exposing students to a variety of epistemologies. In undergraduate programs, the absence of foundational coursework on indigenous or cultural psychology perpetuates a Eurocentric bias that prevents students from engaging meaningfully with their cultural heritage during their formative educational years (Torres, 2019; Matasci et al., 2020).

Through deferred introductions, the colonial narrative imprinted on the educational landscape is not only sustained but intensified. In the absence of foundational coursework, students are effectively insulated from the richness of their cultural and epistemological heritage for a longer period of time. Due to this, a critical period of formative development, where students could otherwise explore diverse perspectives, is marred by a Eurocentric bias, leading to an environment of epistemic alienation (Mukherjee, 2015).

A systematic lack of consideration for indigenous and cultural perspectives in both curricular design and instructional practices illustrates the enduring colonial legacy within Indian psychology education. Discourse separation coupled with the deferral of the introduction of diverse perspectives perpetuates a distorted epistemological landscape that hinders the development of a holistic understanding of psychology. It is imperative that conscientious efforts are made to dismantle hierarchical structures, integrate diverse perspectives into curricula, and initiate a paradigm shift toward a more inclusive and culturally sensitive pedagogy within Indian psychology in order to address this multifaceted issue.

Decolonization Initiatives and Prospects

Indian psychology has been characterized by historically biased teachings, which have led to a nascent but robust movement towards decolonization. Through this transformative initiative, historical imbalances will be rectified by promoting a pedagogy that is more culturally sensitive and inclusive (Sinha & Fox Lee, 2017). Several noteworthy efforts exemplify this paradigm shift:

1. *Course Development*: In some Indian universities, indigenous and cultural psychology courses are being integrated into the curricula. Through this curriculum diversification, students will be able to engage critically with diverse cultural perspectives, thereby developing a more comprehensive understanding of psychology (NCERT, 2022).
2. *Textbook Revisions*: Since textbooks have discursive implications, there is a discernible trend toward revising existing Indian psychology textbooks in order to ensure a more balanced representation of indigenous and cultural perspectives. This remedial approach represents an affirmative step towards dismantling the historical biases embedded in educational materials (NCERT, 2022).
3. *Innovative Pedagogical Approaches*: Educators are actively experimenting with culturally appropriate teaching methods in order to align pedagogical methods with the intrinsic nature of Indian psychology. The use of storytelling and experiential learning, for instance, are gaining traction as pedagogical tools that are more closely aligned with the narrative-rich fabric of Indian psychological thought (Mukherjee, 2019).
4. *Advocacy for Indigenous Psychologists*: There is a concerted effort underway within the organization to increase the visibility and contribution of indigenous and cultural psychologists. Platforms dedicated to showcasing their scholarly endeavors are emerging, contributing to a diversified and representative landscape within the discipline (O'Keefe et al., 2021).

It is clear from the analysis of colonial influence in the teaching of Indian psychology that historical, epistemological, and pedagogical factors interact in a complex manner. A decolonized pedagogy is an ongoing process, with an awareness and commitment to addressing historical biases and fostering an approach that is more inclusive and culturally sensitive. Taking into account the intricate terrain of colonial legacies, Indian psychology education has the potential to transform into a dynamic, culturally relevant discipline that authentically reflects indigenous psychological narratives.

5. CASE STUDY AND PRACTICAL APPLICATIONS

Indian psychology has proven its practical relevance across diverse domains, showcasing success in real-world applications. One notable example involves the application of Indian psychology principles to national leaders like Lokamanya Tilak, Sri Aurobindo, and Mahatma Gandhi (Krishnan, 2022). These leaders acknowledged the influence of the Bhagavad Gita on their understanding of human existential crises, utilizing Indian psychology principles to navigate complex challenges in their roles.

In mental health services for American Indian children and families, the application of Indian psychology addresses cultural gaps that non-Indian psychologists may face (Everett et al., 1983). Culturally sensitive approaches become essential to understand the values, practices, and needs of American Indian clients, preventing conflicts and frustrations that might hinder the delivery of appropriate mental health services.

Indian psychology's practical applications extend to identity formation and learning styles in virtual worlds, where traditional social psychology theories may fall short (Junglas et al., 2007). The unique norms and dynamics of virtual environments shape identity exploration and learning, offering insights for the design and implementation of educational and social virtual platforms.

Additionally, Indian psychology has been instrumental in understanding psychological adaptation to extreme environments, exemplified by a study on Indian expeditioners in Antarctica (Khandelwal et al., 2017). This research assessed various psychological factors, shedding light on the challenges faced by individuals in extreme conditions and informing strategies for well-being and adaptation.

Building upon these applications, Indian psychology has demonstrated success in mental health interventions for American Indians and Alaska Natives (Gone & Alcántara, 2007). Culturally appropriate interventions have proven effective in addressing mental health problems specific to these populations, enhancing overall well-being. Exploring the concept of resilience among California Indian tribal leaders further showcases the practicality of Indian psychology (Ramirez & Hammack, 2014). The leaders' adoption of a narrative of survivance serves as a buffer against psychosocial stress, contributing to their resilient narrative identity and informing interventions for similar challenges faced by indigenous communities.

In the healthcare sector, Indian psychology has been applied to improve the quality of life and treatment outcomes for tuberculosis patients (Peddireddy, 2016). Psychological interventions complement medical treatments, addressing psychological distress and promoting holistic healthcare. During the COVID-19 pandemic, Indian psychology has played a pivotal role in understanding and addressing psychological responses in India (Gopal et al., 2020). Longitudinal studies have examined the dynamics of psychological distress, revealing gender inequalities that require immediate attention.

The practical applications of Indian psychology also extend globally, with its use in China to assess psychological distress and provide policy recommendations during the COVID-19 epidemic (Qiu et al., 2020). This nationwide survey emphasizes the importance of understanding and addressing psychological well-being in the general population during crisis situations. These examples collectively underscore the practical relevance and positive outcomes of applying Indian psychology across various contexts.

By incorporating cultural perspectives and understanding unique challenges, Indian psychology offers valuable insights and approaches to promote well-being and address psychological issues effectively.

6. CONTEMPORARY RESEARCH AND TRENDS

The Indian psychology education field is undergoing a discernible shift towards an enriched paradigm, characterized by a deliberate integration of indigenous and cultural perspectives. This transformative endeavor is evidently manifested in the development of curricular frameworks and educational programs, in which an intricate exploration of traditional practices intrinsic to Indian cultural heritage, such as yoga, meditation, Ayurveda, and indigenous healing modalities, is given due consideration. The goal of this is to develop psychological education that is rooted in the profound philosophical and spiritual underpinnings inherent in the Indian culture as opposed to a Western-centric orientation (Salagame, 2011).

Furthermore, an inclination towards pragmatism is discernible, as evidenced by an increased emphasis on practical skills and applications within the scope of Indian psychology education. In support of this trajectory, a growing number of programs are offering internships and clinical training opportunities in a strategic manner. This evolution addresses the imperative of preparing students for effective engagement with the multifaceted challenges presented in real-world situations by imparting both theoretical and practical knowledge (McQuaid & Spirito, 2012; Mishra & Padalia, 2021; Dwivedi et al., 2023).

Additionally, the integration of technology into pedagogical methodologies has become an important feature of contemporary Indian psychology education. A concerted effort has been made to create a dynamic and interactive educational environment through the use of online learning platforms, educational games, simulations, and virtual reality. With the integration of technology, Indian psychological landscape is aligned with broader global trends, enhancing the accessibility and effectiveness of the educational apparatus (Dwivedi et al., 2023).

There has been a notable evolution in Indian psychology research characterized by a nuanced synthesis of Western and indigenous perspectives. In both theoretical constructs and empirical investigations, this synthesis reflects an intellectual convergence that seeks to construct theories and models relevant to Indian sociocultural contexts. It represents an attempt to transcend the limitations of conventional psychological paradigms and emphasize the contextual relevance that is integral to a comprehensive understanding of psychological phenomena in the Indian context (Mishra & Padalia, 2021).

In addition, it is noteworthy that emerging issues in the field are given a high degree of attention. Researchers are increasingly focused on contemporary challenges, focusing scholarly inquiry on topics such as mental health and well-being in the digital age, the psychological impacts of climate change, and the interrelationship between mental health and social justice. Throughout this research agenda, a commitment is made to understanding and mitigating contemporary psychosocial challenges in Indian communities (Thoma et al., 2021; Hwong et al., 2022).

In terms of methodology, there is a discernible trend towards methodological pluralism in Indian psychology, with researchers increasingly adopting mixed methods approaches. It is through this judicious triangulation of quantitative and qualitative approaches that we are able to gain a more nuanced and comprehensive understanding of the multifaceted nature of psychological phenomena. In acceptance of the multidimensional nature of the human experience, this methodological diversification aligns with the broader global trajectory of psychological research (Mishra & Padalia, 2021).

A burgeoning field of positive psychology occupies a prominent position within Indian psychology. Researchers within this field are actively engaged in developing interventions tailored to Indian populations, with the overarching goal of strengthening mental health and fostering holistic wellbeing (Ghosh & Deb, 2016).

Moreover, cross-cultural psychology is becoming a prominent research area, as scholars conduct comparative analyses to discern universal and culturally specific characteristics of mental health and well-being. In addition to contributing to the global discourse, this cross-cultural inquiry offers a nuanced understanding of the culturally contingent nuances shaping psychological phenomena in the Indian context (Antić, 2021).

At the same time, community psychology is gaining prominence as a crucial field of inquiry. Using contextually attuned interventions, researchers engage collaboratively with community members to address mental health concerns. Research and community involvement are converging to underscore the importance of culturally sensitive and contextually grounded approaches to promoting mental health in Indian communities (Ghosh & Deb, 2016; Townley et al., 2018).

Contemporary patterns in Indian psychology highlight a dynamic and developing scene. The combination of local perspectives, the practical approach towards real-world implementations, the smooth integration of technology, and the acceptance of various research methodologies together epitomize the field's commitment to significance, adaptability, and intellectual progress in unraveling the intricacies of the human mind within the unique fabric of the Indian environment.

7. CONCLUSION

It is a dynamic, evolving field that draws deeply from the rich tapestry of Indian culture, philosophy, and ancient scriptures. However, Indian psychology has often been overshadowed by Western paradigms and Euro-American norms despite its historical roots and valuable contributions. There have been many challenges faced by Indian psychology, including a lack of documentation, linguistic barriers, and a preference for Western education. In spite of this, there is increasing recognition of the importance of integrating Indian perspectives into the global discourse on psychology. In addition to theoretical considerations, Indian psychology also includes practical applications and contemporary research. Whether it is influencing national leaders or addressing mental health gaps in diverse populations, Indian psychology has demonstrated its relevance in real-world settings. Cultural sensitivity and inclusivity have become increasingly important in addressing biases within mainstream psychology, particularly when teaching and learning Indian psychology.

While challenges persist, emerging trends in research are emphasizing cultural context and sensitivity. Developing culturally sensitive mental health services, exploring cultural psychology, and incorporating indigenous perspectives underscore a paradigm shift towards a more inclusive approach to psychological research and practice in India. As Indian psychology continues to develop, it is imperative that we overcome biases, promote research collaboration, and promote the value of indigenous knowledge systems. An understanding of the mind-body connection, consciousness, and spirituality within Indian psychology may contribute to a more comprehensive understanding of human behavior on a global scale. Ultimately, Indian psychology's future lies in nurturing a balance between tradition and modernization, fostering a deep appreciation for the diverse cultural fabric from which it draws its inspiration.

REFERENCES

Adams, G., Kurtiş, T., Ordóñez, L. G., Molina, L. E., & Oropeza, I. D. (2018). Decolonizing Knowledge in Hegemonic Psychological Science. In N. N. Wane & K. L. Todd (Eds.), *Decolonial Pedagogy: Examining Sites of Resistance, Resurgence, and Renewal* (pp. 35–53). Springer International Publishing. doi:10.1007/978-3-030-01539-8_3

Aishe. (2021). Rise in Number of Foreign Students Studying in India, BTech Most opted Course. *News18*. https://www.news18.com/news/education-career/rise-in-number-of-foreign-students-studying-in-india-rises-btech-most-opted-course-3863621.html

Antić, A. (2021). Transcultural Psychiatry: Cultural Difference, Universalism and Social Psychiatry in the Age of Decolonisation. *Culture, Medicine and Psychiatry*, *45*(3), 359–384. doi:10.100711013-021-09719-4 PMID:33905076

Avasthi, A., Kate, N., & Grover, S. (2013). Indianization of psychiatry utilizing Indian mental concepts. *Indian Journal of Psychiatry*, *55*(6, Suppl 2), S136–S144. doi:10.4103/0019-5545.105508 PMID:23858244

Avasthi, A., Kate, N., & Grover, S. (2013). Indianization of psychiatry utilizing Indian mental concepts. *Indian Journal of Psychiatry*, *55*(6, Suppl 2), S136–S144. doi:10.4103/0019-5545.105508 PMID:23858244

Chaudhary, N., Misra, G., Bansal, P., Valsiner, J., & Singh, T. (2022). Making Sense of Culture for the Psychological Sciences. *Review of General Psychology*, *26*(4), 399–415. doi:10.1177/10892680211066473

Clay, R. A. (2002). *A renaissance for humanistic psychology*. APA. Https://Www.Apa.Org. https://www.apa.org/monitor/sep02/renaissance

Cornelissen, M. (2013). *Foundations and applications of Indian psychology* (G. Misra, Ed.; 2nd ed.). Pearson.

Dalal, A. K. (2011). A journey back to the roots: Psychology in India. In *Foundations of Indian Psychology* (p. 39). https://www.ipi.org.in/texts/ajit/dalal-joureny-to-the-roots.pdf

Dalal, A. K., & Misra, G. (2010). The Core and Context of Indian Psychology. *Psychology and Developing Societies*, *22*(1), 121–155. doi:10.1177/097133360902200105

Daniels, R. J., Trebilcock, M. J., & Carson, L. D. (2011). The Legacy of Empire: The Common Law Inheritance and Commitments to Legality in Former British Colonies. *The American Journal of Comparative Law*, *59*(1), 111–178. doi:10.5131/AJCL.2010.0015

Dwivedi, Y. K., Kshetri, N., Hughes, L., Slade, E. L., Jeyaraj, A., Kar, A. K., Baabdullah, A. M., Koohang, A., Raghavan, V., Ahuja, M., Albanna, H., Albashrawi, M. A., Al-Busaidi, A. S., Balakrishnan, J., Barlette, Y., Basu, S., Bose, I., Brooks, L., Buhalis, D., & Wright, R. (2023). “So what if ChatGPT wrote it?” Multidisciplinary perspectives on opportunities, challenges and implications of generative conversational AI for research, practice and policy. *International Journal of Information Management*, *71*, 102642. doi:10.1016/j.ijinfomgt.2023.102642

Everett, F., Proctor, N., & Cartmell, B. (1983). Providing psychological services to american indian children and families. *Professional Psychology, Research and Practice*, *14*(5), 588–603. doi:10.1037/0735-7028.14.5.588

Ghosh, A., & Deb, A. (2016). Positive Psychology Progress in India: Accomplishments and Pathways Ahead. *Psychological Studies*, *61*(3), 113–125. doi:10.100712646-016-0367-5

Gone, J., & Alcántara, C. (2007). Identifying effective mental health interventions for american indians and alaska natives: A review of the literature. *Cultural Diversity & Ethnic Minority Psychology*, *13*(4), 356–363. doi:10.1037/1099-9809.13.4.356 PMID:17967104

GopalA.SharmaA.SubramanyamM. (2020). Dynamics of psychological responses to covid-19 in india: a longitudinal study. doi:10.1101/2020.06.12.20129791

Grassini, S. (2023). Shaping the Future of Education: Exploring the Potential and Consequences of AI and ChatGPT in Educational Settings. *Education Sciences*, *13*(7), 7. doi:10.3390/educsci13070692

Gupta, A. (2015). pedagogy of third space: A multidimensional early childhood curriculum. *Policy Futures in Education*, *13*(2), 260–272. doi:10.1177/1478210315579540

Heylighen, F. (1992). A cognitive-systemic reconstruction of maslow's theory of self-actualization. *Behavioral Science*, *37*(1), 39–58. doi:10.1002/bs.3830370105

Hoshmand, L. T. (2007). Cultural–Ecological Perspectives on the Understanding and Assessment of Trauma. In J. P. Wilson & C. S. Tang (Eds.), Cross-Cultural Assessment of Psychological Trauma and PTSD (pp. 31–50). Springer US. doi:10.1007/978-0-387-70990-1_2

Huppes, N. (2011). *Teaching Indian Psychology—Challenges and Prospects An application-oriented paper.* Indian Psychology Institute. https://www.ipi.org.in/texts/neeltje/nh-teaching-indian-psychology.php

Hwang, K.-K. (2004). *The Epistemological Goal of Indigenous Psychology: The Perspective of Constructive Realism* [National Taiwan University]. https://scholarworks.gvsu.edu/iaccp_papers?utm_source=scholarworks.gvsu.edu%2Fiaccp_papers%2F265&utm_medium=PDF&utm_campaign=PDFCoverPages

Hwong, A. R., Wang, M., Khan, H., Chagwedera, D. N., Grzenda, A., Doty, B., Benton, T., Alpert, J., Clarke, D., & Compton, W. M. (2022). Climate change and mental health research methods, gaps, and priorities: A scoping review. *The Lancet. Planetary Health*, *6*(3), e281–e291. doi:10.1016/S2542-5196(22)00012-2 PMID:35278392

Jabin, N., Wohra, S., & Das, A. (2022). Education in India and the Post- Colonial Perspective. *Analysis*, 487–498.

Jaiswal, Y. S., & Williams, L. L. (2016). A glimpse of Ayurveda – The forgotten history and principles of Indian traditional medicine. *Journal of Traditional and Complementary Medicine*, *7*(1), 50–53. doi:10.1016/j.jtcme.2016.02.002 PMID:28053888

Junglas, I., Johnson, N., Steel, D., Abraham, D., & Loughlin, P. (2007). Identity formation, learning styles and trust in virtual worlds. *The Data Base for Advances in Information Systems*, *38*(4), 90–96. doi:10.1145/1314234.1314251

Juntunen, C., Barraclough, D., Broneck, C., Seibel, G., Winrow, S., & Morin, P. (2001). American indian perspectives on the career journey. *Journal of Counseling Psychology*, *48*(3), 274–285. doi:10.1037/0022-0167.48.3.274

Krishnan, R. (2022). The bhagavad gita as the epitome of indian psychology vis-à-vis modern psychology. *Mind & Society*, *11*(01), 62–66. doi:10.56011/mind-mri-111-20228

Malviya, S. (2021, September 12). Influence of western culture on Indian society. *The Times of India*. https://timesofindia.indiatimes.com/readersblog/know-your-rights/influence-of-western-culture-on-indian-society-37332/

Manickam, L. (2008). Research on Indian Concepts of psychology: Major Challenges and Perspectives for future action. In *Handbook of Indian Psychology* (pp. 492–505). https://www.researchgate.net/publication/312056622_Research_on_Indian_Concepts_of_psychology_Major_Challenges_and_Perspectives_for_future_action

Mason, R., & De la Torre, M. (2000). Heritage conservation and values in globalizing societies. In *World culture report 2000: Cultural Diversity, Conflict and Pluralism*. UNESCO PUBLISHING, UNESCO Digital Library. https://unesdoc.unesco.org/ark:/48223/pf0000121094

Matasci, D., Jerónimo, M. B., & Dores, H. G. (Eds.). (2020). *Education and Development in Colonial and Postcolonial Africa: Policies, Paradigms, and Entanglements* (pp. 1890s–1980s). Springer International Publishing., doi:10.1007/978-3-030-27801-4

Mathew, V. G. (2001). *A Short History of Indian Psychology*. Psychology4All. https://www.psychology4all.com/HistoryI.htm

McCarty, T. L., Borgoiakova, T., Gilmore, P., Lomawaima, K. T., & Romero, M. E. (2005). Indigenous Epistemologies and Education—Self-Determination, Anthropology, and Human Rights. *Anthropology & Education Quarterly*, *36*(1), 1–7. doi:10.1525/aeq.2005.36.1.001

McQuaid, E. L., & Spirito, A. (2012). Integrating Research Into Clinical Internship Training Bridging the Science/Practice Gap in Pediatric Psychology. *Journal of Pediatric Psychology*, *37*(2), 149–157. doi:10.1093/jpepsy/jsr114 PMID:22286345

Miller, C. J., McNear, J., & Metz, M. J. (2013). A comparison of traditional and engaging lecture methods in a large, professional-level course. *Advances in Physiology Education*, *37*(4), 347–355. doi:10.1152/advan.00050.2013 PMID:24292912

Miranda, A., & Gutter, P. (2002). Diversity research literature in school psychology: 1990-1999. *Psychology in the Schools*, *39*(5), 597–604. doi:10.1002/pits.10051

Mishra, A. K., & Padalia, D. (2021). Re-envisioning Psychology: A Critical History of Psychology in India. In G. Misra, N. Sanyal, & S. De (Eds.), *Psychology in Modern India: Historical, Methodological, and Future Perspectives* (pp. 163–201). Springer. doi:10.1007/978-981-16-4705-5_10

Mukherjee, M. (2015). Indian education at the crossroads of postcoloniality, globalization and the 21st century Knowledge Economy (Part 1). *Policy Futures in Education*, *13*(2), 165–170. doi:10.1177/1478210314568180

Mukherjee, M. (2019, January 1). *Culturally Responsive Teaching Learning in Indian Multicultural Context: Review of Contemporary Policy & Practice*. 25th International Multi-disciplinary Conference On Arts, Social Science, Management and Technology. Research Gate.

Müller, F. M. (1879). *Taittiriya Upanishad. The sacred books of the East* (Vol. 15). Oxford University Press. https://holybooks-lichtenbergpress.netdna-ssl.com/wp-content/uploads/15.SacredBooksEast.Va-rOrSch.v15.Muller.Hindu_.Mull_.Upanishads.p2.KathMundTait.Mait_.Oxf_.1884.pdf

NCERT. (2022). *National Curriculum Framework for Foundational Stage, 2022*. Government of India.

O'Keefe, V. M., Cwik, M. F., Haroz, E. E., & Barlow, A. (2021). Increasing Culturally Responsive Care and Mental Health Equity With Indigenous Community Mental Health Workers. *Psychological Services*, *18*(1), 84–92. doi:10.1037er0000358 PMID:31045405

Olkin, R., & Pledger, C. (2003). Can disability studies and psychology join hands? *The American Psychologist*, *58*(4), 296–304. doi:10.1037/0003-066X.58.4.296 PMID:12866396

Paranjpe, A. C. (2002). Indigenous Psychology in the Post- Colonial Context: An Historical Perspective. *Psychology and Developing Societies*, *14*(1), 27–43. doi:10.1177/097133360201400103

Paranjpe, A. C. (2011). Indian Psychology and the International Context. *Psychology and Developing Societies*, *23*(1), 1–26. doi:10.1177/097133361002300101

Peddireddy, V. (2016). Quality of life, psychological interventions and treatment outcome in tuberculosis patients: The indian scenario. *Frontiers in Psychology*, *7*. doi:10.3389/fpsyg.2016.01664 PMID:27833578

Pedersen, P. (2003). Culturally biased assumptions in counseling psychology. *The Counseling Psychologist*, *31*(4), 396–403. doi:10.1177/0011000003031004002

Phiri, P., Sajid, S., & Delanerolle, G. (2023). Decolonising the psychology curriculum: A perspective. *Frontiers in Psychology*, *14*, 1193241. https://www.frontiersin.org/articles/10.3389/fpsyg.2023.1193241. doi:10.3389/fpsyg.2023.1193241 PMID:37388662

Pickar, D. (2008). Countertransference bias in the child custody evaluator. *Journal of Child Custody*, *4*(3), 45–67. doi:10.1300/J190v04n03_04

Qiu, J., Shen, B., Zhao, M., Wang, Z., Xie, B., & Xu, Y. (2020). A nationwide survey of psychological distress among chinese people in the covid-19 epidemic: Implications and policy recommendations. *General Psychiatry*, *33*(2), e100213. doi:10.1136/gpsych-2020-100213 PMID:32215365

Ramirez, L., & Hammack, P. (2014). Surviving colonization and the quest for healing: Narrative and resilience among california indian tribal leaders. *Transcultural Psychiatry*, *51*(1), 112–133. doi:10.1177/1363461513520096 PMID:24459128

Rao, S. K. R. (1979). *Consciousness in Advaita*. IBH Prakashana for Sri Abhinava Vidyatheerta Swamigal Scientific Research Academy.

Salagame, K. K. K. (2011). Indian Psychology. In *The Encyclopedia of Cross-Cultural Psychology* (pp. 695–698). John Wiley & Sons, Ltd. doi:10.1002/9781118339893.wbeccp283

Sayegh, P., Vivian, D., Heller, M., Kirk, S., & Kelly, K. (2023). Racial, cultural, and social injustice in psychological assessment: A brief review, call to action, and resources to help reduce inequities and harm. *Training and Education in Professional Psychology*, *17*(4), 366–374. Advance online publication. doi:10.1037/tep0000451

Schaffer, J., & Rodolfa, E. (2020). Reflecting on reflective practice. *Clinical Psychology : a Publication of the Division of Clinical Psychology of the American Psychological Association*, *27*(4). Advance online publication. doi:10.1111/cpsp.12361

Sedlmeier, P., & Srinivas, K. (2016). How Do Theories of Cognition and Consciousness in Ancient Indian Thought Systems Relate to Current Western Theorizing and Research? *Frontiers in Psychology*, *7*, 343. doi:10.3389/fpsyg.2016.00343 PMID:27014150

Sharma, M. (2021). *Indian Psychology-Exploring the Historical Roots*. Emerging Trends and Future Implications., doi:10.25215/0902.168

Sharma, S. (2006). Psychiatry, colonialism and Indian civilization: A historical appraisal. *Indian Journal of Psychiatry*, *48*(2), 109–112. doi:10.4103/0019-5545.31600 PMID:20703396

Sinha, C., & Fox Lee, S. (2017). Note on "History of psychology in India: Problems and prospects.". *History of Psychology*, *20*(1), 126–128. doi:10.1037/h0101578 PMID:28150967

Sivananda, S. S. (1999). *Guru Tattva – The Divine Life Society* (6th ed.). The Divine Life Society. https://www.dlshq.org/download/guru-tattva/

Thoma, M. V., Rohleder, N., & Rohner, S. L. (2021). Clinical Ecopsychology: The Mental Health Impacts and Underlying Pathways of the Climate and Environmental Crisis. *Frontiers in Psychiatry*, *12*, 675936. doi:10.3389/fpsyt.2021.675936 PMID:34093283

Torres, S. (2019). *Beyond Colonizing Epistemicides: Toward a Decolonizing Framework for Indigenous Education.* [Thesis, LMU]. https://digitalcommons.lmu.edu/etd/895

Townley, G., Brown, M., & Sylvestre, J. (2018). Community Psychology and Community Mental Health: A Call for Reengagement. *American Journal of Community Psychology*, *61*(1–2), 3–9. doi:10.1002/ajcp.12225 PMID:29315707

Wilson, J. P. (2007). The Lens of Culture: Theoretical and Conceptual Perspectives in the Assessment of Psychological Trausma and PTSD. In J. P. Wilson & C. S. Tang (Eds.), Cross-Cultural Assessment of Psychological Trauma and PTSD (pp. 3–30). Springer US. doi:10.1007/978-0-387-70990-1_1

Chapter 2
An Overview of Mindfulness Based on Practical Rationality

Damini Saini
https://orcid.org/0000-0001-5734-5067
Indian Institute of Management, Raipur, India

Shashwat Ranjan
Indian Institute of Management, Raipur, India

ABSTRACT

Though there has been an increase in the studies on mindfulness in organizations, the studies around its process have been scant. Most of the studies use only quantitative methods by collecting data based on scale-based questionnaires and doing further analysis to assess the impact of mindfulness on the organizational effectiveness as a whole. This chapter is an effort to explore the concept of mindfulness so that we can utilize it most effectively. The authors tried to connect several theories to the phenomena of mindfulness, for example, trait activation theory and broad and build theory. They present an alternate theoretical lens based on 'practical rationality,' which can substantiate the use of qualitative methods for collecting data on mindfulness and help develop a higher orientation of experience among individuals. The authors concluded that mindfulness is an individual-level process that workplace factors and systems can influence. In addition, the purpose of initiating mindfulness should not be towards more 'hedonic' reasons like stress management. Instead, the purpose should be more 'eudemonic.'

1. INTRODUCTION

Recently, mindfulness has received significant attention in psychology, spirituality and management studies. This is due to the general recognition that mindfulness can be the primary determinant of well-being, meaningfulness, and organisational effectiveness. Some studies have reported strong correlations of mindfulness with brain connectivity (Kilpatrick et al., 2011). 'Mindfulness' has been described as a "moment-to-moment experience of one's judgement" (Brown & Ryan, 2003). Mindfulness in Western practices finds its roots in the Buddhist traditions of 'Vipassana' and 'Mahayana' (Kornfielf, 2011).

DOI: 10.4018/978-1-6684-9778-4.ch002

The word 'Sati', a 'Pali' word from the Buddhist text, is from where mindfulness derives its meaning. 'Sati' means 'to remember' and 'awareness' (Bodhi, 2011). Most recent studies have dived deeper by applying mindfulness to behavioural science, neuroscience, and clinical studies. They have tried to understand the role of mindfulness in better regulation of thoughts and emotions. Mindfulness in the organisational context has been looked at from two sides – the 'Well-being perspective' (Saini, 2020), which includes 'emotional exhaustion, 'affective states', 'psychological detachment' 'job satisfaction' and the 'Functioning' perspective, which includes 'work engagement' 'creativity' etc. (Garg & Saini,2023; Reb et al.,2020). All of these have tried to look at from the viewpoint of 'impact' by using some existing theoretical explanations. Also, most have analysed mindfulness as a quantitative variable recorded through questionnaires, mapping them with appropriate scales like MAAS (Brown & Ryan, 2003) and FFMQ (Baer et al.,2006). Studies around the 'process' of mindfulness have been scant. Mindfulness is essentially a subjective phenomenon and thus requires a deeper qualitative lens and is looked upon.

In this chapter, we would like to present an overview of mindfulness by critically evaluating some of the recent studies on mindfulness and analysing whether they have been able to explain the process of mindfulness and its importance in the workplace setting(Saini,2020). We have also proposed an alternate theoretical lens, ' practical rationality' (Sandberg & Tsoukas, 2011), which can support qualitative mechanisms to record and analyse mindfulness in an organisational setting. In addition, we have justified using mindfulness not just for temporary benefits but to develop a higher orientation of experience.

2. LITERATURE REVIEW

As mentioned above, mindfulness as a topic finds its roots in Eastern knowledge and traditions, which have been adopted and tailored to be applicable in a workplace setting. So, various clinical and non-clinical researchers have supported that being mindful is suitable for the individual, and the impact of it can be seen in various interrelated areas. This has been increasing over the period due to an increase in 'attention overload', 'stressors', and 'increased connectivity,' i.e., people can sit and conduct meetings anytime and from any location after the digital wave, and also an increase in multi-tasking (Reb et al., 2020). Most of the studies around mindfulness have looked at individual-level factors. Some individual-level factors studied as mediators include – 'empathy', 'paranoid cognition', 'sleep quality', 'creative process engagement', 'emotional stability', 'self-esteem' etc. Some moderators include – 'perceived leader humility', 'work engagement', and 'work experience'. Workplace factors like 'situational demands', 'job control', 'on-task attentional pull', 'off-task attentional pull', 'organisational caring climate', 'external challenges ', 'supervisor support', etc., have been studied as antecedents to mindfulness. From the perspective of outcomes, the factors have been both organisational and workplace levels, which include – 'job satisfaction', 'turnover intention', 'anxiety', 'burnout', 'emotional exhaustion' ', self-compassion, 'employee creativity', 'job performance', 'task performance' 'prosocial behaviour', 'work engagement' etc.

Interestingly, whether the factors are antecedents, mediators, moderators or outcomes, they consider mindfulness an individual characteristic (Shahbaz & Parker, 2021). No recent studies have examined the possibility of group or team mindfulness (Liu et al., 2020). Even the organisational level factors like the role of HR in ensuring the systems are in a proper place wherein the HR needs to act as a 'business partner' in order to implement the work designs, listen to employee's voices and lead to their improved performance has not been looked upon in detail (Arrowsmith & Parker, 2013). Organisational level factors are essential because if the systems are not in place, then mindfulness would be impacted. Any intervention would fall short in such cases. Another precise observation from studies has been that the focus has been only towards benefits. E.g., The role of mindfulness in facilitating constructive conflict management (Kay & Skarlicki, 2020). The assumption that mindfulness only leads to benefits somehow dilutes the proper questioning into what is the very genesis of mindfulness.

Two possibilities have been observed for mindfulness – 'within-person-level' vs. 'between-person-level'. Within-person is a scenario wherein the same person experiences different states like conscientiousness or neuroticism, whereas in between-person scenarios, different persons go through the same state like conscientiousness. Let me illustrate with an example from a study on antecedents of mindfulness. If a person is conscientious and his sudden state of being more conscientious leads to an increase in his or her mindfulness, it is an example of a within-person state. Suppose this would have been the case among many other individuals, i.e., if people who tend to be more conscientious are also more mindful than it is a between-person state (Reina & Kudesia, 2020).

In recent studies, models have experimented with mindfulness within-person and between-person cases by making it operational as a state, trait, practice or an added intervention. State mindfulness refers to a temporary state that a person may experience in some situation, which makes it a within-person case. In contrast, trait mindfulness is more stable and observed among many individuals, making it a between-person case. The practice-based approaches include simple observations like focusing on breathing, eating, walking, etc. Higher-order practices, i.e., training-based activities to make it more inherent, are called interventions. These operationalisations improve people's state or trait mindfulness (Shahbaz & Parker, 2021).

There are predominantly two sides of mindfulness that have been observed – "orientation to experience" and "self-regulation of attention" (Bajaj et al.,2018). Many observational-based practices, like focusing on breathing, thoughts, and body sensations, come under the 'self-regulation of awareness'. 'Orientation to experience' comes with a need for something higher order. E.g., qualities like enthusiasm, curiosity or even openness to experience where the purpose is to experience something new would fall under 'orientation to experience'. Positive individual outcomes like 'happiness' and 'psychological well-being' find their way into these approaches. Many self-regulation-based practices directed towards individual, organisational outcomes like 'job satisfaction' or 'employee creativity' are goal and achievement-driven, making them 'hedonic'.

Additionally, findings from studies suggest an indirect association between mindfulness and employee creativity via creative process engagement (Cheung et al., 2020). It is because there is an underlying assumption that mindfulness leads to better attentional focus. It can be associated with employee creativity.

On the contrary, if we see people looking for higher enlightenment, they are more oriented towards experiences. All the subsequent practices, like yoga and meditation, are directed towards such experiences. The literature says this is a 'eudaimonism' form of happiness wherein the individual finds greater happiness in self-actualisation self-actualisation. The purpose of mindfulness changes here and becomes oriented towards higher experience.

2.1 Theoretical Basis

Studies around mindfulness, which have looked into either antecedents or individual-level factors, have used some existing theories to explain the basis of their study research. They include – 'The Conservation of Resource Theory' (Hobfoll, 2001), 'Trait-Activation Theory' (Tett & Burnett, 2003), 'Broaden & Build Theory' (Fredrickson, 2001), 'Self-Determination Theory (Ryan et al., 2008), 'Mindfulness to

Meaning Theory' (Garland et al., 2015), 'Affective-Events Theory' (Weiss & Cropanzano, 1996) and 'Metacognitive Theory' (Kudesia, 2019). Let us analyse each of these theories to understand whether they substantiate the process of mindfulness.

2.1.1 Conservation of Resource Theory

The theory posits that when an individual acquires more resources, such an acquisition would cause him or her to acquire more. In contrast, when resources are scarce, the individual will tend to deplete more resources. For example – If a person is given too much of a workload, the capacity to focus would drain, which would eventually lead to the draining of psychological health (Hobfoll, 2001). So, if an individual is more focused, he or she can be more stressed, provided the pressure is high based on work. This would lead him or her to focus less and eventually lose concentration strength. Another critical thing the COR theory says is that if the initiative is taken to acquire some beneficial resources, they would also protect the previously necessary acquired resources. Findings (Liu et al.,2020) suggest that individual mindfulness is an essential tool to restore and lead to better work engagement. This is also in line with the findings (Brown & Ryan, 2003), which specified that people who practice mindfulness stand differently than others because they can evaluate their circumstances well and avoid unnecessary perceptions. However, what if the individual consistently loses resources due to mental fatigue? Does a self-regulation-based approach aid an individual's rescue? This is where we cannot proceed with an explanation from COR.

2.1.2 Trait-Activation Theory

Trait activation theory is relevant to the trait mindfulness functionality discussed in the literature section. Traits are more stable characteristics among individuals. The trait activation theory (Tett & Burnett, 2003) posits that certain traits arise due to situational cues, which can be task, social or organisational. In theory, they have stated that job demands (charges and duties in one's jobs), distractors (presence of sociable people in the team), and releasers (outside work events) are 'trait activators' because they aid the already existing traits whereas constraints (responsibly neglecting) is a trait deactivator and facilitator (which help the already existing situation) is a mix of both. These traits are impacted by situation specificity. If we look into 'trait mindfulness', situations can impact it. Therefore, does the situation impact a person's mindfulness, or is it the other way round, as past research (Brown & Ryan, 2003) suggests that mindfulness can facilitate more situational control?

2.1.3 Broaden and Build Theory

Broaden and Build Theory posits a framework of positive emotions as per which a person may eliminate the automatic arousal of negative emotions by widening their experience of positive emotions (Fredrickson, 2001). Such positive emotions would widen their "momentary thought-action repertoire". The theory of Broaden and Build furthers the argument of attention and situational cues. Moreover, findings from one of the recent studies on transgenders (Thoroughgood et al., 2020) which considered 'trait mindfulness' as a moderator with 'paranoid cognition' as a mediator and their impact on 'emotional exhaustion' highlight the relevance of 'trait mindfulness' in making people handle a situation positively. Paranoid cognition refers to experiences or situations that initiate a paranoid thinking process in people's minds. The study found that those high on 'trait mindfulness' during everyday interaction with coworkers could respond to their paranoid discrimination. They were also able to recover from their perceptions of discrimination. Better mindfulness could be an addition to experiencing positive emotions. However, the study also highlights the role of an organisational system in fostering greater belongingness and casting out all prejudices. So, we can say that state or trait mindfulness would enhance one's experience of positive emotions within an organisational setting.

2.1.4 Self-Determination Theory

In addition to awareness and its role in creating positive affect, (Ryan et al.,2008) have stated the 'self-determination theory' from an 'eudaimonia' perspective wherein they have discussed in depth the principles of living in eudaimonia, which includes – following intrinsic values for own self, living in 'clear awareness', satisfying the basic psychological needs and being mindful and controlled throughout. The original SDT focused more on the intrinsic motivation that drove people towards any action. However, looking from an extrinsic point of view also became relevant over the period, leading to the coming up of 'basic psychological needs'. These include – the 'need for autonomy', which refers to independence in making one's own choices; the 'need for competence', which refers to the belief in an individual about his or her capabilities; and the 'need for relatedness', which refers to a feeling of being cared. Some studies, like (Walker & Colosimo, 2011), which looked into the relationship between 'mindfulness', 'self-compassion' and 'psychological well-being', have used SDT to formulate their basic framework. SDT highly emphasises the environmental factor, which again brings the question of proper systems within the organisation.

2.1.5 Mindfulness to Meaning Theory

In our above discussion on theories, we learned the importance of attention, traits, and positive emotions. The process of how the state of mindfulness could lead to higher-order actualisation has been explained by the Mindfulness to Meaning theory (Garland et al.,2015), which posits that there is a 'positive reappraisal' which occurs because of an awareness mode which in turn makes an individual view his or her thoughts from a metacognitive perspective. The transactional model states that given any situation, be it joyous or stressful, it is an individual's appraisal that makes him or her react. Usually, the stress-based reactions are spontaneous because they are perceived as threats. "Cognitive reappraisal refers to an adaptive form of self-regulation by which people shift their view of a situation and its perceived meaning before it elicits an emotional reaction in them, thereby generating a more adaptive response" (Garland et al.,2009). If stress is appraised as controllable, it could result in positive affect and even better self-efficacy. A study (Weinstein et al.,2009) found that mindfulness could lead to appraising exams as a challenge rather than a threat. Mindfulness can create open-mindedness so the individual can observe the present moment, leading to widening cognitive resources and ignoring unnecessary reactions. More recently, (Coo & Salanova, 2017) used Mindful Interventions (MBI) like guided meditations and teaching components in their study on the psychological health of workers. The results indicated that a Mindful Program improved the workers' trait of mindfulness, happiness and performance and validated the role of positive affect.

2.1.6 Affective-Events Theory

In the mindfulness-to-meaning theory, we discussed the role of positive affect. The theory of affective-events theory becomes relevant in such cases because it posits that individuals' affective states have further implications on their behaviours at work. In their study (Chong et al.,2020) looked into the impact that 'respite' activities, i.e., relaxation-based practices that people take while in the middle of their work, which may include a mild stroll, chatting with coworkers, etc., can have on their job performance. Respite activities distract people from any stress during work.

These generate positive or negative effects and have implications like work engagement and emotional exhaustion. Therefore, they also checked for any role of trait mindfulness in generating positive or adverse effects. Emotions like 'inspiration', 'excitement' and 'enthusiasm' come under the bracket of positive affect, whereas emotions like 'fear', 'upset' and 'distress' come under the adverse affect. A significant finding from this study was that respite activities could generate positive effects. AET also postulates that there can be possible short-lived reactions which would induce affective states. This matches the 'state' mindfulness, which certain situations can influence. Focused breathing can also be a respite activity used for relaxation during the middle of the work. It is a more practice-based approach which can help bring more positive affective states.

2.1.7 Metacognitive Theory

If we see any mindfulness-based studies (Cheung et al.,2020; Thoroughgood et al.,2020; Brown & Ryan, 2003), the critical discussion about the process has been that mindfulness is about "awareness of the present moment". Even in the above discussion on theories, we saw the relevance towards regulation, awareness, and affective states. The Metacognitive theory (Kudesia, 2019) presents mindfulness as a 'metacognitive process'. 'Metacognition' is how people monitor and adjust their information processing. The theory presents two models of information processing – the 'linear model' and 'alternate model'. Let us expound with examples – When a person faces negative situations often and then 'self-limits' by declaring oneself worthless, which leads to him or her entirely giving up, this is a linear model because there is a sequential pattern. Mindful attention here may act as a remedy to stop any such negative perceptions.

Another end of the linear model is 'mindful conceptualisation', wherein people use their experience of having faced negative situations to form concepts. Example – A person sees that whenever he or she smiles too much during any conversation, the response is not favourable from the other end. So, the person conceptualises that smiling too much is not good. This is called 'mindful conceptualisation'. The 'alternate model' suggests that perceptions and concepts are intertwined. It follows a more practice-based approach wherein people, after having faced certain negative situations, develop some experience and then devise a solution. Example – The person in the above case may try to hold on more to his or her lips when the conversation extends. There are two ways by which alternate model functions – 'absorbed engagement', i.e., when people respond to such situations spontaneously and 'deliberate engagement', i.e., when people use their formed concepts to understand and repair such adverse situations.

The metacognitive theory also presents three beliefs in the metacognitive practice, which include – the 'virtue of monitoring,' i.e., the self is valuable, 'attentional sufficiency,' i.e., our attention does not get depleted by more use and 'map-terrain-differentiation,' i.e., "one's map of situation does not reflect the terrain on which they act". The concept of 'attentional sufficiency' as a belief system can explain why being more aware helps overcome certain situations. It says that our attention will never deplete if we firmly believe (Jensen et al.,2012).

To understand the role of 'metacognitive beliefs', 'cognitive resources' and 'features of the situation', an exploratory and confirmatory study was conducted by (Reina & Kudesia, 2020). The proposed model tried to discover the various antecedents to mindfulness at specific situational levels. The underlying assumption was that 'cognitive resources', i.e., the amount of information power a person can allocate to mental tasks, would reduce mental fatigue. 'Metacognitive beliefs' mean an individual's belief about how their mind works. The 'cognitive resources can also be impacted by the 'metacognitive belief' of the individual. Situational appraisals that they considered included – 'On-task attentional pull', i.e., making presentations for office work and 'Off-task attentional pull', i.e., use of social media emails during work. The findings clearly stated that metacognitive beliefs help compensate for any mental fatigue. They have a stronger association with mindfulness than cognitive resources. These findings suggest that metacognitive beliefs motivate people to provide cognitive resources for self-regulation.

This is an essential finding as it has given a clear picture of the paradox that negative situations which lead to the generation of stress and then lead to fatigue should ideally lead to a reduction of cognitive resources and less attentional focus and mindfulness. Instead, the metacognitive belief of an individual can motivate and help the individual not feel scarcity through depletion but appraise (Lazarus & Folkman, 1984) and generate those necessary cognitive resources by self-regulation.

2.2 Existing Methodologies

Some widely used methods include – survey studies, longitudinal field experiments, one-day field experiments, lab experiments, experience sampling studies, etc. (Reb et al., 2020). These studies would be supported by training-based interventions in which the participants would be induced into a mindfulness condition through guided meditations, motivational talks or daily lectures. The data collection happens once during the beginning and then in the end. In the case of ESM studies, if the independent variable needs to predict a dependent variable, the DV is measured at a different time of the day when the intervention would have been administered.

For, Hafenbrack et al. (2020), in their study on the impact of mindfulness on prosocial behaviour, administered their intervention during the morning on the active group and then recorded the prosocial behaviour during the afternoon. Similarly, (Thoroughgood et al.,2020), in their study on trait mindfulness as a moderator, recorded the mediator paranoid cognition and the DV emotional exhaustion the following day. This kind of data collection is called the interval contingent strategy. Studies like (Walker & Colosimo, 2011; Bajaj et al.,2018) have collected data based on self-reporting without administering interventions.

The categorical classification of intervention design includes (Eby, et al., 2019) –

1- Pre-Test/Post-Test – The same group would undergo different training to assess change.
2- Randomised or Non-Randomized Waitlist Control Group – Two groups will be divided randomly or non-randomly into an active experiment group and a waitlist group as a control group. The active experiment group would receive training first, followed by the waitlist group.
3- Randomised or Non-Randomized Pre-Test/Post-Test – Two groups would be randomly or non-randomly divided into active and control groups. The control group would not receive any training, or if they received it would be training for comparing both results.

4- Randomised Switching replication designs – In the beginning, a pretest is followed by one of the groups as an active experimentation group and the other as a control group. The roles get switched, and further comparisons are made.
5- Multiple Baseline – The group is checked on their behaviour stability, and then a sequence of training-based interventions is administered.

Out of all the methods mentioned above, 'Pre-Test/Post-Test' has been used the most, followed by 'randomised waitlist group' and 'randomised pre-test/post-tests. Most training interventions are designed to reduce stress, like MBSR, i.e., Mindfulness-Based Stress Reduction; MBCR, i.e., Mindfulness-Based Cognitive Therapy Training; and Yoga-Based and meditation-based techniques. Additionally, if we look at how these training interventions have been delivered, it is mostly by 'lectures' followed by 'audio recordings', 'group discussion', 'written materials', 'retreats' and even 'online modules. It is important to note that mindfulness is not only about stress reduction. Our previous discussion highlights that such attention can also lead to higher orientation.

Coming to the scales used to measure mindfulness, items from MAAS, i.e., Mindfulness Attention Awareness Scale (Brown & Ryan, 2003) and FFMQ, i.e., Five Facets Mindfulness Questionnaire (Baer et al., 2006) have been used widely. Some of these items include "I find myself occupied with the future or the past", "I find myself doing things without paying attention", "I pay attention to how my emotions affect my thoughts and behaviour", "I can usually describe how I feel at the moment in considerable detail", "I perceive my feelings and emotions without having to react to them", "I find myself listening to someone with one ear, doing something else at the same time" etc.

One interesting thing to note from these items is that even though they are being used to measure a variable, these questions demand deeper level information processing, which can be termed 'reflection'. For example – Suppose I am part of an experiment's active group and undergo a focussed breathing meditation; it might develop a 'state mindfulness' behaviour in me, but what is the guarantee that it would stay with me for a long time? Most of the time in the experimental design studies, people have been tested on mindfulness by being given an intervention for stress reduction. Sometimes, the participants were unaware that they were being tested for mindfulness. All of these studies have hardly ever questioned the qualitative nature of mindfulness. This poses the question of whether all the short-term programs yield the proper benefit (Eby et al., 2019).

3. 'PRACTICAL RATIONALITY' AS AN ALTERNATE THEORY AND WAY FORWARD

If we look from a philosophical standpoint, what most of the studies have followed is a positivist stance wherein both epistemologies, as well as ontology have been objectivist. Both can be subjective based on individual beliefs (Reina & Kudesia, 2020). Example – It is not necessary that the everyday practice of meditation would undoubtedly increase my cognitive resources to a large extent and make me live positively. It is also not necessary that such practices would always help me reduce stress. The cause of stress can be manifold. Focused breathing might induce a 'state of mindfulness' but may not stand for long as a permanent redressal. What if mindfulness-based positivity leads me to such a selfless acceptance that it may hamper my personal growth? Questions that surround a person's mindfulness are often contextual. In contextualism (Tsoukas, 1994), facts assumed are loosely structured. Historical events are assumed to lie at the intersection. The construction of narratives and stories is emphasised, and the conclusions are left open-ended. Therefore, loose frameworks are purposely put forward. E.g., Mintzberg's concept of strategic management wherein Mintzberg calls strategy a 'creative process' which would lose its distinctiveness if put into models. In this sense, putting mindfulness within the framework of practising and achieving benefits would dilute its purpose. Instead, an orientation towards higher experience fills it with the required curiosity.

Therefore, we would like to introduce the applicability of 'practical rationality'.

Management under scientific rationality followed an entity-based view, i.e., to look at organisations as one single entity. Practical Rationality was introduced as an alternative to scientific rationality (Sandberg & Tsoukas, 2011). Two things come under this theory – 'entwinement' and 'breakdowns'. 'Entwinement' refers to being connected with whatever we encounter. Heidegger's Existential Ontology posits that, as human beings, we are never separated; instead, we are entwined with others. E.g., Take the case of an apprenticeship worker. There could be some specific description in the job, but when practically working, the person may discover much more. Therefore, an apprentice as a learner would experience much more during the practice and perhaps need to learn more.

While performing our duties, we are usually in 'absorbed coping' mode. It is only when some uncertainty comes that 'breakdowns' would occur. E.g.- While teaching an offline class, if there is a power shutdown, it is a 'temporary breakdown' because the distraction caused is minimal. Nevertheless, if the classes are happening online and power cuts happen, in that case, the class has to stop, which is a 'complete breakdown'. People need to search for breakdowns. The first-order breakdown would involve realising the need for change while absorbing coping. Second-order breakdown is deliberately trying to create a breakdown, e.g., scenario planning.

Taking the context of mindfulness, the problem with putting the practice of mindfulness within a framework prevents the very nature of the practice. In addition, putting a more scholastic attitude disconnects from the social context. Therefore, if we see mindfulness in this context, sudden negative situations cause 'temporary breakdowns' in our routine, which can be a cup of tea falling and spilling over. A total breakdown can be caused by organizational-level outcomes like pressure to get targets, layoffs, or the sudden emergence of bad news. Focused breathing, which enhances the mindfulness of an individual, does help in these situations (Hafenbrack et al., 2020). It is because mindfulness starts with training on neutral stimuli like breath, which then gets cultivated and aids us during emotionally charged and demanding situations (Jha et al.,2010). Therefore, we posit that mindfulness should not be recorded by mere surveys or be enabled by training or stress reduction-based interventions. Researchers can ascertain individuals' mindfulness by asking them to search for breakdowns while entwined in their daily activities. In this sense, (Forjan et al.,2020) were unique in their study as they collected data based on diary entries and then did further analysis. On similar lines, we suggest that more such subjective approaches based on practical rationality shall be undertaken to understand individuals' mindfulness. Below, we outline an example of the same by incorporating the Socratic style of questioning.

Drawing upon the metacognitive theory, people can be tested on their beliefs by following the MBM, i.e., Metacognitive Beliefs in Mindfulness Scale (Reina & Kudesia, 2020), which includes items to check on their 'attentional sufficiency', 'virtue of monitoring', and 'map-terrain differentiation'. However, we propose following the Socratic questioning principles to enhance their higher orientation. Socratic style of questioning is an inductive dialectic means of asking progressive series of questions that are answered by the client (Corsini, 2002). It is assumed that the client knows the answer already. The discussion happens in a more abstract manner (Padesky,1993a). Therefore, individuals can be asked the same questions as presented in these popular scales like MBM, MAAS or FFMQ, but not in a survey. Instead, there can be an addition of 'Why' in those questions. For instance, items like - "I find myself doing things without paying attention" and "I find myself occupied with the future or the past" can be replaced and asked as "Why do I find myself doing things without paying attention?" or "Why I find myself occupied with the future or the past". Some more modifications can be like instead of "I can usually describe how I feel at the moment in considerable detail", asking "Can I usually describe how I feel at the moment in considerable detail?" would put the person in some deeper cognition. Individuals in their diary entries can record these questions or even be self-recorded in audio mode, which can subsequently be analysed qualitatively. Thus, a proper qualitative approach to derive individual mindfulness would justify the presence of subjectivity among individual's perceptions.

4. DISCUSSION AND CONCLUSION

The arguments in the above sections state the following – 1) Evaluating the process of mindfulness from existing literature and theories, 2) The importance of an organisational system in enhancing the process, 3) Applying a more qualitative approach to record and measure mindfulness to enhance a higher orientation towards experience. We understood that 'Mindfulness' is an individual-level process that workplace factors and systems can influence. In addition, the purpose of initiating mindfulness should not be towards more 'hedonic' reasons like stress management. Instead, the purpose should be more 'eudemonic'. Happy people would make the organisation happy.

This will, in turn, improve the organisational outcomes. Therefore, a more systematic approach towards improving 'intrinsic motivation' and 'extrinsic rewards' can be helpful. From the part of the organisation, existing theories like the 'upper echelons theory', which postulates that it is the leadership which would help implement a ground-level strategy, can be more helpful in developing the strategic viewpoint (Nahavandi & Krishnan, 2017). Implementation of mindfulness requires a long-term orientation; thus, it should happen more thoughtfully. From a strategic lens, for organisations, there can be enormous challenges of increased cost due to allocation of resources, availability of employee's time, presence of good trainers, revamping the organisational mission, etc., which could deter them from the required competitiveness (Krishnan, 2021).

Therefore, there would be an additional requirement from the leadership lens to exhibit more kindness, authenticity, humility, accountability and generosity (Nahavandi & Krishnan, 2017). Irrespective of the challenges, implementing the requisite work setting and enhancing mindfulness may show little impact, but it would surely do so in the long run. Especially post-COVID-19, wherein most people got used to working at home, there needed to be more regular face-to-face connection among people. New mindfulness-based initiatives can counter this.

Another Eastern perspective of mindfulness that has not been discussed in the literature is the 'Bhagawad Gita'. Chapter 4, Verse 29 of Bhagwad Gita says, "apane juhvati pranam prane panam tathapare pranapana-gati ruddhva pranayama-parayanah apare niyataharah pranan pranesu juhvati" which means "people who are inclined to the process of breath restraint to remain in trance, practice by offering the movement of the outgoing breath into the incoming, and the incoming breath into the outgoing, and thus, at last, remain in trance, stopping all breathing. Others, curtailing the eating process, offer the outgoing breath into itself as a sacrifice". The context here is 'pranayama', which means controlling the breath. These methods were presented in the 'Hatha Yoga' system, whose processes help control the senses and advance towards higher self-realization. Even in our above discussion on recent studies, we came across that the practice of focused breathing does help in enhancing metacognition. On a concluding note, we would say that if we ease the means to achieve mindfulness for an individual in any way, it can be further implemented for a broader group of people. Many organizational employees can benefit from the higher orientation of mindfulness practice, which leads to a higher orientation of organizations towards serving society.

REFERENCES

Arrowsmith, J., & Parker, J. (2013). The meaning of 'employee engagement' for the values and roles of the HRM function. *International Journal of Human Resource Management*, *24*(14), 2692–2712. do i:10.1080/09585192.2013.763842

Baer, R. A., Smith, G. T., Hopkins, J., Krietemeyer, J., & Toney, L. (2006). Using self-report assessment methods to explore facets of mindfulness. *Assessment*, *13*(1), 27–45. doi:10.1177/1073191105283504 PMID:16443717

Bajaj, B., Gupta, R., & Sengupta, S. (2018, October 19). Emotional Stability and Self-Esteem as Mediators Between Mindfulness and Happiness. *Journal of Happiness Studies*. Advance online publication. doi:10.100710902-018-0046-4

Bodhi, B. (2011). What does mindfulness really mean? A canonical perspective. *Contemporary Buddhism*, *12*(1), 19–39. doi:10.1080/14639947.2011.564813

Brown, K. W., & Ryan, R. M. (2003, April). The benefits of being present: Mindfulness and its role in psychological well-being. *Journal of Personality and Social Psychology*, *84*(4), 822–848. doi:10.1037/0022-3514.84.4.822 PMID:12703651

Cheung, S. Y., Huang, E. G., Chang, S., & Wei, L. (2020, July). Does being mindful make people more creative at work? The role of creative process engagement and perceived leader humility. *Organizational Behavior and Human Decision Processes*, *159*, 39–48. doi:10.1016/j.obhdp.2019.12.003

Chong, S., Kim, Y. J., Lee, H. W., Johnson, R. E., & Lin, S.-H. (2020, July). Mind your own break! The interactive effect of workday respite activities and mindfulness on employee outcomes via affective linkages. *Organizational Behavior and Human Decision Processes*, *159*, 64–77. doi:10.1016/j.obhdp.2019.11.001

Coo, C., & Salanova, M. (2017, May 31). Mindfulness Can Make You Happy-and-Productive: A Mindfulness Controlled Trial and Its Effects on Happiness, Work Engagement and Performance. *Journal of Happiness Studies*, *19*(6), 1691–1711. doi:10.100710902-017-9892-8

Corsini, R. J. (2002). *The dictionary of psychology*. Brunner-Routledge.

Eby, L. T., Allen, T. D., Conley, K. M., Williamson, R. L., Henderson, T. G., & Mancini, V. S. (2019, June). Mindfulness-based training interventions for employees: A qualitative review of the literature. *Human Resource Management Review*, *29*(2), 156–178. doi:10.1016/j.hrmr.2017.03.004

Forjan, D. N., Tuckey, M. R., & Li, Y. (2020, January 20). Problem solving and affect as mechanisms linking daily mindfulness to task performance and job satisfaction. *Stress and Health, 36*(3), 338–349. doi:10.1002mi.2931 PMID:31957967

Fredrickson, B. L. (2001). The role of positive emotions in positive psychology: The broaden-and-build theory of positive emotions. *The American Psychologist, 56*(3), 218–226. doi:10.1037/0003-066X.56.3.218 PMID:11315248

Garg, N., & Saini, D. (2023). Workplace spirituality to cultivate innovative work behaviour: The moderating role of perceived working conditions. *The International Journal of Sociology and Social Policy*. doi:10.1108/IJSSP-03-2023-0050

Garland, E., Gaylord, S., & Park, J. (2009). The role of mindfulness in positive reappraisal. *Explore (New York, N.Y.), 5*(1), 37–44. doi:10.1016/j.explore.2008.10.001 PMID:19114262

Garland, E. L., Farb, N. A., Goldin, P. R., & Fredrickson, B. L. (2015, November 24). Mindfulness Broadens Awareness and Builds Eudaimonic Meaning: A Process Model of Mindful Positive Emotion Regulation. *Psychological Inquiry, 26*, 293–314. doi:10.1080/1047840X.2015.1064294 PMID:27087765

Hafenbrack, A. C., Cameron, L. D., Spreitzer, G. M., Zhang, C., Noval, L. J., & Shaffakat, S. (2020, July). Helping People by Being in the Present: Mindfulness Increases Prosocial Behavior. *Organizational Behavior and Human Decision Processes, 159*, 21–38. doi:10.1016/j.obhdp.2019.08.005

Hobfoll, S. E. (2001, December 21). The Influence of Culture, Community, and the Nested-Self in the Stress Process: Advancing Conservation of Resources Theory. *Applied Psychology, 50*(3), 337–421. doi:10.1111/1464-0597.00062

Jensen, C. G., Vangkilde, S., Frokjaer, V., & Hasselbalch, S. G. (2012). Mindfulness training affects attention—Or is it attentional effort? *Journal of Experimental Psychology. General, 141*(1), 106–123. doi:10.1037/a0024931 PMID:21910559

Jha, A. P., Stanley, E. A., Kiyonaga, A., Wong, L., & Gelfand, L. (2010). Examining the protective effects of mindfulness training on working memory capacity and affective experience. *Emotion (Washington, D.C.), 10*(1), 54–64. doi:10.1037/a0018438 PMID:20141302

Kay, A. A., & Skarlicki, D. P. (2020, July). Cultivating a conflict-positive workplace: How mindfulness facilitates constructive conflict management. *Organizational Behavior and Human Decision Processes, 159*, 8–20. doi:10.1016/j.obhdp.2020.02.005

Kilpatrick, L. A., Suyenobu, B. Y., Smith, S. R., Bueller, J. A., Goodman, T., Creswell, J. D., Tillisch, K., Mayer, E. A., & Naliboff, B. D. (2011). Impact of mindfulness-based stress reduction training on intrinsic brain connectivity. *NeuroImage, 56*(1), 290–298. doi:10.1016/j.neuroimage.2011.02.034 PMID:21334442

Kornfielf, J. (2011). *Teachings of the Buddha*. Shambala Publications.

Krishnan, H. A. (2021). Mindfulness as a strategy for sustainable competitive advantage. *Business Horizons, 64*(5), 697–709. doi:10.1016/j.bushor.2021.02.023

Kudesia, R. S. (2019). Mindfulness as Metacognitive Practice. *Academy of Management Review, 44*(2), 405–423. doi:10.5465/amr.2015.0333

Lazarus, R., & Folkman, S. (1984). *Stress, appraisal, and coping*. Springer.

Liu, S., Xin, H., Shen, L., Hi, J., & Liu, J. (2020, January 21). The Influence of Individual and Team Mindfulness on Work Engagement. *Frontiers in Psychology, 10*, 2928. doi:10.3389/fpsyg.2019.02928 PMID:32038356

Nahavandi, A., & Krishnan, H. A. (2017). Indo-European Leadership (IEL): A Non-Western Leadership Perspective. *Global and Culturally Diverse Leaders and Leadership (Building Leadership Bridges*, (PP. 105-123). Emerald. doi:10.1108/S2058-880120170000003006

Padesky, C. A. (1993a). *Socratic Questioning: Changing minds or guiding discovery?* Keynote address to European Congress of Behavioural and Cognitive Therapies, London.

Reb, J., Allen, T., & Vogus, T. J. (2020, July). Mindfulness arrives at work: Deepening our understanding of mindfulness in organizations. *Organizational Behavior and Human Decision Processes, 159*, 1–7. doi:10.1016/j.obhdp.2020.04.001

Reina, C. S., & Kudesia, R. S. (2020, July). Wherever you go, there you become: How mindfulness arises in everyday situations. *Organizational Behavior and Human Decision Processes, 159*, 78–96. doi:10.1016/j.obhdp.2019.11.008

Ryan, R. M., Huta, V., & Deci, E. L. (2008). Living well: A self-determination theory perspective on eudaimonia. *Journal of Happiness Studies, 9*(1), 139–170. doi:10.100710902-006-9023-4

Saini, D. (2020). Does Mindfulness & Happiness Predict Job Satisfaction among Indian Employees? *Indian Journal of Industrial Relations, 56*(1).

Sandberg, J., & Tsoukas, H. (2011, April 1). Grasping the Logic of Practice: Theorizing Through Practical Rationality. *Academy of Management Review, 36*(2), 338–360. doi:10.5465/amr.2009.0183

Shahbaz, W., & Parker, J. (2021, June 26). Workplace mindfulness: An integrative review of antecedents, mediators, and moderators. *Human Resource Management Review*. doi:10.1016/j.hrmr.2021.100849

Tett, R. P., & Burnett, D. D. (2003). A personality trait-based interactionist model of job performance. *The Journal of Applied Psychology, 88*(3), 500–517. doi:10.1037/0021-9010.88.3.500 PMID:12814298

Thoroughgood, C. N., Sawyer, K. B., & Webster, J. R. (2020, July). Finding calm in the storm: A daily investigation of how trait mindfulness buffers against paranoid cognition and emotional exhaustion following perceived discrimination at work. *Organizational Behavior and Human Decision Processes, 159*, 49–63. doi:10.1016/j.obhdp.2019.02.004

Tsoukas, H. (1994). Refining Common Sense: Types of Knowledge in Management Studies. *Journal of Management Studies, 31*(6), 761–780. doi:10.1111/j.1467-6486.1994.tb00638.x

Walker, L. H., & Colosimo, K. (2011, January). Mindfulness, self-compassion, and happiness in non-meditators: A theoretical and empirical examination. *Personality and Individual Differences, 50*(2), 222–227. doi:10.1016/j.paid.2010.09.033

Weinstein, N., Brown, K. W., & Ryan, R. M. (2009, June). A multi-method examination of the effects of mindfulness on stress attribution, coping, and emotional well-being. *Journal of Research in Personality*, *43*(3), 374–385. doi:10.1016/j.jrp.2008.12.008

Weiss, H. M., & Cropanzano, R. (1996). Affective events theory: A theoretical discussion of the structure, causes and consequences of affective experiences at work. *Research in Organizational Behavior*, *18*, 1–7.

Chapter 3
Atman's Awakening:
Bhagavad Gita's Path to Moksha Through Karma Yoga and Atmabodha

Shreya Chawla
Christ University, India

Madhu Giri
https://orcid.org/0009-0008-7950-4821
Christ University, India

ABSTRACT

Indian psychology is characterized by its diverse and rich traditions that have evolved over several centuries. This chapter tries to fulfill four objectives: 1) To provide a brief overview of the concept of self in Bhagavad Gita; 2) to give a brief overview of the two frameworks for moksha given in the Bhagavad Gita with the help of empirical evidence of current research; 3) to propose a conceptual model using Triguna Framework and Trimarg Framework; and 4) to provide the implications of the proposed model. The chapter begins with an explanation of the Indian philosophical understanding of self from the lens of Bhagavad Gita. In the second section, an effort has been made to compare and contrast the two frameworks given in Bhagavad Gita for Moksha. The last section introduces a conceptual model to enhance sattva guna and reduce the rajas and tamas gunas to attain atmabodha that can have positive psychological implications in modern times.

INTRODUCTION

The Bhagavad Gita was written between 2500 and 5000 BC. Chapters 25–42 of the epic Mahabharata, which has 100,000 shlokas, are represented by the Gita. Bhagavad Gita is considered a scripture of utmost importance in the Sanātana Dharma (eternal religion). The fundamental ideas addressed in the Bhagavad Gita are deconditioning, dismantling the ego, and consciousness. These ideas are thought to be the necessary prerequisites for a person's transformation. The Bhagavad Gita, translated as the 'Song of God,' is a 700-verse scripture divided into 18 chapters penned by Lord Ganesha as told by Sage Ved Vyasa.

DOI: 10.4018/978-1-6684-9778-4.ch003

The Bhagavad Gita is a revered body of knowledge that cuts across time and culture in the large body of Vedic literature, which principally explains the nature and experience of the inner Self or Atman. The nature of atman is among the most important psychological issues summarized in Bhagavad Gita.

It is based on a discourse between the two protagonists of the Mahabharata, Pandava prince Arjuna and Lord Krishna, an incarnation of Lord Vishnu. The conflict between the Kauravas and Pandavas, two groups of cousins, is portrayed in the Mahabharata. On the battlefield of Kurukshetra, the Pandavas and their allies defeated the Kauravas with Lord Krishna's assistance. A man of integrity, a person with clarity of thought, and someone with compassion, Arjuna, the best archer of his day, falls into a condition of complete despair prior to the start of the battle on the battlefield of Kurukshetra. Due to his feelings of remorse, uncertainty, and loyalty to his family, Arjuna is reluctant to participate in the battle because he worries about losing his relatives and teachers. As a result, he considers leaving the battle. In this crucial moment, Lord Krishna revealed Arjuna which path to take in order to fulfil his duty in the war and achieve victory and righteousness against evil.

All the chapters emphasize a wide range of topics such as ignorance in the form of desires, attachment (vasanas), raag, dwesha, creation of the universe as an interplay of trigunas-sattva, rajas and tamas, paths(margas) to attain moksha, brahamna, etc. Based on the content analysis of the Bhagavad Gita, this chapter tries to fulfill the following objectives:

- To propose different stages of how a sādhak can move from ignorance to brahmana.
- To propose an application-based model based on the constructs discussed in Bhagavad Gita

BACKGROUND

Casebeer (1952) observed that the holy text emphasizes the existence two selves within an individual, which are referred to as:

- **Brahman**: The Absolute, the Supreme Reality, or the supreme self. It is considered to be beyond the laws of life and death, changeless, and persists throughout all the experiences. The shloka in the Bhagavad Gita that supports this are:

śhrī bhagavān uvācha

akṣharaṁ brahma paramaṁ svabhāvo 'dhyātmam uchyate

bhūta-bhāvodbhava-karo visargaḥ karma-sanjñitaḥ

Bhagavad Gita 8.13

This shloka, as translated by Swami Adidevananda, "The Supreme Imperishable (Aksara), according to the Lord, is brahman.' It cannot be destroyed and is the sum total of all individual selves. One's own material nature (the body) is known as Adhyatma or that which dwells with the self." This shloka further clarifies that the brahman can be known only through self-knowledge, an action (karma) just like the offering (to the gods) that causes beings' existence, manifestation, and sustenance of beings. Another shloka

evaṁ buddheḥ paraṁ buddhvā sanstabhyātmānam ātmanā

jahi śhatruṁ mahā-bāho kāma-rūpaṁ durāsadam

Bhagavad Gita 3.43

In this shloka the self is being referred to as Atman as highlighted by Swami Sivananda "The higher self ought to regulate the lower self. The foe of desire must be subdued."

- **Atman**: It is also known as the individual self, which may be impacted by mind, ego, or personality; in other words, the atman is brahman within the sheath of personality (Casebeer, 1952). Brahman is atman lodged within the individual being. Prabhavananda & Isherwood (1947). These alternate realities present a more thorough and fulfilling comprehension of the atman.

The Bhagavad Gita considers individuals as divine and spiritual. In an Indian context, Dr. Sangeetha Menon reflects on the role of the Bhagavad Gita in strengthening the mental faculty. Based on shlokas 8.13 and 3.43, the three types of selves according to Bhagavad Gita are presented in Figure 1.

Figure 1. depicts the selves and how individuals perceive them. The lower self, or the physical body, is the only self. After a rigorous process, the sādhak can perceive the atman or Individual self beyond

Figure 1. Types of self

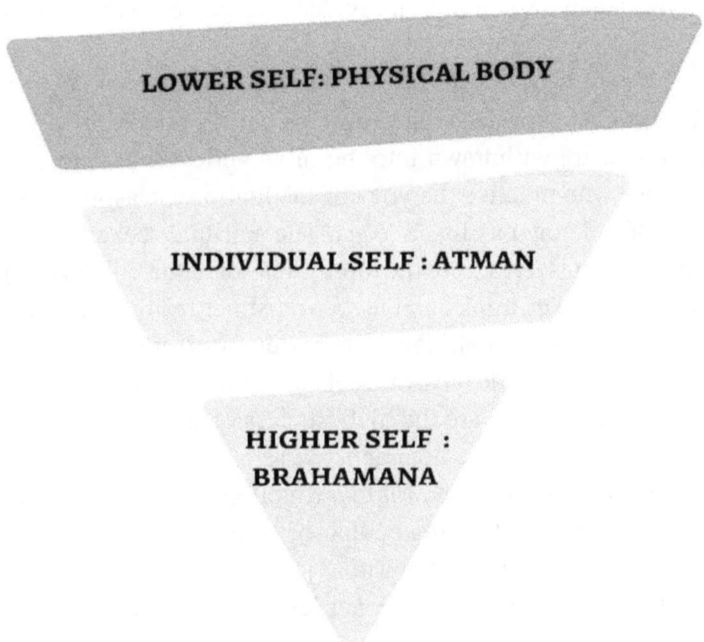

the lower self. Moreover, a few people like ascetics, rishis, or sometimes householders like Raja Janak could perceive the higher self or Brahmana.

Some significant concepts essential in awakening the atman discussed in the Bhagavad Gita are self-knowledge (Atmabodha), Karma Yoga, and Moksha. They are highlighted in the following shlokas:

.jñānena tu tad ajñānaṁ yeṣhāṁ nāśhitam ātmanaḥ

teṣhām āditya-vaj jñānaṁ prakāśhayati tat param

Bhagavad Gita 5.16

This shloka, as comprehended by Swami Sivananda, is that self-knowledge annihilates ignorance, which is considered the root cause of human suffering. In this shloka, the term self-knowledge is represented by ātmanaḥ jñānaṁ. However, long after the composition of the revered text Bhagavad Gita, Adi Shankaracharya, an Indian teacher, composed a text known as Atmabodha, which refers to self-knowledge or self-awareness. The text consists of sixty-eight verses that describe the path to Self-knowledge or the awareness of Atman. (Dalal, 2010; Isaeva,1993). There are several paths to attain Atmabodha, which are indicated in the following shloka.

dhyānenātmani paśhyanti kechid ātmānam ātmanā

anye sānkhyena yogena karma-yogena chāpare

Bhagavad Gita 13.25

As per Swami Shivananda's commentary on the shloka, an individual can achieve atmabodha through any of the following paths, depending on their individual nature, temperament, and capacity:

a) **Raja Yoga:** The first path is Maharshi Patanjali's Raja yoga, also known as the yoga of meditation. Patanjali. Raja yogins experience the supreme self in buddhi by a sanctified mind, as with concentration, all senses are withdrawn into the mind and are not permitted to run towards their sensuous things. Those who practice the yoga of meditation are aspirants of the middling class.
b) **Sankhya Yoga:** It is also known as Jnana Yoga. The spiritual seekers do vichara, i.e., analysis or reflection, and separate themselves from the three gunas of nature. The three gunas are sattva, rajas, and tamas. The spiritual seeker thinks and feels as distinct from the three alities, being the silent unattached witness who is a non-doer, nonenjoyer, immortal, eternal, self-existent, self-luminous, indivisible, unborn, unchanging, and thus, the seeker identifies himself/herself with the Atman(Self). Those who practice Sankhya Yoga are the highest class of spiritual aspirants.
c) **Karma Yoga:** The spiritual aspirant who practices karma yoga surrenders his/her actions and their fruits to the Lord. They have *Isvarapana Buddhi* (intelligence that offers everything to God). This results in mental purity, leading to Atmabodha, or self-knowledge. Those who practice Karma Yoga are considered as the beginners of spiritual journey. Through rigorous Sadhana, or spiritual practises, the sādhak of the middle and beginner levels soon become sādhak of the highest level.

The following shloka emphasizes on the importance of karma yoga.

śhrī bhagavān uvācha

sannyāsaḥ karma-yogaśh cha niḥśhreyasa-karāvubhau

tayos tu karma-sannyāsāt karma-yogo viśhiṣhyate

Bhagavad Gita 5.2

This shloka, as explained by Swami Sivananda, propagates that for an individual who wants to attain moksha but does not have atmabodha yet, the practice of karma yoga is accessible and superior to the practice of karma sannyasa, i.e., renunciation of action. In another shloka

yāmimāṁ puṣhpitāṁ vāchaṁ pravadanty-avipaśhchitaḥ

veda-vāda-ratāḥ pārtha nānyad astīti vādinaḥ

kāmātmānaḥ swarga-parā janma-karma-phala-pradām

kriyā-viśheṣha-bahulāṁ bhogaiśhwarya-gatiṁ prati

Bhagavad Gita 2.42

The karma kanda of the Vedas, which lays down particular rules for specific actions to obtain definite fruits in the form of fulfilling desires, is deeply enamoured by the foolish people in expectation of sensuous enjoyments in Svarga (heaven), according to Swami Sivananda's interpretation. Swami Sivananda further states that moksha can only be attained by atmabodha but not by performing a thousand and one sacrifices.

Based on the shlokas 5.16, 13.25, 5.2, 2.42, and 3.4, we want to depict how the sādhak, which is translated as a seeker or spiritual aspirant, takes the journey from the state of ignorance, i.e., identification with the physical body (lower self) to the state of brahmana (higher self) or samadhi. The process is depicted in Figure 2.

Fig. 2 depicts the four stages: ignorance, atman wakening, transition, and samadhi, which a sādhaka needs to go through to reach from the lower self (physical body) to the higher self (brahmana). This chapter will only focus on the first three stages.

These concepts are usually considered essential for spiritual aspirants but are not considered to have any practical and psychological significance, which is not valid. Through this chapter, we will delve into the aspects of different stages depicted in Fig 2. and understand how these concepts can be used in day-to-day living to improve the quality of life of individuals. Some of the applications of these constructs of Bhagavad Gita are discussed here briefly.

Figure 2. Journey of a sādhak from ignorance to samadhi

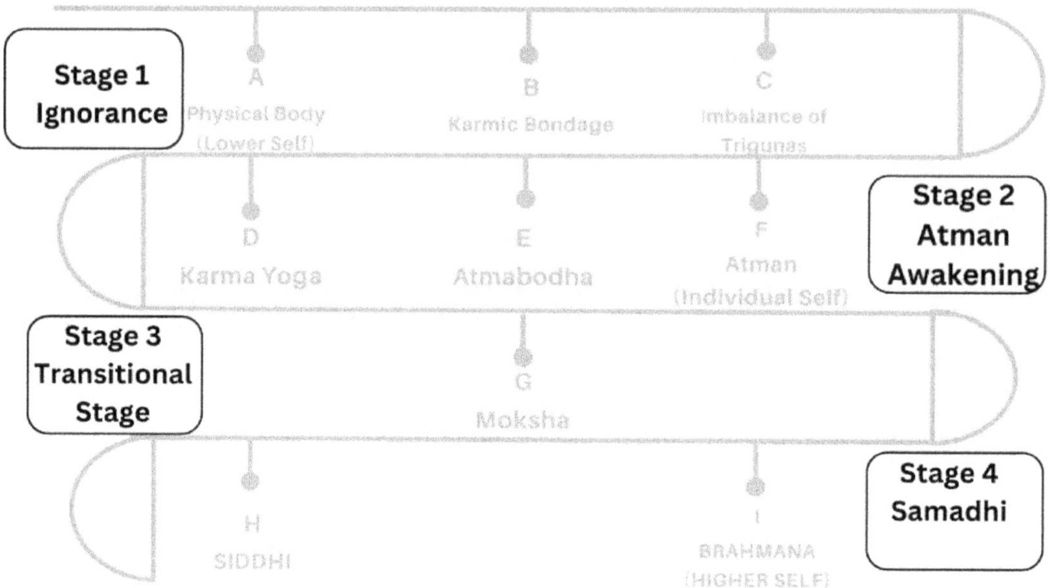

THE APPLICATIONS OF BHAGAVAD GITA IN THE REALM OF PSYCHOLOGY

Until recently, the Bhagavad Gita has been largely perceived as a religious and philosophical text. However, the paradigm, knowledge, and concepts from works like the Bhagavad Gita have received widespread acceptance as a tool for learning or knowledge generation across academic disciplines, particularly in the social sciences like psychology, due to a greater awareness of Indian social reality. Due to the immense amount of research that has been conducted, it is practically impossible to include all the applications of the Bhagavad Gita in a psychological context, but some applications are discussed here:

1. The interaction between Lord Krishna and his disciple Arjuna depicts many psychotherapeutic principles (Bhatia et al., 2013), Cognitive Behaviour Therapy principles (Sharma,2014) in the Bhagavad Gita. Phogat et al. (2020) compared the Bhagavad Gita to humanistic-existential therapy by suggesting that just like the humanistic and existential approaches focus on the importance of self-awareness and self-understanding to achieve personal growth, the Bhagavad Gita talks about self-knowledge (Atmabodha) that leads to the attainment of peace.
2. The Bhagavad Gita's central theme also outlines a procedure for resolving Arjuna's disputes with the three gunas, tamas, rajas, and sattva, which are analogous to the ideas of id, ego, and superego. Like the Id, Tamas represents self-centeredness and a lack of regard for consequences. The other two gunas, Rajas and Sattva, are analogous to the ego and superego. Like Freudian psychoanalytic theory, the trigunas are the source of conflict and engage in a never-ending struggle for dominance that causes anxiety. Interventions can be designed for balancing these gunas, which could help the client.

3. The Asakti Model (Roy & Kumar, 2023) focuses on how asakti (attachment) can lead to insecurity, aggression, possessiveness, and a high need for recognition and frustration, leading to psychological problems. This model further emphasizes how spiritual asakti brings a balance of mind and body and allows individuals to attain mental, spiritual, and emotional well-being.
4. The Triguna theory in Bhagavad Gita offers a useful framework for understanding mindful leadership. Sattvic leaders have been found to have a better sense of balance, a higher level of positivism in the face of difficulties and crises, and tend to be more innovative and creative than rajasic and tamasic leaders (Sathiyaseelan et al., 2022).

The management of *trigunas* is vital in the sādhak's transformational journey. Triguna imbalance is the primary cause of ignorance in stage 1, which is discussed here in detail.

STAGE ONE: IGNORANCE

The Upanishads clearly show that material richness cannot bring spiritual enlightenment. In contrast, a spiritually enlightened (rich) person will not experience poverty as materialists would define it. Materialists are considered as ignorant in the Bhagavad Gita. The reason is that from the spiritual point of view, the poorest person has unlimited desires. However, the needs of a spiritually enlightened person are very few, and desires are minimal. Hence, the Upanishads declare that 'one who realizes the self attains all the worlds (lokas) and all the desires (kamas).' There is no limit to desires; hence, it is the need of the hour to make people realize its negative consequences. The actions (karmas) performed using the physical body to fulfill all the desires are full of attachment for the fruits and desirable consequences, which leads to the karmic bondage in the individual, which further imbalances the trigunas, i.e., sattva, rajas, and tamas. It has cognitive and affective implications for an individual.

It should be noted that not all individuals walk down the path to reach moksha. Most individuals never come out of their ignorance and spend their whole lives in the effect of attachments and fulfilling their desires, considering the outward reality as the ultimate truth. However, on the other hand, some individuals seek spiritual enlightenment and try to discover the higher self. Such individuals are also known as spiritual aspirants/ seekers. In this chapter, such individuals will be referred to as sādhak. In contrast, individuals who identify with their physical body or lower self and are not seeking atmabodha or moksha will not be considered sādhak.

Identification With Physical Body

In the first stage, an individual is just aware of his/ her physical body and considers it to be the ultimate truth, which is also considered as the state of ignorance in the Bhagavad Gita as discussed here:

nādatte kasyachit pāpaṁ na chaiva sukṛitaṁ vibhuḥ

ajñānenāvṛitaṁ jñānaṁ tena muhyanti jantavaḥ

Bhagavad Gita 5.15

The shloka emphasizes that ignorance envelopes knowledge. The individuals live in delusion that they will enjoy the rewards for their meritorious acts. Hence, as Swami Sivananda explains, they identify with the body and senses, which hinders attaining moksha.

Karmic Bondage

The enjoyment of various sensory experiences is possible because of the actions of the sense organs, which create passion and attachment to worldly objects. To satiate their passion, individuals under the sway of likes and dislikes perform further actions that strengthen the karmic bondage of individuals in this world. The following shloka also emphasizes this:

adhaśh chordhvaṁ prasṛitās tasya śhākhā

guṇa-pravṛiddhā viṣhaya-pravālāḥ

adhaśh cha mūlāny anusantatāni

karmānubandhīni manuṣhya-loke

Bhagavad Gita 15.2

The shloka, as discussed by Swami Sivananda, "The trigunas of nature nourish this tree of Samsara. Individuals who live under the influence of passion and attachment are controlled by their likes and dislikes; the sense objects are their buds, and the roots that grow downward are the bonds of Karma. This magnificent tree's sprouts appeal to the senses with their qualities of sound, touch, color, taste, and fragrance. The roots of Karma on this earth are produced by the karmic tendencies from previous lives—that grow downward. These roots strengthen the karmic bondage of individuals by further actions."

Imbalance in Trigunas

Triguana Framework

The Bhagavad Gita states that the entire creation is the interplay of the three gunas collectively held to be subtle principles of nature responsible for the universe's creation, maintenance, and dissolution. (Maharishi, 1967). This framework emphasizes attaining moksha using the material body as the medium. The three gunas together make up the material body sattva, rajas, and tamas.

i) **Sāttva:** The word "sattva" comes from the root verb "as," which means "to be," and is related to the word "Asti," which means "is." That which promotes evolution and positive life-supporting qualities is termed "sattva guna." In Bhagavadgita, Sattva is associated with peacefulness, serenity, happiness, and wisdom(Agarwal, 2021).

According to Uma et al. (1971), Sattvic personalities are more likely to be introverted, have clear perceptions and cognitions (Sitamma et al., 1995), tend to be less verbally hostile (Wolf, 1998), be able to experience PSI and ESP (Sebastian & Mathew, 2002), and prefer self-growth (Sharma, 1999). One attains sattva, a peaceful mental state, via development and mastery. (Tikhe and others, 2012) Furthermore, increasing sattva guna is associated with many positive psychological outcomes, such as connectedness and oneness with others, psychological well-being, and happiness.

ii) **Rājas:** The word "rājas" comes from the root "ranj." Rajas guna balances sattva and tamas. Rajas, is categorised as tejas, denotes activity, urgency, and variability (Williams, 1964).In the Bhagavad Gita, rajas are associated with desire, greed, attachment, craving, ambition, and aggressiveness. (Agarwal, 2021)

Rajsic personalities exhibit high verbal aggression and low life satisfaction (Wolf, 1998), are extraverted (Uma et al., 1971), have explicit cognitions and keen perceptions, and are less satisfied with their jobs. Similar to ego function, rajas guna induces goal-directed action with an anticipation of reward (Bhatia et. al., 2013). Further, rajas are closer to sattva than tamas in the hierarchy of the gunas (Das, 1987).

iii) **Tāmas**: The term tamas has the root 'tam.' In the Bhagavad Gita, the term for life's harmful or destructive elements is "tamas guna." It also indicates a lack of activity. Tamas guna's characteristics are anger, greed, ignorance, confusion, inertia, darkness, and brutality (Kaur & Sinha, 1992), lethargy (Khemka, 2011), inertia, and resistance, obstinacy, stupidity, and helpless despair (Anuradha,2015).

In the Bhagavad Gita, tamas is characterized as being born of ignorance, which leads to poor attention, carelessness, lack of interest in work, inertia. (Agarwal, 2021), which causes suffering. Tamas Guna is maximizing pleasure and fulfilling desires by choosing the path that will bring both short-term delight and long-term sorrow. (Agarwal,2020). Tamas was associated with a disparity between the authentic and ideal selves. (Rani,2007). Psychoticism inclinations (Mohan & Sandhu, 1986); poor cognition, memory problems, and delusions (Sitamma et al., 1995); lower life satisfaction (Wolf, 1998); and low ESP abilities (Rao, 1979) are characteristics of tamasic personalities.

Various researchers who have conceptualised trigunas differently—as "three aspects or dimensions of human temperament and personality" (Marutham et al., 1998), as "temperamental conditions of an individual" as "types of personality" (Wolf, 1998), or as "three broad behavioural tendencies" (Mathew, 1995)—have all supported the co-existence of three gunas. The statistical results does not view them as separate dimensions because they indicate some correlation between the three gunas. Sattva guna has been considered the most desirable, leading to worldly peace and spiritual progress (Bhagavad Gita, 14.18). The three gunas are conceptualized as a progressive development from tamas to rajas to sattva (Mohan & Sandhu, 1986).

Therefore to attain the moksha it become imperative for the sādhak to transcend these gunas as highlighted in the following shloka

guṇān etān atītya trīn dehī deha-samudbhavān

janma-mṛityu-jarā-duḥkhair vimukto 'mṛitam aśhnute

Bhagavad Gita 14.20

One achieves immortality by transcending the three gunas of material nature connected to the body and freed from birth, death, old age, and suffering.

The Bhagavad Gita offers a more advanced path to success than only cultivating Sattvic qualities. It endorses transcending trigunas and attaining a superior unperturbedness or human perfection (moksha) by having a steady mind, peace, and bliss. (Bhatia.et.al., 2013). The same is depicted in Figure 3.

Transcending the Trigunas

Transcendence is not an 'experience' in the ordinary sense because transcendence implies no experiencer or experienced. In Eastern cultures, the conception of a transcendental self is more prevalent than in Western cultures. The technique of "transcending" the activity of the mind to directly experience the innermost self, or Atman, is used in Vedic Therapy (Pomfrey, 2002).

This mental procedure allows the individual to settle to finer and finer levels of the lower self. It starts from the level of the senses and settles through the mind, intellect, finest feeling, and ego. From time to time during this process, the mind spontaneously slips beyond the finest aspect of the lower self and experiences the most settled state of the individual self, i.e., the Atman. This process in Vedic psychology is known as transcending (Maharishi, 1963). Transcending is that which increases the life-supporting influence of the sattva most effectively. (Maharishi, 1967).

Figure 3. Triguna framework for Moksha
(Bhagavad Gita 14.20)

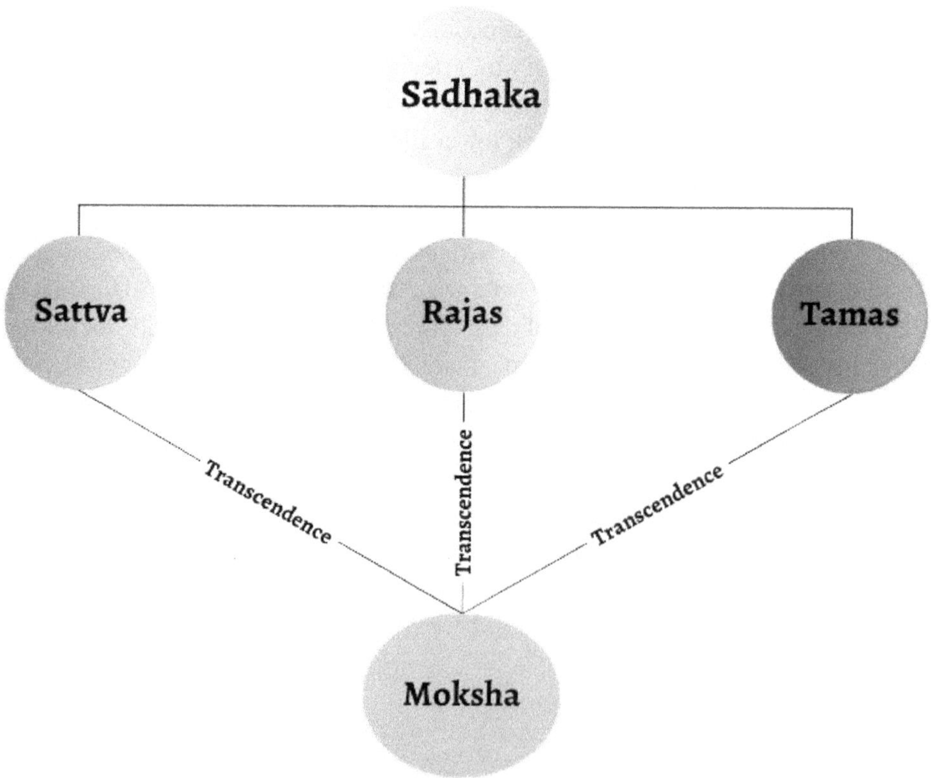

According to Vedic psychology, a split within the individual is initiated in stressful situations, either between cognition and affect or the unconscious and conscious mind, or heart and mind, which is the source of psychopathology.

A widening gap between cognition and affect (or conscious and unconscious) signals anxiety in the individual that further strains the ego resources of the client. The Bhagavad Gita indicates that in this weakened position of severe anxiety, the individual's defenses inevitably "slip." The fall of the defenses weakens one's sense of self and leaves the ego unprotected on the intrapsychic battlefield, thereby vulnerable to psychopathology. Ironically, though the defenses are viewed as critical to the development and protection of the ego, ultimately, they are seen in Vedic psychology as preserving and protecting the lower self.

Lord Krishna has taught the art of transcending in the Bhagavad Gita by providing Arjuna with a technique to transcend the mind and its limitations, which will facilitate Arjuna's ability to move beyond his "lower self' with its restricted thoughts, beliefs, and actions and establish him in his (Madahavananda, 1982). This realm of the self is independent of conditioning, not only from internalized objects but also from consciousness's entire waking, sleeping, and dreaming states (Gambhirananda, 1965).

Transcending is effortlessly accomplished through "dhyana," Sanskrit for "meditation" (Shearer, 1982). The technology provided by the Vedic Tradition of Knowledge and offered today by Vedic psychology is known as Transcendental Meditation (TM) (Dillbeck, 1991). The purpose of Arjuna's therapy and the primary focus of the Bhagavad Gita is to allow Arjuna to experience more evolved states of the human nervous system, known as higher states of consciousness. In these higher states, the self, transcendental consciousness, is not lost in the activity of waking, sleeping, or dreaming states of consciousness (Maharishi, 1963). This mental technique allows one to directly experience pure consciousness, known by physiologists as a unique fourth state of consciousness called "restful alertness," transcendental consciousness or the Atman (Travis & Wallace, 1977). According to Maharishi (1963), pure consciousness provides the individual with a profound state of rest for the body while the mind gains a heightened awareness. The rest allows the body to "spontaneously heal itself' or divest itself from the impressions of past stressful impressions.(Brooks and Scarano(1989).

The repeated experience of restful alertness, the fourth state of consciousness, systematically eliminates stress from the nervous system. The profound level of rest experienced by sādhak practicing the Transcendental Meditation(TM) technique has been shown to have striking effects on a broad range of disorders. The study, titled Neurohumoral Correlates of Transcendental Meditation (Subrahmanyam & Porkodi, 1980), indicated significant effects of TM on neurochemistry and the resulting behavioral changes in patients with aggressive behavior, moderate mental retardation, or epilepsy.

The transcendence of the three gunas is not effortless as the interplay of gunas always keeps the sādhak attached to the outworldy situations. So, to transcend the three gunas, sādhak can utilize any of the paths suggested in the Trimarg framework for attaining moksha.

The trimarg framework includes the path of karma yoga also forms the beginning of stage II, as depicted in Fig.2.

STAGE TWO: ATMAN AWAKENING

Stage II focuses on the practice of karma yoga, which will lead to atmabodha and, hence, to experiencing atman. Before understanding karma yoga, it is imperative to discuss the Trimarg framework of Bhagavad Gita.

Trimarg Framework (Flood, 1996)

The Bhagavad Gita teaches the integration of values with lifestyle, relationships, education, and spirituality to avoid physical and psychological ailments, achieve positive well-being, and attain the final goal of human life, i.e., moksha, through the three paths of yoga. Yoga means yog or to unite. Traditionally, yoga is the uniting of the individual self (Atman) with the universal self (Brahamna) (Singh, 2018). According to Gita, a sādhak can follow any one of the paths from the threefold path, or Trimarg framework to attain moksha, as shown in Fig. 4.

i) **Jñāna-mārga or Jnana Yoga-the path of knowledge**: Jnana Yoga is the path to attaining self-awareness that "flattens" the ego. Jnana yoga's primary goal is to help practitioners break free from

Figure 4. Trimarg Framework for Moksha
(Bhagavad Gita)

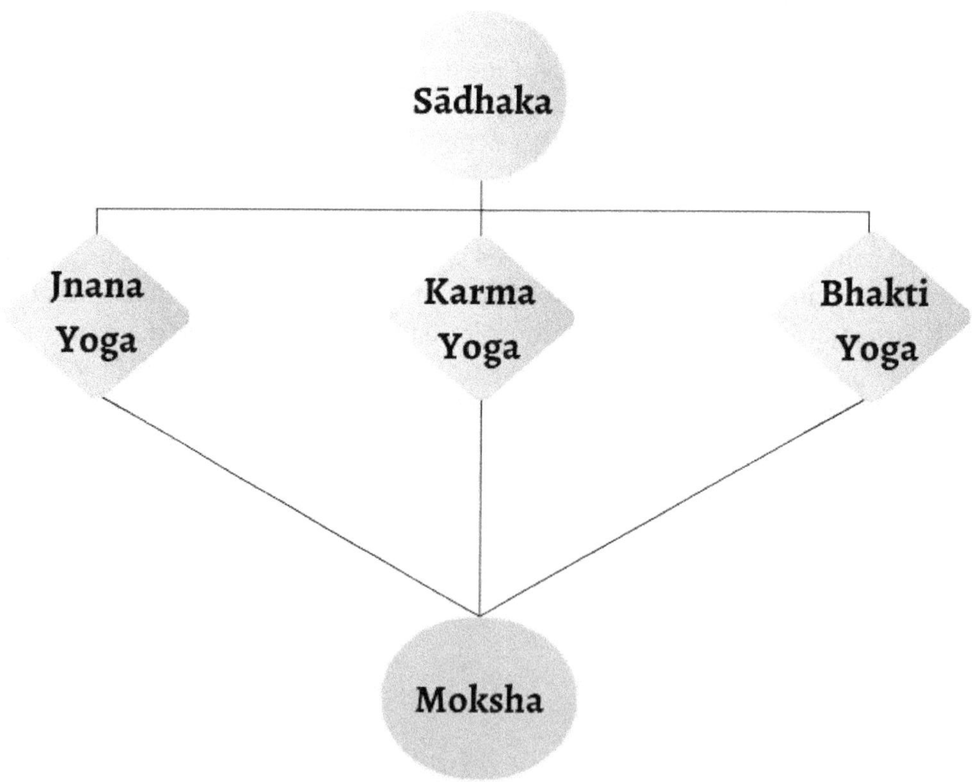

the ego's constrained perspective and cultivate an awareness of their place within a greater, more universal self.

ii) **Bhakti-mārga or Bhakti yoga-the path of devotion:** Bhakti Yoga, the path of faith, which includes rituals like "Japa," "Homa," "Archana," and "Vandana," can also be of therapeutic importance (Balodhi, 1984). The Bhagavad Gita's Bhakti Yoga is a spiritual philosophy emphasizing loving devotion to an unnamed higher power or principle, which may or may not be a personal deity.

iii) **Karma-mārga or karma yoga the path of action:** Karma Yoga is a selfless action that detaches emotion and desire from action (Keshavan, 2020). Karma yoga is about taking action without thinking, "What is in it for me?" As such, it seeks to let go of one's desire or attachment, acting in Karma yoga's spirit. Such an action would be detached, unmotivated by self-interest, and unconcerned with success or failure. This chapter illustrates the role of karma yoga in attaining atmabodha and, hence, moksha.

Karma Yoga

In the Bhagavad Gita, Lord Krishna advises the person to follow the 'Karma Yoga,' the 'path of detached action' to attain moksha. Similarly, sādhak can practice karma yoga to attain spiritual goals like moksha. Karma yoga can be practiced by renouncing selfishness and being indifferent to the fruits of action rather than the action itself (Rao & Paranjpe, 2016). The following shloka also presents this thought:

Shrī bhagavān uvācha

asanśhayaṁ mahā-bāho mano durnigrahaṁ chalam

abhyāsena tu kaunteya vairāgyeṇa cha gṛihyate

Bhagavad Gita 6.5

Swami Sivananda advised that sādhak should repeatedly try to control the wandering mind by continuous Abhyasa or practise. Vikshepa, the fluctuation of the mind and wants, is destroyed by this continuous repetition, which makes it steady and one-pointed. Karma yoga reveals the secret of work, one that allows one to live in the world while also finding their actual selves through their work. Karma yoga is "a technique for performing actions in a manner that the effects of the action do not bind the individual" (Tilak, 2000).

Karma yoga can be practiced by performing four categories of actions: unselfish actions, actions without attachment, actions originated by svadharma (one's right, duty, or nature; one's role in the social and cosmic order), and actions permeated by sattva guna (Vivekananda, 2009).

In the Bhagavad Gita, Arjuna struggles with guilt and displays several other cognitive biases that prevent him from achieving moksha. Lord Krishna addresses Arjuna's dilemma with the knowledge of Karma Yoga. Karma Yoga is a unique concept where actions are performed in the Lord's service without expecting or attaching themselves to results. It encourages action but discourages the individual's attachment to the result. Any potential pain or guilt linked with the action is alleviated by detachment from the result. This understanding dispels the myth that one should not retaliate against family members, no matter how bad they may be, and significantly lightens Arjuna's burden.

People highly misunderstand the meaning of karma yoga. Karma yoga should not be confused with most people's work because the latter is viewed as an aimless, passion-driven, semi-conscious scramble for name, fame, and enjoyment. The goal of karma-yoga is not worldly success. Karma-yoga aims not to change the world but to change oneself. (Bhajanananda, 2006).

Moreover, karma yoga is usually confused with leaving all the things and doing nothing or altogether forgoing action or complete inaction, which, however, is not valid. The complete renunciation of action is known as Karma sannyasa, which is different from karma yoga. The clear distinction is given in the following shloka.

Śhrī bhagavān uvācha

sannyāsaḥ karma-yogaśh cha niḥśhreyasa-karāvubhau

tayos tu karma-sannyāsāt karma-yogo viśhiṣhyate

Bhagavad Gita 5.2

According to Swami Adidevananda, the Lord declared that both renunciation of actions—that is, karma sannyasa and karma yoga—lead to moksha. However, of the two, karma yoga is better than the karma sannyasa." Moreover, Swami Sivananda emphasizes that Karma Sannyasa is suitable only for those with atmabodha. In contrast, those who have not attained atmabodha should practice karma yoga as it is easy and, therefore, suitable for all.

Mulla and Krishnan (2006), in a content analysis of the Bhagavad Gita, found that karma yoga has three components: a duty-oriented mindset, a lack of interest in rewards, and equanimity between pleasure and discomfort. Duty orientation is the belief that one must perform the roles assigned to him/her in society honestly. This is a practical way to attain moksha (Mulla & Krishnan, 2006).

A person high on karma yoga is a self-starter, disciplined, and quality-conscious. Karma-Yoga is the path to reach moksha through work. Karma yoga is a healthier way to carry out deliberate deeds. It has multiple aspects from a) selection of goals, not for materialistic benefits but for inner perfection or more significant social well-being; b) initially not clinging to preferred outcomes and later, as one develops, not clinging to the process of action itself; c) treating all outcomes and then all moments, good and bad, with a sense of equality; d) offering all one's work to the highest consciousness, the Divine or the wisdom and optimal order inherent in things (Sri Aurobindo, 1997).

One can seek the path of Karma Yoga while navigating the demands and pressure of a materialistic society by motivating oneself against the tendency of inaction, which underlies the fear of failure.

Karmanyevadhikaraste ma phaleshu kadachana

Ma Karmaphalaheturbhurma Te Sangostvakarmani

Bhagavad Gita 2.47

Lord Krishna asserted that "the results do not enter under your purview; only the work does. One should not let the rewards of action or the connection to inaction be one's driving force."

Anxiety occurs because of the need for a result to get in the way. When emotions are strong, work is impeded, and sādhak is distracted. Giving up the desire and the outcome are identical. The future of the labor done in the present is the expectation of a result. Because planning is already in place, we should consider it for the future. Lord Krishna emphasizes concentrating on the present rather than the past or the future.

There can be an inconsistency in attitude and behavior when one decides to follow the path of Karma Yoga, as one may need to learn the first step to understanding how to bridge this inconsistency. The path of Karma yoga is fit for sādhak who have a tendency or inclination for work and a desire for moksha. The following shloka emphasizes this:

śhrī bhagavān uvācha

loke 'smin dvi-vidhā niṣhṭhā purā proktā mayānagha

jñāna-yogena sāṅkhyānāṁ karma-yogena yoginām

Bhagavad Gita 3.3

The shloka, as explained by Swami Adidevananda, talks about two-fold paths: Jnana yoga for the Sankhyas and karma yoga for the yogins. Swami Sivananda further emphasizes that this shloka highlights the four ways of practicing karma yoga: i) discrimination, ii) dispassion, iii) sixfold virtues, and iv) longing for moksha. A sādhak might achieve sixfold virtues via karma yoga: i) mental control; ii) sense control; iii) fortitude or endurance; iv) turning away from worldly objects; v) faith; and vi) tranquilly. Swami Adidevananda further clarifies this as sādhaks whose Buddhi is agitated by objects of senses are qualified for karma yoga, which acts as a means to an end. Karma yoga is a means of purifying the heart and preparing the sādhak for Jnana Yoga.

Hence, the sādhak can adhere to the discipline of self-knowledge or Atmabodha.

Atmabodha

According to Vedānta philosophy, Karma yoga serves as a preamble to Atmabodha. It makes it clear that karma yoga purifies the mind and prepares it to receive the wisdom of Atmabodha (Dhiman, 2019), which alone directly leads to human perfection or moksha. The Vedantic process for moksha is depicted in Figure 5.

Figure 5. Vedānta process for Moksha

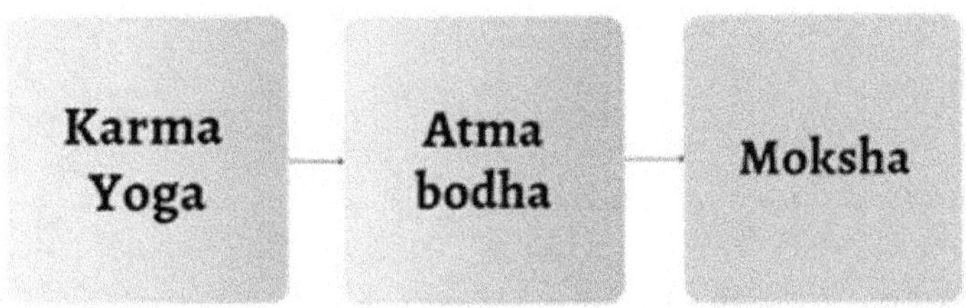

As depicted in Fig. 2 and Fig. 5, attaining atmabodha is possible after the continuous practice of karma yoga. The following shloka indicates the same:

karma-jam buddhi-yukta hi phalam tyaktva manishinah

janma-bandha-vinirmuktah padam gachchhanty-anamayam

Bhagavad Gita 2.51

According to Swami Sivananda, this shloka conveys that knowledge of the Self or atmabodha, which dawns when Karma Yoga purifies the mind.

The Bhagavad Gita is the pinnacle text on human Atmabodha. (Balodi & Raina, 2014). Atmabodha is translated as self-knowledge. According to the Bhagavad Gita, people are attached to the sensuous, material conception of life, but Atmabodha can immediately eradicate this conception. The fundamental tenet of Atmabodha is that a person's emotions and behavior are significantly affected by their thoughts or whatever they are committed to. Atmabodha helps with self-analysis and self-introspection.

Naess (1986) observed that the current capitalist economy is egocentric. Everyone is structured to satisfy the individual's needs. For society to start taking care of itself and the entire ecosystem, there needs to be a more profound shift in consciousness. This shift in consciousness is possible only when everyone has 'self-knowledge,' which denotes the awareness of organic wholeness and some 'rectification' of ourselves.

According to Swami Nikhilananda (1996), atmabodha, or SK (self-knowledge), is vital, and all other forms of knowledge are of secondary importance. One's actions, feelings, reasoning, and thinking depend on one's idea of the self. One's view of life will be either materialistic or spiritual according to one's conception of oneself". Adolescents' levels of aggression were significantly reduced by Yoganidra, group counseling, Bhramari Pranayam, and Atma Bodha & Tatva Bodha ki Sadhana, as was found in a study on adolescents by Saraf (2016). Atma Bodha ki Sadhna includes Atma Chintan, Atma Sudhara, Atma Nirman, and Atma Vikasa.

The idea of emotional intelligence originated in ancient Indian scriptures such as the Bhagwad Gita, according to a comparison of the Western and Indian models (Ray, 2020). Emotional Intelligence in the Indian context focuses on higher levels of self. Indians are taught the concept of emotional intelligence and social values through ancient Indian texts that reiterate concepts like "Atmabodha," which refers to aligning oneself with the universe in order to participate in social outcomes rather than materialistic goals (Gopraj & Sharma, 2011)

Such an individual is known as the sthithapragnya, who has the knowledge that distinguishes between the 'real' self (the permanent; the atman) and the 'unreal' self (the impermanent; the materialistic world). (Gayathri & Meenakshi 2012). Atmabodha enables one to detach oneself from this 'unreal' world and steer one's thoughts toward the 'real,' the Atman.

Atman

Yastvātmaratireva syādātmatṛptaśca mānavaḥ,

ātmanyeva ca santuṣṭastasya kāryaṃ na vidyate

Bhagavad Gita 3.17

Swami Sivananda translates this shloka as "But for the one who rejoices only in the self, who is satisfied with the self, and who is content in the self alone, verily has no duty."

The shloka emphasizes the importance of concentrating and finding contentment within the self, as only a person will perform all his/her actions not as a duty but as a part of the self.

In the following shloka, Swami Sivananda highlights that the atman is one homogeneous essence. The six modifications or changes (Shad Bhava Vikaras) that the body experiences—namely, existence, ii) birth, iii) growth, iv) modification, v) decay, and vi) death—have no impact on atman.

tribhir guṇa-mayair bhāvair ebhiḥ sarvam idaṁ jagat

mohitaṁ nābhijānāti māmebhyaḥ param avyayam

Bhagavad Gita 7.13

The self has been studied as "an ontological entity" in the Indian worldview. (Bharati, 1985). The Indian concept of self includes:

- **Physical self** is the physical body in which the metaphysical self is embodied
- The **psychological self** includes the mind, intellect, and ego; in Indian conceptions of the self, these components appear to be just as concrete as the other organs. (Bhawuk,2011)
- Both independent and interdependent ideas of selves are included in the **social self**. Individualists' independent conception of self is limited to physical or psychological characteristics. In contrast, the interdependent concept of self for collectivists has a social self, including social relationships and identity descriptors. Indians portray independent and interdependent social selves (Sinha & Tripathi, 1994). Beyond the social self, the Indian conception of the self also includes the metaphysical self, or atman. (Bhawuk,2011).
- The **metaphysical self** is the core or the authentic self (Bhawuk, 2011), and realizing the authentic self is the goal of human life. Most people think of the metaphysical self as atman, which is in the living being because of previous karma.

The Indian conceptualization of Self is depicted in Figure 6.

The åtman, or true self, is described in the Bhagavad Gita as incomprehensible, unknowable, and eternal. Its attributes include not being destroyed and not being subject to change. The åtman transcends time, never gives birth, or experiences death, neither kills nor is killed. The åtman is immortal, unborn, enduring, ancient, and separate from the body. The human body is compared to the "åtman" by using the clothing analogy; just as we discard worn-out clothing, the "åtman" departs from the human body.

The term "åtman" refers to something that cannot be broken by force (also known as "unbreakable" or "unpierceable"), burned by fire, submerged in water (also known as "insoluble"), or dried by wind. The åtman is further characterized as all-pervading, stable, immobile, and eternal; unmanifest, beyond perception, and unmodifiable; and described as simply amazing to see, talk about, and listen about. The material body and the åtman are the two distinct facets of human existence, as explicitly stated in these verses; the material body is temporary, and the åtman is eternal.

Figure 6. The concept of the Indian Self adapted from Bhawuk (2011)

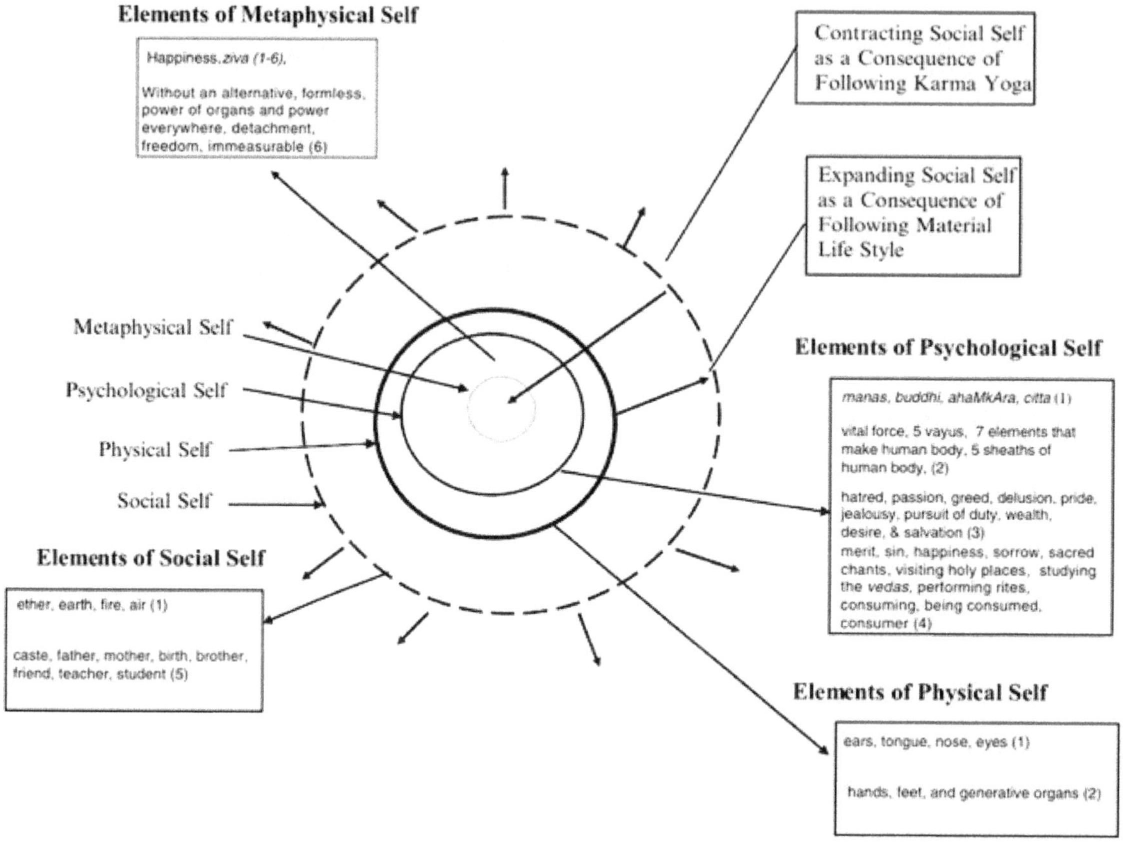

However, the elements of growing self like professional success, acquisition of wealth, property, technological gadgets, and conspicuous consumption to gratify various needs constantly are a source of ego enhancement which leads to endless, perhaps infinite, growth of social self. Whenever these desires are not fulfilled, it leads to anger, anger to delusion, and indiscriminate action, which in turn leads a person to their ruin. This state of individuals is visible in today's era of consumerism and competitiveness. The journey into the self is only possible by psychologically disengaging oneself from worldly affairs. Freedom of the mind from such concerns is essential for experimenting with and getting the knowledge of the true self (Osho, 2005).

From immemorial times, most technological advancements are seen in today's world. Human life has not been known to be as comfortable as it is today. Even after that, people are distressed and suffer from many physical and psychological ailments, and their levels of satisfaction and contentment know no bounds. Today, when everything is available online or just a click away, the instant gratification of our desires leads to the formation of new desires, which is an endless loop. This web that ensnares a person in this materialistic world is called 'Maya.' The concept of Maya highlights that this world is nothing but an illusion that blinds a person and prevents him/ her from realizing the 'Atman' or attaining Atmabodha (Deshmukha,2021), considered the objective of human life in Indian thought, which further hinders in attaining moksha.

STAGE THREE: TRANSITIONAL STAGE

The third stage is the transitional stage, as in attaining moksha, the individual is freed from the karmic bondage, also referred to as the liberation from the effects of karma(Casebeer, 1952). Moksha in the Bhagavad Gita is a delight in the self, contentment with the self, self-realization (Deshmukh, 2021), and self-fulfillment. (Bora, n.d.).

Moksha

Moksha (derived from the root muc) is 'to let loose,' to let go,' or 'to unleash.' Many people consider the true meaning of moksha to liberate oneself from the worldly cycle of birth and death. The following shlokas depict the concept of moksha from the lens of Bhagavad Gita.

yāmimāṁ puṣhpitāṁ vāchaṁ pravadanty-avipaśhchitaḥ

veda-vāda-ratāḥ pārtha nānyad astīti vādinaḥ

kāmātmānaḥ swarga-parā janma-karma-phala-pradām

kriyā-viśheṣha-bahulāṁ bhogaiśhwarya-gatiṁ prati

Bhagavad Gita 2.42 and 2.43

Explaining these shlokas, Swami Sivananda states that moksha can only be attained by knowledge of the self, i.e., atmabodha.

Moreover, "Arjuna Vishad Yoga," the very first chapter of the Bhagavad Gita, depicts the sadness and anguish of the Pandava prince Arjuna. The 18th chapter "Moksha Sanyas Yoga," in contrast, describes renunciation and liberation from fear, grief, and pain. Of all the living beings, humans are believed to be the only ones who can pursue moksha (or liberation), enlightenment, jnana (or knowledge), or self-realization. (Bhawuk,2011)

Moksha can be attained while living in the physical body (Casebeer, 1952). It has been supported by Radhakrishnan (1948) as he emphasizes that one can, while living in a world of time, "possess the immortality of timeless self-existence."

According to Mishra (2013), moksha is not an "otherworldly" reality but relates to the present world and encompasses all aspects of human existence. Pursuing moksha can aid in establishing positive interpersonal and intergroup relationships. Furthermore, it enables one to thrive in both personal and professional spheres. Many Indians pray for moksha (getting out) from miserable and highly threatening life circumstances. Individuals with long-term illnesses also discuss and pray for moksha or getting rid of the illness.

According to Kuppuswamy (1977), moksha is something that one aspires to achieve in life rather than a condition of freedom that one experiences after death. To attain moksha, the sādhak should know that wealth and sensual desire will likely distract the sādhak. Therefore, the experience of wealth and sensual desire is necessary for the sādhak, enabling the sādhak to revert his or her focus back to the primary goal of moksha. (Narayanan,2010)

Moksha is considered one of the vital purusharthas, i.e.' the goal or purpose of human life. The other three purusharthas are Dharma, Artha, and Kāma. According to the Purusharath model, the pursuits of life must be physically pleasant and morally sound. Artha and Kama represent material pursuits; Dharma represents moral pursuits, and moksha represents the category of spiritual pursuits. Artha and Kama purusharths are considered physically pleasant, while dharma and moksha are considered morally good. This conceptualization implies that pursuing only physically pleasant goals by rejecting morally good goals tends to reduce human beings to the level of animals. On the other hand, pursuing only morally good goals, disregarding physically pleasant goals, does not look practical.

In the purushartha model, these goals are fully integrated into the ultimate goal of human life, called moksha. In this sense, moksha is regarded as the highest goal (parampurushartha) of human life. (Mishra,2013) Thus, moksha strengthens us not only spiritually but also materially.

Moksha may be realized while the individual lives in his present body. He is to continue to work and to find realization in ordinary living, but his activity must no longer be motivated by the desire for the results; he must acknowledge that Brahman is the Doer, which is the central tenet of karma yoga as well. Bhagavad Gita mentions

karmaṇaiva hi sansiddhim āsthitā janakādayaḥ

loka-saṅgraham evāpi sampaśhyan kartum arhasi

Bhagavad Gita 3.20

Swami Sivananda explains that the above shloka states that King Janaka and others had atmabodha and attained moksha, yet they performed actions, i.e., they kept on practicing karma yoga to set an example to the masses. They worked for the guidance of men. This shloka indicates that moksha can be attained while living in the world. So, moksha is a prerequisite for attaining samadhi or uniting with the brahman, which is the final stage for the sādhak.

STAGE FOUR: SAMADHI

This stage can be the ultimate goal for the sādhak, which is freedom from the cycle of birth, death, and rebirth. Here, the atman finally unites with the brahmana, the absolute or supreme self. Samadhi refers not merely to mental discipline but to a state of calm and bliss, which may also be called ananda or siddhi satchianada. More discussion on samadhi is out of the scope of this chapter.

Based on stages I, II, and III discussed above, we propose the karmayoga and atmabodha model for moksha.

KARMAYOGA AND ATMABODHA MODEL FOR MOKSHA

This chapter intentionally focuses on integrating Bhagavad Gita's teachings in lifestyle, relationships, education, and spirituality to achieve Atmabodha for attaining the final goal of human life, i.e., moksha (yoga of perfection or human perfection or self-realization) through karma yoga by enhancing the sattva and rajas gunas and diminishing tamas guna. The proposed model is depicted in Fig. 7.

Methods Used in Model Development

The present model was developed using the following methods:

1. **Hermeneutical Inquiry:** This process was adopted to achieve understanding by interpreting the phenomena under study. In this inquiry, the Bhagavad Gita was interpreted to describe and explain the concepts of atman, karmayoga, trigunas, atmabodha, and moksha, as suggested by Allen and Jensen (1990).
2. **Heuristic Inquiry:** After an exhaustive reading of the Bhagavad Gita, immersion, self-dialogue, self-exploration, and then exploring the nature of others' experiences was undertaken by the authors. This process was conducted to rigorously analyze and transform the subjective data(in the form of direct reports and observations) into objective accounts of reality, as suggested by Douglass and Moustakas (1985).
3. **Content Analysis:** The thorough analysis of the Bhagavad Gita yielded the themes of atman, karma yoga, trigunas, atmabodha, and moksha. It provided the background and context of the verses, which led to an in-depth understanding of each verse.
4. **Model Mining:** From the steps mentioned above, raw models were mined as depicted in Fig 3, 5, and 6. It further led to the emic-embedded model in which the emic perspective provided theoretical insights into the existing indigenous thoughts. Construction and model mining as a methodological approach has been successfully used by several scholars (Bhawuk, 1999; 2010).

The researches that can support the karma yoga and atmabodha model for moksha are discussed below.

Figure 7. Path of Karmayoga, Triguna & Atmabodha for attaining Moksha

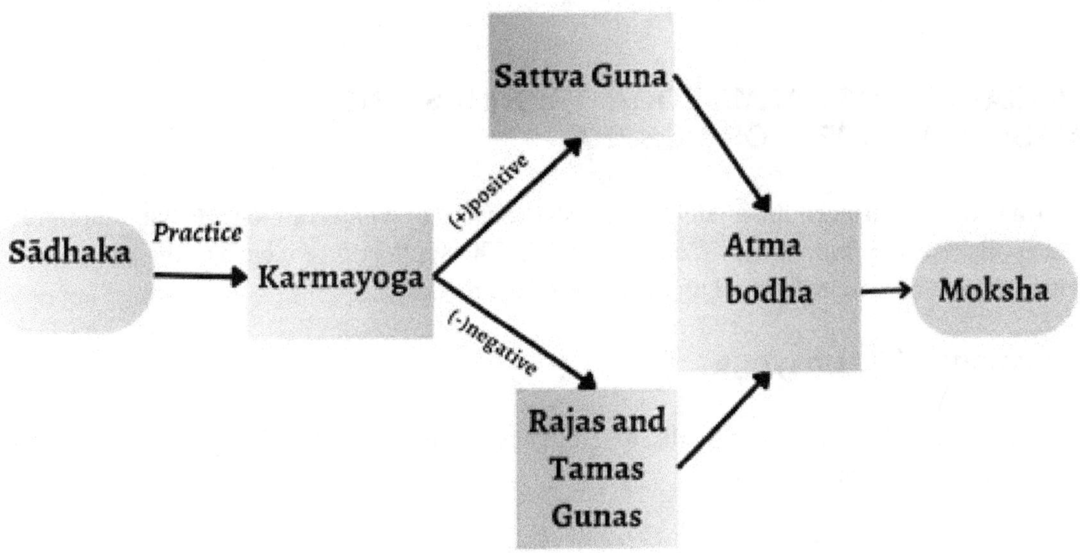

Research Evidence for the Model

The karma yoga and atmabodha model for moksha postulates that sādhak by practicing karma yoga will increase the sattvic guna and reduce the rajas and tamas gunas, thereby purifying the mind of the sādhak for attaining atmabodha, which will further pave the way for attaining moksha.

Swami Vivekananda (2009) states that sādhak is unable to catch even a glimpse of the infinite freedom beyond unless sādhak gives up the intense attachment to this fleeting conditioned existence. With practice and mind training, worldly disengagements begin to occur spontaneously, allowing sādhak to perceive realities differently. This disengagement can be brought about by practicing karma yoga. When sādhak detaches himself/herself from the fruits of one's actions, sādhak finally realizes that all external events (that can be perceived) are merely the gunas acting on each other and that with the practice of karma yoga and increased sattva guna, sādhak can gain atmabodha which will in turn, brings them one step closer to attaining moksha..

A suggested developmental trajectory and an implied hierarchy exist: individuals evolve through developing sattva and reducing tamas and rajas (Mulla & Krishnan, 2019). Though they both have advantages and disadvantages, Rajas and Tamas are symbolic of a violent mental state where illogical emotions and impulsive behaviour are uncontrollable. (Deshpande & colleagues, 2008). While Rajas and Tamas guna had negative correlations with attention and atmabodha, Sattva guna demonstrated a significant positive correlation with both.

Sri Aurobindo (1997) has suggested that although sattvik happiness is not the highest state, given that the influence of ego and desire is still present, with increasing inner freedom from these, it may culminate into the yoga of perfection or moksha (Sri Aurobindo, 1997). To attain moksha, it becomes imperative that the authentic and ideal selves of the individual are in congruence, which is possible only when the person first has Atmabodha. After attaining atmabodha by enhancing sattva guna, the individual seems to be in an in-between stage of well-being, especially of the eudemonic kind (Agarwal,2021) and moksha. Moksha can be considered as freedom from karmic bondage. Moksha represents a psychological state with no desires or wants, and the mind experiences absolute silence (shoonyata). A psychological state that frees anyone from individualistic limitations and allows functioning at a higher level of consciousness can never be irrelevant. (Mishra, 1994).

APPLICATIONS OF KARMA YOGA, TRIGUNAS, AND ATMABODHA MODEL FOR MOKSHA

The karma yoga and atmabodha model for Moksha consists of many components with multiple psychological applications for individuals in day-to-day life. The applications of each of the components of the model will contribute to the overall applications of the model.

Applications of Karmayoga

Karmayoga is one of the most widely discussed topics of Bhagavad Gita. Its applications are multifold. Some of them are discussed below:

- **Coping Strategy:** In keeping with the behaviorist tenet, Karma Yoga holds that overt behavioral changes must first be produced, and then complementary cognitive and affective change will follow. In behavior therapy, "action" (karma) is used as a tool for the treatment of depression. (Wolpe, 1973). Singh & Oberhummer (1980) reported that the Karma Yoga teaching enabled the patient to work in the face of her fear sort of escape-response prevention technique by inhibiting the patient's escape into their obsessive thoughts and fantasies or their compulsory actions in the treatment of obsessive-compulsive disorders in the initial sessions of behavior therapy and also propelled her to go on working for the benefit of her children during the long follow-up period.
- **Leadership**: The duty-orientation and indifference to rewards aspects of karma yoga presuppose an altruistic motive, a predictor of transformational leadership. (Singh and Krishnan 2005a). Leaders high on Karma Yoga are likely to be perceived as more transformational by their followers. (Mulla and Krishnan, 2014). The virtues of universal morality, such as selflessness, compassion, desirelessness, forbearance, peace, and harmony, can be found in karma yogis and servant leaders (Dhiman, 2019).
- **Moral Development:** The three dimensions of Karma-Yoga, which are duty orientation, indifference to rewards, and equanimity, are related to the four components of moral development, i.e., moral sensitivity, moral judgment, moral motivation, and moral character(Mulla & Krishnan, 2014)
- **Empathy:** Karma yoga has been found to be strongly related to empathic concern (an affective domain) among individuals with low personal distress. (Mulla & Krishnan, 2008)

Applications of Trigunas

The trigunas include sattva, rajas, and tamas. All the gunas have different characteristics, which can have various psychological implications for individuals. The theory of trigunas can be applied in a variety of contexts:

- **Emotional Regulation:** Sattva guna is associated with self-control and mental balance or stability. (Kumar et.al., 2022) Those with sattvic personality can regulate their emotions well, i.e., they foster positive emotions and manage negative ones.
- **Addiction Recovery:** Manipulation of the guṇas is critical to healing from pain, injury, and addiction. (Britton,2018). In a study by Nedungottil et al. (2021), it was found that males without alcohol dependence were higher on Sattva guna conscientiousness, extraversion, life satisfaction, and positive affect. In contrast, males with alcohol dependence were higher on Tamas guna, neuroticism, and negative affect.
- **Menatal health constructs:** Sattvic personalities tend to be relatively less verbally aggressive (Wolf, 1998) and prefer self-growth (Sharma, 1999), while Rajasic tend to show high verbal aggressiveness and less satisfaction with life (Wolf,1998) and experience less job satisfaction (Sharma,1999) and tamasic have poor cognition, defective memory and experience less satisfaction with life (Wolf, 1998).

Applications of Moksha

- **Sense of Unity:** The Bhagavad Gita points out that a person who has attained moksha becomes one with all, and therefore, he/she always keeps doing good for all. These texts suggest the need to change our way of looking at others.

Unless a sense of 'unity' or feeling of 'oneness' with others is developed, such as in moksha, relationship problems experienced at the individual or group level are highly likely to surface and remain unsolved. All activities and pursuits based on love for and relatedness with others can offer solutions not only to individual problems but also familial, social, political, and professional problems. In this sense, moksha seems to carry great potential for success in worldly life in general and dealing with problems of human relationships in particular. (Mishra,2013).

- **Social Welfare:** According to the Bhagavad Gita, a person can achieve moksha or yoga of perfection by reflecting on one's life and identifying ways to serve others and contribute to the well-being of oneself and society. Moksha seems an individualistic concern; however, the task cannot be achieved in isolation from society. It must be accomplished in the context of one's interpersonal relationships and social obligations. (Dasgupta,2015). Many people use collectivistic means (e.g., welfare activities) to achieve this valued goal (Mishra, 1994).

Therefore, the karma yoga and atmabodha model for moksha is a holistic model as it can have multifarious applications in an individual's life, from social, emotional, behavioral, and organizational to psychological aspects. All are impacted by the constructs discussed in this model.

FUTURE RESEARCH DIRECTIONS

The karma yoga and atmabodha model for moksha presented above invites scholars from other countries to examine the concepts of karma yoga, trigunas,atmabodha, and moksha in their cultural context using local languages. For instance, Singh et al. (2016) found that Trigunas accounted significantly for well-being dimensions. Sattva accounted for 48% variance in Czechs, 56% in Indians, and 55% in Americans; Rajas accounted for 21% variance in Czechs, 08% in Indians, and 54% in Americans and Tamas accounted for 50% variance in Czechs, 20% in Indians and 64% in Americans.

Moreover, the concept of moksha is prevalent in other Indian traditions; for instance, in Jain tradition, moksha necessitates the eradication of all karmas (actions), whether good or negative, because if karma is left behind, it will bear fruit. In Jainism, moksha and nirvana are regarded as the same (Carrithers & Humphrey, 1991; Jaini, 2000). Nirvana is 'the highest happiness' (ananda) and the final destination of human life, according to one school of Buddhism. While in the Sikh tradition, the moksha concept appears as mokh dwar (the door of salvation). It is regarded as the 10th door in the human body, which is invisible. All these traditions agree that moksha is a state of life in which there are no desires or wants (vasanas) and a state of cognition in which there are no frames or images. This state, called shoonyata, represents a psychological state with no desires or wants, and the mind experiences absolute silence. Hence, based on all the available conceptions regarding the concept of moksha, various dimensions of moksha should be researched. Further research studies should be carried out on how moksha can be a goal for all individuals irrespective of their age, gender, socioeconomic status, caste, race, and professional affiliations. Its therapeutic implications can also be explored in counseling and clinical settings.

CONCLUSION

Indian philosophy highlights that truth should be realized rather than known intellectually. It further emphasizes and clarifies spirituality as the way of living to not merely know the truth but become one with it (Sheldon, 1951). By realizing our true selves or attaining moksha, we can give equal rights to every ecosystem species to live freely in this biosphere. (Barman, 2020). This chapter offers a thorough understanding of the path of moksha through the lens of the Bhagavad Gita, emphasizing the triguna framework, karma yoga, and atmabodha for their contributions to attaining moksha. The chapter highlights the value of practicing Karma Yoga in order to enhance sattva guna and reduce Rajas and Tamas gunas, which will help the individual in attaining atmabodha and catalyze the process of moksha. This chapter provides a more nuanced understanding of the intricacies of the human psyche..

Moreover, this chapter highlights the importance of atmabodha and cultivating higher qualities, such as compassion and wisdom, to live a meaningful and fulfilling life in modern times. By recognizing and understanding the interplay of Sattva, Rajas, and Tamas within oneself, sādhak can make conscious choices to align their actions with their higher nature and move closer towards moksha. This understanding can help sādhak navigate the complexities of modern life and find a sense of purpose, fulfillment, and inner peace. Additionally, the chapter offers a valuable perspective on the concept of duality and the interconnectedness of all things. By recognizing that the gunas exist within oneself and in the world around them, sādhak can cultivate empathy, gratitude, and a sense of unity with others, fostering harmonious relationships and collective well-being. The Triguna theory provides a framework for sādhak to understand and transcend their lower tendencies towards materialistic desires and inertia and instead focus on developing clarity and higher consciousness. This understanding of the Triguna theory and Karma Yoga can bring about a shift in perspective and behavior, allowing individuals to navigate the challenges of modern life with a greater sense of living.

REFERENCES

Agarwalla, S., Seshadri, B., & Krishnan, V. R. (2015). Impact of Gunas and Karma Yoga on Transformational Leadership. *Journal of Human Values*, *21*(1), 11–22. doi:10.1177/0971685815569590

Agrawal, J. (2021). Sattva enhancement therapy: An illustrative report. *Indian Journal of Clinical Psychology*, *48*(2), 3–6.

Agrawal, J., & Cornelissen, R. M. (2020). *Yoga and positive mental health.* OSF.

Allen, M. N., & Jensen, L. (1990). Hermeneutical inquiry meaning and scope. *Western Journal of Nursing Research*, *12*(2), 241–253. doi:10.1177/019394599001200209 PMID:2321377

Anuradha, M. V., & Kumar, Y. L. N. (2015). Trigunas in organizations: Moving toward an east-west synthesis. *International Journal of Cross Cultural Management*, *15*(2), 195–214. doi:10.1177/1470595815594636

Apte, V. S. (Ed.). (1975). The practical Sanskrit–English dictionary. (4th Ed.). Delhi: Motilal Banarsidass.

Balodhi, J. P. (Ed.). (1984). *Relationship of Ithihasa and Puranas to Vedas: Our Vedic Heritage* (pp. 64–68). Chinmayanada Mission.

Balodi, G., & Raina, D. (2014). A comparative study of emotional maturity and values in Bhagavad Gita readers and non-readers. *Indian Journal of Positive Psychology*, *5*(4), 415.

Benfey, T. (Ed.). (1982). Sanskrit English dictionary. New Delhi: Milan.

Bhajanananda, S. (2006). *Selfless work: Its basis, methods, and fulfillment. Belur Math*. Ramakrishna Mission Vivekananda University Press.

Bhatia, S. C., Madabushi, J., Kolli, V., Bhatia, S. K., & Madaan, V. (2013). The Bhagavad Gita and contemporary psychotherapies. *Indian Journal of Psychiatry*, *55*(6, Suppl 2), S315–S321. doi:10.4103/0019-5545.105557 PMID:23858274

Bhawuk, D. P. (2010). Methodology for building psychological models from scriptures: Contributions of Indian psychology to indigenous and universal psychologies. *Psychology and Developing Societies*, *22*(1), 49–93. doi:10.1177/097133360902200103

Bhawuk, D. P., & Bhawuk, D. P. (2011). Indian concept of self. *Spirituality and Indian Psychology: Lessons from the Bhagavad-Gita*, (pp. 65-91). Springer.

Britton, A. (2018). Applied Yogic Wisdom: Ancient Science, Contemporary Recovery [Doctoral dissertation, Loyola Marymount University].

Brooks ; Scarano. (1989). Transcendental Meditation in the treatment of post-vietnam adjustment. *Journal of Counseling and Development*, *64*, 212–215.

Carrithers, M., & Humphrey, C. (1991). *The assembly of listeners: Jains in society*. Cambridge University Press. doi:10.1017/CBO9780511896637

Casebeer, A. J. (1952). *"Philosophy, Religion and Theology". Concepts of self-realization (a comparison of the concept of self-realization in the "Bhagavadgita" with that concept in the Pauline Epistles)* [Thesis, University of Southern California]. ProQuest LLC. doi:10.25549/usctheses-c40-1215

Chinmayananda, S. (1982). *ATMABODHA*. Central Chinmaya Mission Trust.

Chinmayananda, S. (2021, September 8). *Bhagavad Gita chapter 3 - verse 17 - 3.17 Yas tvatma-ratir*. Shlokam. https://shlokam.org/bhagavad-gita/3-17/

Dalal, R. (2010). *Hinduism: An Alphabetical Guide*. Penguin Books.

Dasgupta, S. D. (2015). (Un) Holy Connections? Understanding Woman Abuse in Hinduism. In *Religion and Men's Violence Against Women* (pp. 371–382). Springer New York. doi:10.1007/978-1-4939-2266-6_23

Dasgupta, S. N. (1975). *A history of Indian philosophy* (Indian ed., Vol. 1–5). Motilal Banarsidass. (Original work published 1922)

Deshmukh, D. S. K. (2021). Effect of Pragya Yoga and Pranakarshan Pranayama (Popounded by Acharya Sriram Sharma) on aggression level of Juvenile delinquents. International Journal of Yogic, *Human Movement and Sports Sciences*, *6*(2), 81–84.

Deshpande, S., Nagendra, H. R., & Raghuram, N. (2008). A randomized control trial of the effect of Yoga on Gunas (personality) and Health in normal healthy volunteers. *International Journal of Yoga, 1*(1), 2–10. doi:10.4103/0973-6131.36785 PMID:21829278

Dhillon, M. (2023). Weaving Together the Ancient and the Contemporary: Intersections of the Bhagavad Gita with Modern Psychology. *Pastoral Psychology, 72*(4), 1–13. doi:10.100711089-023-01070-2 PMID:37359496

Dhiman, S. (2019). Karma Yoga: The Path of Enlightened Action. In: Bhagavad Gītā and Leadership. Palgrave Studies in Workplace Spirituality and Fulfillment. Palgrave Macmillan, Cham. doi:10.1007/978-3-319-67573-2_5

Dillbeck, M. C. (1991). The Bhagavad-Gita: A case study. *Modern Science and Vedic Science, 4*, 96–134.

Douglass, B. G., & Moustakas, C. (1985). Heuristic inquiry: The internal search to know. *Journal of Humanistic Psychology, 25*(3), 39–55. doi:10.1177/0022167885253004

Gambhirananda, S. (1965). *Brahma sutra bhasva*. Calcutta, India: Sun lithographing Co.

Gavin, D. (1996). *Flood, An introduction to Hinduism*. Cambridge University Press.

Gayathri, N., & Meenakshi, K. (2012). Emotional intelligence through the Bhagavad-Gita. *International Journal of Research Studies in Psychology, 1*(2), 73–80. doi:10.5861/ijrsp.2012.v1i2.83

Gopalacharya, C. S. (Ed.). (1967). *Shabdārthakausthubha* [Sanskrit- Kannada Dictionary]. Vol. 1–6). Bangalore Press.

Isaeva, N. V. (1993). *Shankara and Indian Philosophy*. SUNY Press.

Jaini, P. (2000). *Collected papers on Jaina studies*. Motilal Banarsidass.

Kaur, P., & Sinha, A. K. (1992). Dimensions of guna in organizational setting. *Vikalpa, 17*(3), 27–32. doi:10.1177/0256090919920303

Keshavan, M. S. (2020). Building resilience in the COVID-19 era: Three paths in the Bhagavad Gita. *Indian Journal of Psychiatry, 62*(5), 459–461. doi:10.4103/psychiatry.IndianJPsychiatry_829_20 PMID:33678824

Khemka, S. S., Ramarao, N. H., & Hankey, A. (2011). Effect of integral yoga on psychological and health variables and their correlations. *International Journal of Yoga, 4*(2), 93–99. doi:10.4103/0973-6131.85492 PMID:22022128

Krishnan, V. R., & Mulla, Z. R. (2022). Karma-yoga: philosophy of moral development and work motivation. In *Indigenous Indian Management: Conceptualization, Practical Applications and Pedagogical Initiatives* (pp. 127–156). Springer International Publishing. doi:10.1007/978-3-030-87906-8_5

Kumar, R. S., Britto, J., Ilavarasu, J., & Rajesh, S. K. (2022). Study of Emotion Regulation Based on Yogic Personality Using Implicit, Explicit, and Eye Tracking Techniques. *International Journal of Yoga, 15*(2), 122–129. doi:10.4103/ijoy.ijoy_36_22 PMID:36329772

Kuppuswamy, B. (1977). *Dharma and Society*. Macmillan.

Macdonell, A. A. (Ed.). (1924). *A Practical Sanskrit Dictionary*. Oxford University Press.

Madahavananda, S. (1982). *Vivekacudamani*. The Indian Press.

Maharishi Mahesh Yogi. (1963). *The science of being and the art of living: Transcendental meditation*. Signet.

Maharishi Mahesh Yogi. (1967). *On the Bhagavad-Gita: A translation and commentary*. Penguin/Arkana.

Marutham, P., Balodhi, J. P., & Mishra, H. (1998). Sattva, Rajas, Tamas (SRT) Inventory. *Nimhans Journal*, 15–19.

Mishra, R. C. (1994). Individualist-collectivist orientations across generations. In U. Kim, H. C. Triandis, C. Kagitcibasi, S. Choi, & G. Yoon (Eds.), *Individualism and collectivism: Theory, method, and practice* (pp. 225–238). SAGE Publications.

Mishra, R. C. (2013). Moksha and the Hindu worldview. *Psychology and Developing Societies*, *25*(1), 21–42. doi:10.1177/0971333613477318

Monier Williams, M. (1964). *A Sanskrit – English Dictionary* (Rev. ed.). Motilal Banarsidass.

Mukundananda, S. (n.d.). Bhagavad Gita, The Song of God – Swami Mukundananda (Chapter 14, Verse 20). *Holy Bhagavad Gita*. https://www.holy-bhagavad-gita.org/chapter/14/verse/20

Mulla, Z. R., & Krishnan, V. R. (2006). Karma Yoga: A conceptualization and validation of the Indian philosophy of work. *Journal of Indian Psychology*, *24*(1/2), 26–43.

Mulla, Z. R., & Krishnan, V. R. (2008). Karma-Yoga, the Indian work ideal, and its relationship with empathy. *Psychology and Developing Societies*, *20*(1), 27–49. doi:10.1177/097133360702000102

Mulla, Z. R., & Krishnan, V. R. (2014). Karma-yoga: The Indian model of moral development. *Journal of Business Ethics*, *123*(2), 339–351. doi:10.100710551-013-1842-8

Mulla, Z. R., & Krishnan, V. R. (2022). Karma-yoga: philosophy of moral development and work motivation. In *Indigenous Indian Management: Conceptualization, Practical Applications and Pedagogical Initiatives* (pp. 127–156). Springer International Publishing.

Murthy, P. K., & Kumar, S. K. (2007). The concept of Triguna: A critical analysis and synthesis. *Psychological Studies*, *52*(2), 103–113.

Narayanan, Y. (2010). Sustainable consumption as a means to self-realization: A Hindu perspective on when enough is enough. *Sustainable Development (Bradford)*, *18*(5), 252–259. doi:10.1002d.476

Nedungottil, C., Agrawal, J., Sharma, M. P., & Murthy, P. (2021). *Men with and without alcohol dependence: A comparative study of Triguna*. Anasakti, Personality and Subjective Well-being.

Osborne, A. (1970). *Ramana Maharshi and the path of self-knowledge*. Rider & Co.

Osho. (2005). *Jeevan kya hai (What is life?)*. New Delhi: Hind Pocket Books.

Pomfrey, P. L. (2002). *The return of the self: Transcendence and transformation. A case study of the Bhagavad-Gita in the light of Vedic psychology* [Doctoral dissertation, The Wright Institute].

Radhakrishnan, S. (1948). *Indian Philosophy* (Vol. I). George Allen and Unwin Ltd.

Rani, J. N. (2007). Impact of yoga training on triguna and self-ideal disparity. Psychological Studies. *Natl Acad Psychol India.*, *52*, 174–177.

Rao, K. R. (2008). Introducing Indian Psychology. In K. R. Rao, A. Paranjpe, & A. K. Dalal (Eds.), Handbook of Indian Psychology (pp. 7–18). essay, Foundation Books.

Rao, P. V. K., & Harigopal, K. (1979). The three gunas and ESP: An exploratory investigation. *Journal of Indian Psychology*, *2*(1), 63–68.

Ravindra, P. N., & Babu, P. (2021). A Correlation Study between Tri-Guna and Emotional Style: A Theoretical Approach toward Developing a Working Model to Integrate Tri-Guna with Affective Neuroscience and Well-Being. *International Journal of Yoga*, *14*(3), 213–221. doi:10.4103/ijoy.ijoy_52_21 PMID:35017863

Roy, G., & Kumar, R. (2023). Construction of Asakti Model from Shrimad Bhagavad Gita: An Understanding of Attachment from Indian Ethos. *Psychological Studies*, 1–11. doi:10.100712646-023-00750-6

Sathiyaseelan, A., Balasundaram, S., & Zirkler, M. (2022). Indian Perspectives of Mindful Leadership. In *International Research Conference on Mindfulness 2022* (IRCM 2022).

Sebastian, K. A., & Mathew, G. V. (2002). Three gunas and PSI experience; a study of PSI experience in relation to inertia, activation, and stability. *Journal of Indian Psychology*, *20*(2), 44–48.

Sharma, N. (2014). Cognitive behaviour therapy in perspective of the Bhagwat Gita. *International Journal of Humanities and Social Science Invention*, *3*(1), 2319–7722.

Sharma, R. (1999). Self-concept and job satisfaction in sattva rajas and tamas personalities. *Journal of Indian Psychology*, *17*(2), 9–17.

Shearer, A. (1982). *(Trans.). Effortless being. The yoga sutras of Patanjali*. Wildwood House Limited.

Singh, C., & Reddy, T. O. (2018). Yoga origin, history and development in India. [IJMEES]. *Indian Journal of Movement Education and Exercise Sciences*, *8*(1), 9–12.

Singh, N., & Krishnan, V. R. (2005a). *Toward a Better Understanding of Transformational Leadership: Differentiating between Altruism and Self-sacrifi ce*. Proceedings of the Australian and New Zealand Academy of Management Conference, Canberra.

Singh, R., & Oberhummer, I. (1980). Behavior therapy within a setting of karma yoga. *Journal of Behavior Therapy and Experimental Psychiatry*, *11*(2), 135–141. doi:10.1016/0005-7916(80)90012-9

Sinha, D., & Tripathi, R. (1994). Individualism in a collectivist culture: A case of coexistence of dichotomies. In U. Kim, H. C. Triandis, C. Kacitçibabi, S. C. Choi & G. Yoon (Eds.), Individualism and Collectivism: Theory, Method and Applications (pp. 123-136). Thousand Oaks, CA: Sage.

Sitamma, M., Sridevi., & Rao, P. V. K. (1995). Three gunas and cognitive characteristics: A study of field dependence independence and perceptual acuity. *Journal of Indian Psychology*, *13*(2), 13–20.

Sotillos, S. B. (2022, December 20). *Book review – Perennial psychology of the Bhagavad Gita*. Academia. https://www.academia.edu/45645129/Book_Review_Perennial_Psychology_of_the_Bhagavad_Gita

Subrahmanyam, S., & Porkodi, K. (1980). Neurohumoral correlates of Transcendental Meditation. *Journal of Biomedicine (Sydney, NSW)*, *1*, 73–88.

Suthren Hirst, J. G. (2005). *Śaṃkara's Advaita Vedānta: A Way of Teaching*. Routledge. doi:10.4324/9780203001929

Tajfel, H. (1981). *Human groups and social categories*. Cambridge University Press.

Tajfel, H. (1982). *Social identity and intergroup relations*. Cambridge University Press.

Talukder, M. M. H. (2016). On "Self-realization" – the Ultimate Norm Of Arne Naess's Ecosophy T. *Symposion (Los Angeles, Calif.)*, *2*(3), 219–235. doi:10.5840ymposion20163217

Tikhe, S. G., Nagendra, H. R., & Tripathi, N. (2012). Ancient science of yogic life for academic excellence in university students. *Ancient Science of Life*, *31*(3), 80–83. doi:10.4103/0257-7941.103179 PMID:23284211

Travis, F. T., & Wallace, R. K. (1977). Autonomic patterns during respiratory suspensions: Proposed markers of transcendental consciousness. *Psychophysiology*, *34*(1), 39–46. doi:10.1111/j.1469-8986.1997.tb02414.x PMID:9009807

Uma, K., Lakshmi, Y. S., & Parameshwaran, E. G. (1971). Construction of a personality inventory based on the doctrine of three gunas. *Research Bulletin (International Commission for the Northwest Atlantic Fisheries)*, *6*, 49–58.

Vivekananda, S. (2009). *Karma-Yoga: The Yoga of action*. Advaita Ashrama.

Wolf, D. B. (1998). The Vedic Personality Inventory: A study of gunas. *Journal of Indian Psychology*, *16*(1), 26–43.

Wolpe, J. (1973). *The Practice of Behavior Therapy*. Pergamon Press.

ADDITIONAL READING

Bhawuk, D. (2011). *Spirituality and Indian psychology: lessons from the Bhagavad-Gita*. Springer Science & Business Media. doi:10.1007/978-1-4419-8110-3

Chinmayananda, S. (1982). *ATMABODHA*. Central Chinmaya Mission Trust.

Rama, S., Ballentine, R., & Ajaya, S. (2007). *Yoga and psychotherapy: The evolution of consciousness*. Himalayan Institute Press.

Rao, K. R. (2008). Introducing Indian Psychology. In K. R. Rao, A. Paranjpe, & A. K. Dalal (Eds.), Handbook of Indian Psychology (pp. 7–18). essay, Foundation Books.

KEY TERMS AND DEFINITIONS

Atmabodha: Knowledge of atman.

Atman: Individual metaphysical self which is in the physical body of an individual due to karmic bondage or as a result of karmas of previous birth.

Brahmana: Brahmana is the absolute self which is omnipresent and is free from the impact of trigunas.

Karma Yoga: Actions performed without any expectations of the results.

Karma: Any actions performed by individuals.

Moksha: It is freedom from karmic bondage which is necessary for atman to free itself from the cycle of birth and death and unite with brahmana.

Sādhaka: Any individual who has realized that the physical body is not the only truth and want to attain spiritual goals.

Triguna: The triguna refers to three gunas from which the whole universe is made. The three gunas are sattva, rajas and tamas.

Chapter 4
Effect of Spiritual Leadership on Intention to Quit:
Mediator Effect of Person–Organization Fit

Elif Baykal
İstanbul Medipol University, Turkey

ABSTRACT

Spiritual leadership is a holistic leadership approach through which organizational members can experience their connection with their spiritual realities. With the help of spiritual leadership, employees can find the inner motivation to show the necessary altruism to serve for the common good and vision. Thus, they find the opportunity to experience meaning in their workplace. This study has focused on spiritual leadership and its possible effects on person-organization fit and turnover intentions among Turkish academicians. Moreover, in this study, the mediator effect of person-organization fit in the relationship between spiritual leadership and turnover intentions has been examined. The research model has been investigated among academicians from various Turkish universities. In the related field research, 190 usable surveys were obtained, and the research data has been examined in SPSS 20. Results showed spiritual leadership has a negative effect on turnover intentions and person-organization fit acts as a mediator in this relationship.

1. INTRODUCTION

Dissatisfaction with materialism and ever increasing number of problems and ills of modern world, gave birth to new expectations regarding corporate managers. Modern people are overwhelmed by many social, psychological and economic problems having their roots in excessive greed and a lack of love and compassion (Cacioppe, 2000). Thus as Moxley (2000) claims a renewed search for integrity in life, harmony and peace in the minds of people, namely a new spiritual journey is quite important for modern individuals. In this point, spiritual leadership theory is seen as a significant help in solving the problems of contemporary business environment and attracts attention of several management scientists (Moxley, 1999; Fry, 2004).

DOI: 10.4018/978-1-6684-9778-4.ch004

The previous leadership models often focus on subordinates' internal motvation and they mostly ignore higher order requirements. Moreover, they often ignore the fit between organizations' value systems and individual kevel values (Fry, 2003; Reave, 2005). In contrast to previous leadership styles, spiritual leaders are good at understanding the relationship between individual values and organziational values, hence, they give importance to integrity.

In this study, spiritual leadership is accepted as the focal point since it acts as an intrinsic motivator motivating employees and making them hopeful and creating alignment with their surrounding (Narcıkara and Zehir, 2016). In this study, we assumed that spiritual leadership behavior of the leaders will effect turnover intentions of followers positevely and this relationship will be mediated by the person-organization fit perceptions of the employees. Without doubt, in order to understand spiritual leadership, understanding the construct of spirituality is very important.

1.1. Spirituality and Spiritual Leadership

Studies regarding spirituality seems to be a kind of upheavel to the corporate greed and oppression of the 1980s. In the extant literature, workplace spirituality is accepted as an intensely philosophical construct related to private lives of individuals. It can also be understood as a perspective of individual and organizational norms and values promoting transcendence through activities at work, contributing to the sense of being connected that results in feelings of compassion and enjoyment (Giacalone and Jurkiewicz, 2003). Most of the academic definitions concerned with spirituality claim that spirituality encompasses a sense of wholeness, a sense of connectedness, and inclination to focus on deeper values of individuals (Milliman, Czaplewski and Ferguson, 2003).

An important aspect of spirituality at work is alignment of employee and company goals and values. It can be regarded as organizational level spirituality. According to spiritual leadership researchers, individuals experiencing a strong sense of alignment of their purposes with their organizations purpose can experience meaning in their work. Aligning organizational values and personal values is possible when one can contribute to other people (Milliman, Czaplewski and Ferguson, 2003). Search for common good is also among the most significant elements of workplace spirituality. Spiritual needs can be fulfilled by acceptance of individuals' responsibility for the common goods. That is why, as Garcia-Zamor (2003) claims experiencing spirituality at work is an important goal of workplace spirituality and necessitates changing organizational climate by transforming the leadership style of leaders and followership styles of employees in order to make humanistic practices and policies of the organization become integral parts of day-to-day functions.

In fact, leaders' inclination to boost spirituality at workplace results in higher integration, serving as a means to make employees more engage in their jobs with both their souls and minds (Narcıkara, 2017). Spiritual leadership model attracts attention to both the importance of succeding organizational goals, and also attaining overall growth of society, through membership and calling (Contrereas, 2016). As defined by Fry (2003), conceptually spiritual leadership has its roots is in an intrinsic motivation model that combines theree important dimension, namely "vision," "hope/faith," and "altruistic love" that describes an effective leader. In his model Fry (2003) incorporated spirituality into leadership.

In this model, three spiritual factors regarding leadership are mediated by the two characteristics of followers to effect positive organizational results. These follower characteristics are: (1) meaning/calling: "the experience of transcendence in work and making a difference through service to others and, thus creating meaningfulness and purposefulness (Hannah, Walumba and Fry, 2011); and (2) membership:

the positive feeling related to being understood and appreciated. Since they meet the higher order requirements of people, such as self-efficacy, freedom, skillfulness, membership and relatedness, spiritual leaders create the necessary atmosphere for strong inner motivation earned by severe task involvement and goal orientedness.

In Fry's model, vision explains setting main direction by creating tactical decisions and by helping coordinate various tasks across the company (Fry and Cohen 2009) and boosts alignment of values across the organization, thus fosters higher levels of engagement and productivity (Fry et al., 2017). Furthermore, hope&faith is the baseline for the belief of the individuals that the company's vision, goals, and targets will be attained. In fact, hope is a powerful wish for the fulfillment of goals and faithfulness contributes to certainity for future goals that are hoped. Lastly, altruistic love should be understood as value congruence, and well-being that can be created by being sensible towards others (Fry, 2003). It designates the rules and the way of thinking that is viewed in the organization as morally right (Schein, 2010). On the one hand, calling explains the situation how individuals makes changes via serving other people and, in doing so, ads meaningfulness and purposefulness (Fry et.al., 2017). Moreover, membership boosts sense of belonging and creates the feelings of being understood and appreciated by the organization and its members.

1.2. Person-Organization Fit

Spiritual leadership approach combines basic organizational values with main values and convictions of employees, ensuring that they fit better with their organization. Person-organization fit can be explained as "the coherence between the individual and workplace occuring: (1) in case at least one of them meets the other's needs or (2) in case both of them have similar properties or (3) both. Person-organization fit is mostly a perception about the congruence between an individual's individual values and organizational culture. Kristof (1996) defines person-organization fit as the fit between the person and the organization that occurs under conditions where needs are met mutually, the parties have similar basic characteristics, or both.When employees think that their own values are coherant with their company's values, they are more prone to be engaged with the broader their organization and serve its mission and vision (Cable and Derue, 2002).

Much of the recent research on person-organization fit (see Kristof, 1996) has its roots in Schneider's model of attraction-selection-attrition (Schneider, 1987), which advocates that individualsand organizations are attracted to each other incase they are quiete similar. Namely, in organization, people having similar values and attitudes with their organizations tend to feel more congruent with their organizations. Anyway, in the extant literature, fit is related to tenure, work engagement, individual job performance, personal satisfaction and turnover intentions (Kristof, 1996; Finegan, 2000) and negatively assiciated with burnout (Kilroy et al., 2016).

People having a good fit with their organization attribute positive properties to their companies (Cable and Derue, 2002) and more likely to work harder for the larger causes of their organization (Cable and Derue, 2002). Similarly, Lauver and Kristof-Brown (2001) claim that high levels of person-organization fit perceived by the employee's result in higher levels of extra-role behaviors. If employees perceive the fact that organizational values are compatible with their own identity, they tend to develop a strong link with their companies making it impossible to leave their organizations (Cable and Derue, 2002). In this point, Cable and Derue's (2002) study on P-O fit perceptions of employees and organizational outputs also showed that person organziation fit perceptions of individuals are good predictors of prominent organizational outcome such as organizational citizenship behaviors, organizaitonal identification, organizational trust and turnover decisions.

1.3. Intention to Quit

Intention to quit can be explained as an employee's intents and plans about a possible quit from the existing job. Organizations give importance to retention owing to the strategic importance of intellectual capital and the results of replacing critic personnel (Podsakoff et al., 2007). Hausknecht and Trevor (2011), claims that among the antecedents of employee turnover we can focus on some organizational characteristics including the leadership style, human resources management implications, organizational culture and social networks in the organization. Extant literature confirms that value congruence between employees' and organizations's values create a proper atmosphere that negatively effects turnover intentions (Peltokorpi, Allen and Froese, 2015:). Moreover, strong social intraorganizational relationships decreases the inclination to quit, due to the fact that employees perceiving high level of organizational support and collegues tend to feel a sense of obligation toward their organization and tend to have lower levels of intention to quit. Furthermore, belonging to an external network also lowers the level of intention to quit since it provides greater information about alternative job opportunities, increasing the mobility of employees (Moynihan and Pandey, 2007). On the one hand, having a job that holds intrinsic value to the individual is also an important factor that satisfies individuals and make them stay in their organizations (Moynihan and Pandey, 2007.

In fact, one of the basic assumptions of person-organization fit literature is the fact that individuals are inclined to be more attracted to their companies and less prone to leave incase they find a match between their values (Elfenbein and O'Reilly 2007; Moynihan and Pandey, 2007).

2. HYPOTHESES

In this study it is assumed that, creating a positive atmosphere that results in high levels of meaning at work and value congruence between employees and the organization, spiritual leadership will have a positive effect on percen organization-fit of employees. Spiritual leaders build harmony between organizational values and core values of employees and make them fit better with their organizations. O the one hand, Narcikara (2018) claims that spiritual leadership contributes to the sense of meaning about the work of the individual, the individual who finds his job meaningful, works with a higher dedication and engagement which creates greater persom-organization fit in time. Moreover, as Singhal and Chatterjee (2006) posits spiritual leadership culminates a consciousness of the self, a consciousness regarding orher people and a a group consciousness that make individual aware of the whole and create interconnectedness that align individuals with their organizations, thus building higher person-organization fit. Sheep (2004) goes one step furher and claims that through spirituality at workplace, individuals experience transendence of self, that is to say, they become an integral part of the whole, indistunguishable from and coherent with the group. Spirituality in workplace creates integrity, meaning and purpose, and culminates the necessary baseline for developing a larger than oneself iden-tity, thus helps individuals to appreciate their person–organization interactions better (Singhal and Chatterjee, 2006). Furthermore, as Ashmos and Duchon (2000) suggests wholeness created by spiritual leadership encompasses the idea of an inner life that encompasses the authentic expression in the workplace, creating the necessary ground for a high quality person-organization fit.

Among previous studies, there is not a specific empirical study addressing to spiritual leadership and person-organization relationship. However, there are some empirical studies confirming the relationship between workplace spirituality and person organization-fit relationship which gives clue for the possibility of spiritual leadership/person-organization fit relationship. For instance; In their empirical study Sheep (2004) also revealed the positive relationship between and workplace spirituality and P-O fit. Later, Afsar and Rehman, (2015) revealed the fact spirituality at work positively effects P-O fit of individuals and person-organization fit acts as mediator in the relationship between spirituality at work and innovativeness. Lastly, Baykal (2019a) examined effects of spirituality on person-organization fit and revealed that this positive relationship gives way to higher performance. Thus, being inspired with these studies we hypothesized:

H1: Spiritual leadership has a significant relationship with person-organization fit perceived by employers

Furthermore, existing P-O fit research shows that compatibility between the properties of an individual and his environment is effective on desirable results, such as greater job satisfaction, stronger organizational commitment, higher job engagement, and lower turnover rates (Kristof-Brown et al., 2005). Employees experiencing poor fit with their companies are less likely to quit their jobs (Schneider et al., 1995). Work adjustment theory has been created as a meaningful approach for explaining the link between P-O fit and turnover intentions (Dawis and Lofquist, 1984). This theory claims the existence of an ongoing process of work adjustment between employees and their environment wherein each other values become congruent in time. Similarly, Cable and De Rue's (2002) study focused on the effect of P-O on turnover rates and showed that P-O fit affects intention to stay. Moreover, according to Hobfoll's (1989) conservation of resources theory, epeople with high levels of P-O fit will possibly prefer to continue to hold this fit as a valued resource as long as they work professionally and will not want to quit their job in their current organization.

In Verquer et al,.'s (2003) meta-analysis of 21 person-organization fit studies, results showed modest correlations between P-O fit and satisfaction and with job satisfaction and intent to leave. Kristof-Brown et al. (2005) also meaningful relationships between P-O fit and job satisfaction and rather weaker relationships between person-organization fit and turnover intentions. In recent years, Jin, McDonald and Park (2018) confirmed the assumptions of the study regarding the mediator roles of P-O fit and employee followership. Consistent with conservation of resources theory, they showed that P-O fit perceptions tend to have lower turnover intentions. Memon et al. (2018) also showed the effect of P-O fit on turnover intention. Being inspired from these studies we hypothesized that:

H2: Person organization fit perceived by employees has a significant relationship with turnover intentions

As it is confirmed in the empirical study of Puni, Agyemang and Asamoah (2016) democratic and supportive leadership styles, as in the case with spritual leadership has a negative effect on intention to quit. In fact, spiritual leadership is an important leadership style in retaining people in the organization owing to its supportive and fair leadership approach. Actually, spiritual leadership has the capacity to create an organic link between one's self and the meaning that one loads to his/her life at workplace. Besides that, meaningfulness at work triggered by spiritual leadership pave the way for coping with work stress (Baykal, 2019c). Thereby, spiritual leadership contributes to better coping mechanisms with the emotional requirements of individuals facing hard times and trying to survive in an organization (Nandram and Bindlish, 2017). Indeed, spiritual leaders can provide service and meanings for workers, help them carry the burden of destructive emotions of fear, anxiety, anger, jeaolusy and arrogance to further increase employees' perceptions of satisfaction (Baykal, 2022) and performance (Narcıkara, 2017), and align altruistic love into their social connections with others to have their followers feel themselves cared and respected (Xiang et al., 2019), thus has a potential to contribute to higher levels of well being, engagement, commitment (Baykal, 2021) leading to lower levels of turnover intentions.

However in the related literature, there is a gap in empirical work explaining the positive effect of spiritual leadership on turnover intentions except a few works confirming the negative effect of spiritual leadership on intention to quit (Lee et al., 2010; Yusof, Zulkiffli and Muda, 2016) and some other studies revealed the negative effect of workplace spirituality on turnover intentions (Rego and Cunha, 2008; Beehner and Blackwell, 2016). But the existing works on spiritual leadership-work engagement relationship (Fachrunnisa and Adhiatma 2014; Sheikh et al., 2019; Baykal, 2019b; Saripudin and Rosari, 2019) and spiritual leadership-organizational commitment relationship (Tsui et al., 2019; Baykal, 2019c) provide us clue for the possible negative effect of spiritual leadership on turnover intentions. Being inspired by these studies we wanted to see if the effect of spiritual leadership on P-O fit. Moreover, we wanted to see if P-O fit perceived by employees have a negative effect on intention to quit and if it mediates the relationship between spiritual leadership and turnover intentions. Thus, our hypothesis of this study are;

H3: Spiritual leadership has a significant relationship with intention to quit
H4: Person-organization fit perceived by employees act as a mediator between spiritual leadership and Intention to quit

3. METHODOLOGY

3.1. Sample and Data Collection

In this study, random sampling methodology has been used in collecting data related to the field resarch of the study. Face to face survey method and online survey methods have been used in collecting data from the applicants. EFA has been used in order to test whether the observed variables have been loaded in the supposed dimensions. And correlation and regression methods have been used in hypothesis tests. Responses of the applicants were assessed with five-point Likert Scale. The field research has been conducted on Turkish academicians from all over Turkey. Suggesting that they may have higher expectations in terms of leadership since the academic staff is more educated compared to many white-collar staff working in other sectors, we decided to implement this study among academics. We supposed that individuals would demand more from their superiors in term of support, care and spirituality when their qualifications are higher. About 800 surveys has been sent to academicians from different universities. After a six months period 190 usable surveys have been obtained. In the study, about %35 of applicants have 0-2 years experiences, %32 2-5 years experienced, %28 5-10 years experienced in their current organization. On the other hand, %20 of the applicants are younger than 30 years old and about %50 of them are between the ages of 30-39 and %22 are between the ages of 40-49 that is to say we have a young sample and lastly most of the participants were male, about %62 of the whole sample.

Furthermore, related data has been analyzed regarding descriptive and inferential statistics. Kaiser-Meyer-Olkin Measure of Sampling Adequacy analysis has been used in order to test if the data was sufficient. The sufficiency coefficient was 0,937 and and Barlett score was under 0,001 which were statistically plausible values to continue with factor analysis.

3.2. Analyses

In our survey questions, 17 items have been barrowed from Fry 's (2003) spiritual leadership scale for measuring spiritual leadership, six items were related to person-organization fit perceptions adapted from Cable and DeRue (2002). 4 questions regarding thoughts of quitting have been barrowed from Epstein (2005). The Cronbach's Alpha values are above 0,70, that confirms the reliability of scales. In the original scale Fry's spiritual scale is composed of three subdimensions encompassing; vision hope/ faith and altruism. But in our sample after factor analysis the items loaded into 2 main subdimension, the first one is composed of hope/faith and altruism questions and the second one is composed of vison questions. The results was not astonishing due to the fact that although placed in different subdimension (faith/hope and altruism) in the original scale many altruism items have similar meanings with faith / hope questions. The factor loadings of the whole items can be seen below in Table 1.

Moreover, correletation analysis also applied between the subdimensions of spritual leadership and intention to quit and person-organization fit. Correlation results are listed in Table 2. As seen in Table 2, there are statistically significant relationships between the two factors for each relationship as shown Table-2 ($\rho <0.01$, $\rho <0.05$ level).

3.3. Findings

In order to test the hypothesis regression analysis has been applied. In Table 3, the regression results regarding H1 and H2 hypothesses have been revealed. In the first part of Table 3, regression results related to spiritual leadership dimensions and person-organization fit have been summarized. Results of regression analyzes for SLHFA (Adjusted R2:,308, Sig:,001, t: 10.961***) and for SLV (Adjusted R2:,308, Sig:,001, t: 5,025***) confirmed the assumption of H1, that is to say the regression results show that when an organization is led by spiritual leadership, employees working in this organization are mostly inclined to stay in the organization, they do not make plans for quitting the job, they do not search for opportunities for changing their organization. Furthermore, in the second part of Table 3, the regression results regarding the relationship between person-organization fit and intention to quit has been summarized (Adjusted R2:,229, Sig:,005, t:-7.4104***) confirming the assumptions of H2. Thus, we can say that, as it is supposed in H2, when people has a good alignment with their organizations they do not tend to think about leaving their jobs.

Furthermore, in Table 4, the regression results regarding the assumptions of H3 and H4 have been summarized. In this part, we wanted to see the possible direct effect of spiritual leadership on turnover intentions and possible mediator effect of person-organization fit in the relationship between spiritual leadership and turnover intentions. In this study, Baron and Kenny's (1986) statistical approach has been applied y for testing mediating effect of person-organization fit with multiple regression. According to this approach, four conditions must be met in order to talk about the existence of mediation effect. First of all, the independent variable (spiritual leadership) must have a significant effect on the mediator variable (person-organization fit). As a second condition, the mediator variable (person-organization fit) must have

Table 1. Factor loadings

	1	2	3	4	CronbachAlfa
SLHF7	0,963				0.958
SLHF3	0,957				
SLA10	0,901				
SLA12	0,865				
SLHF8	0,847				
SLHF2	0,839				
SLHF4	0,829				
SLHF6	0,784				
SLA11	0,777				
SLHF5	0,722				
SLHF1	0,716				
SLHF9	0,628				
SLV17		0,929			0.835
SLV16		0,732			
SLV15		0,511			
PO83			0,897		0.894
PO81			0,794		
PO82			0,793		
PO85			0,771		
PO88			0,765		
PO86			0,738		
TITQ74				0,933	0.918
TITQ73				0,923	
TITQ75				0,899	
TITQ76				0,768	
*SLHF=Spiritual Leadership Hope /Faith					
** SLA=Spiritual Leadership Altruism					
***SLV=Spiritual Leadership Vision					
****PO=Person-Organization Fit					
*****TITQ=Turnover Intention to Quit					

a significant effect on the dependent variable (turnover intentions). As a third condition, the independent variable (spiritual leadership) must have a significant effect on the dependent variable (Turnover intentions). Lastly, the effect of the independent variable (Spiritual leadership) should not be significant if it is a full mediation) or ought to be reduced in strength (if it is a partial mediation) after being controlled by the mediator variable (Person-organization fit). The results of H1 and H2 hypothesis fulfilled the first two conditions of testing mediation. Hence, regarding the first and second conditions, we can say that spiritual leadership has a significant effect on person organization fit, and Person-organization fit

Table 2. Correlation results

		SLHFA	SLV	PO	TITQ
SLHFA	Pearson Correlation	1			
SLV	Pearson Correlation	,755**	1		
PO	Pearson Correlation	,558**	,467**	1	
TITQ	Pearson Correlation	-,402**	-,325**	-,483**	1
*SLHFA=Spiritual Leadership Hope /Faith/Altruism					
***SLV=Spiritual Leadership Vision					
****PO=Person-Organziation Fit					
*****TITQ=Turnover Intention to Quit					

Table 3. Regression analyzes for spritiual leadership/person-organization fit and person-organization fit/turnover intentions relationships

	SL-PO		PO-Intention to Quit	
Independent Variable	Beta	T	Beta	T
Constant	1.819	10.961***	-4.667	-14.842***
SLHFA	0,483	5,025***		
SLV	0,099	1,03		
PO			-0.483	-7.4104***
F	41.304		54.810	
Adjusted R Square	0.308		0.229	
Sign.	0.001		0.005	

has a significant effect on turnover intentions (Table 3). Finally, we ought to examine whether spiritual leadership has a significant effect on turnover intentions, and whether these effect has been reduced or disappeared after the effect of person-organization fit has been taken into account.

In the first part of Table 4, we have given the results of regression results explaining the direct effect of spiritual leadership on turnover intentions. From these results we can conclude that the results (Adjusted R2:1,154, Sig:,000, -3.501***) related to the first dimension (SLHFA) and intention to quit, and the results (Adjusted R2:1,154, Sig:,000, t: -0.527*) explaining the relationship between the second dimension (SLV) and ıntention to quit supports H3. That is to say, with its both dimensions spiritual leaders has an important effect on preventing intention to quit but this effect is more powerful through the first dimension, through hope & altruism dimension in comparasion to vision dimension.That means, the aspects of spiritual leaders that instill hope and strengthen love and respect in the organization are more effective in people's intention to stay within the organization when compared to the visionary aspect. Moreover, as it is seen in the second part of Table 4 we tested the H4 hypothesis which claims that person organization fit acts as a mediator in the relationship between spiritual leadership and intentions to quit. In order to talk about mediation effect of person organization fit, the effect of spiritual leadership on turnover intentions, which is seen in the first part of the table below should diminish in

Table 4. Regression analyzes for spiritual leadership/turnover intentions relationships without mediator and with mediator

	SL-Intention to Quit (Without Mediator)		SL-PO-Intention to Quit (With Mediator)	
Independent Variable	**Beta**	**t**	**Beta**	**t**
Constant	**-3.785**	**-13.994******	**-4.790**	**-14.228******
SLHFA	-0.355	-3.501***	-0,19	-1,779**
SLV	-0.057	-0.527*	-0,006	-0,057
PO			-0,552	-4,678***
F	17.526		20.374	
Adjusted R Square	1.154		0.245	
Sign.	0.000		0.000	

the second part when both spiritual leadership dimensions and person-organization dimension put into the model simultaneously.

As summarized in the second part of Table 4, when all spiritual leadership dimensions (SLHFA and SLV) and person-organization fit put into the model together in order to test the mediator effect of person-organization fit, we can see that the effects of spiritual leadership dimesions diminishes but do not disappear. The significant effect of SLHFA on intention to quit continues but also diminishes (t=-1,779**), on the other hand, the effect of SLV on intention to quit becomes statistically insignificant (-0,0579). Hence, we can talk about a partial mediation of person-organization fit in the relationship between spiritual leadership and intention to quit.These results, denotes that the effect of spiritual leadership on intention to quit mostly occurs through person-organization fit in the organizational setting.

3.4. Discussion

As mentioned before, spiritual leadership theory (Fry, 2003) is based on an intrinsic motivation model which incorporates vision, hope/faith, and altruistic love, workplace spirituality, and spiritual well-being concepts (Fry, 2003, Fry and Cohen 2008). By binding individuals to other employees in the organization and and to a transcendent high power, spiritual leaders contribute to wholeness of people and encourage them to search for meaningful work, directing them to a higher purpose and meaning (Hudson, 2014) and contributes to higher levels of person-organization fit. Search for meaning and search for value congruece is a central point in spiritual leadership and workplace spirituality literature. In spiritual leadership literature it is believed that individuals in organizational settings will feel more comfortable and engaged if their search for meaning is met by the organizations. And this mostly possible through value congruence between the organization and the individual. Furthermore, spiritual leaders encourage their followers to be altruistic by taking into consideration the needs and concerns of their organization, other stakeholders, and nature which also contributes to value congruence between employee and his organization. Although there is not any previous study in education sector, there are some existing studies confirming this relationship. For example, in their work Singhal and Chatterjee claimed that it is possible to measure the person organziation fit in spirituality at work terms by assessing employees' preferences about spirituality at work although their model is quiet similar to the model of our study it lack the necessary empirical study, namely field research confirming their suggestion. On the other hand, although scarce in numbers, in the extant literature there are studies regarding negative effects of spirituality on intention to quit. For example Chawla, & Guda, (2010) investigated effects of workplace spirituality on turnover intentions amaong sales representatives and found that workplace spirituality has a negative effect on intentions to quit. Similarly, Beehner, & Blackwell (2016) found negative relationships between workplace spirituality and intention to quit. And Lee, Chen, Wang, and Dadura (2010) also found similar results in their study investigating effects of spiritual management on turnover intentions of employees.

In this study, similar to the studies mentioned above we investigated our model among Turkish academicians and found a positive effect of spiritual leadership on person organization-fit and we confirmed the mediating effect of person-organization fit in the relationship between spiritual leadership and turnover intentions. Interestingly in our study this positive effect accured through the hope/faith & altruism subdimensions of spiritual leadership rather than vision subdimension. Hope/faith and altruism items of spiritual leadership scale are mostly the kind of questions that touch to individuals' values, convinctions and beliefs so it is normal and acceptable to expect such a result. But in vision subdimension, items are mostly the kind of questions asking long term orientation, ambition, commitment to higher goals etc. In this point it will be meaningful to remember properties of our sample. We applied this study on academicians. Individuals belonging to this profession more prone to work individually and can set individual visions and ideals regarding their professional life. Academicians have the chance to work individually or in small groups in order to reach their professional goals. We think the irrelevance between *vision* subdimension of spiritual leadership and person organization-fit perceptions and turnover intentions of employees stems from the fact that sometimes academicians can be more focused on their personal visions and goals rather than organizational ones due to the nature of their profession.

3.4.1 Managerial Implications

The harmony of the individual with the organization she works for and the job she does is at a key point in both maintaining the current employment and increasing the overall success of the organization. Person-organization fit play a decisive role in the work attitudes of individuals. It is thought that the emotional effects of employees' harmony with the organization may have more decisive effects in developing eastern countries compared to western countries. As a matter of fact, in countries such as Turkey, which has a more collectivist view in the cultural context, cohesion is one of the leading factors in ensuring organizational commitment. So, according to the results of this study we believe that creating P-O fit can be used as a managerial tool for retention of Turkish employees.

3.4.2 Limitations and Further Studies

This study shows that spiritual leadership negatively affects employees' intention to leave, that is, it enables employees to stay in their organizations longer. Our study specifically points to the importance of person-organization fit with the organization. In further studies, different mediators can be tested or different sectors can be choosen so that the applicability of the model can be examined. Moreover, cross cultural studies can be conducted to see whether the model is applicable in different cultures.

REFERENCES

Ashmos, D. P., & Duchon, D. (2000). Spirituality at Work: A Conceptualization and Measure. *Journal of Management Inquiry*, *9*(2), 134–145. doi:10.1177/105649260092008

Baykal, E. (2019a). Person Organization Fit: Spiritual Way to Boost Performance. *Asya Studies*, *3*(9), 31–43. doi:10.31455/asya.597151

Baykal, E. (2019b). Effect of Workplace Spirituality on Work Engagement Mediator Effect of Altruistic Love. *PressAcademia Procedia*, *9*(1), 61–64. doi:10.17261/Pressacademia.2019.1066

Baykal, E. (2019c). Creating Organizational Commitment Through Spiritual Leadership: Mediating Effect Of Meaning At Work. *Business & Management Studies: An International Journal*, *7*(2), 837–855. doi:10.15295/bmij.v7i2.1113

Baykal, E. (2021). Understanding Religion As a Phenomenon in Workplace Sprituality: A Durkheimian Approach. *Spiritual Psychology and Counseling*, *6*(2), 27–41. doi:10.37898pc.2021.6.2.134

Baykal, E. (2022). The Relationship Between Spiritual Well-Being and Life Satisfaction During COVID-19. In Handbook of Research on Interdisciplinary Perspectives on the Threats and Impacts of Pandemics (pp. 425-443). IGI Global.

Beehner, C. G., & Blackwell, M. J. (2016). The impact of workplace spirituality on food service worker turnover intention. *Journal of Management, Spirituality & Religion*, *13*(4), 304–323. doi:10.1080/14766086.2016.1172251

Chawla, V., & Guda, S. (2010). Individual spirituality at work and its relationship with job satisfaction, propensity to leavand job commitment: An exploratory study among sales professionals. *Journal of Human Values*, *16*(2), 157–167. doi:10.1177/097168581001600203

Chen, C. Y., & Li, C. I. (2013). Assessing the spiritual leadership effectiveness: The contribution of follower's self-concept and preliminary tests for moderation of culture and managerial position. *The Leadership Quarterly*, *24*(1), 240–255. doi:10.1016/j.leaqua.2012.11.004

Finegan, J. E. (2000). The impact of person and organizational values on organizational commitment. *Journal of Occupational and Organizational Psychology*, *73*(2), 149–169. doi:10.1348/096317900166958

Fry, L., & Kriger, M. (2009). Towards a theory of Being-centered Leadership: Multiple Levels of Being as Context for Effective Leadership. *Human Relations*, *62*(11), 1667–1696. doi:10.1177/0018726709346380

Fry, L., & Nisiewicz, M. (2013). *Maximizing the Triple Bottom Line through Spiritual Leadership*. Stanford University Press.

Fry, L. W. (2003). Toward a theory of spiritual leadership. *The Leadership Quarterly*, *14*(6), 693–727. doi:10.1016/j.leaqua.2003.09.001

Fry, L. W., & Cohen, M. P. (2009). Spiritual leadership as a paradigm for organizational transformation and recovery from extended work hours cultures. *Journal of Business Ethics*, *84*(S2), 265–278. doi:10.100710551-008-9695-2

Fry, L. W., & Matherly, L. L. (2006). *Spiritual leadership and organizational performance: An exploratory study*. In Annual Meeting of the Academy of Management, Atlanta-Georgia. http://www. tarleton. edu/~ fry/sltorgperf. pdf

Fry, L. W., & Slocum, J. W. Jr. (2008). Maximizing the triple bottom line through spiritual leadership. *Organizational Dynamics*, *37*(1), 86–96. doi:10.1016/j.orgdyn.2007.11.004

Giacalone, R., & Jurkiewicz, C. (2003). Toward a science of workplace spirituality. In R. Giacalone, & C. Jurkiewicz (Eds.), Handbook of workplace spirituality and organizational performance (pp. 3–28). Armonk, NY7 Sharpe.

Gould-Williams, J. S., Mostafa, A. M. S., & Bottomley, P. (2015). Public service motivation and employee outcomes in the Egyptian public sector: Testing the mediating effect of person-organization fit. *Journal of Public Administration: Research and Theory*, *25*(2), 597–622. doi:10.1093/jopart/mut053

Hausknecht, J. P., & Trevor, C. O. (2011). Collective turnover at the group, unit, and organizational levels: Evidence, issues, and implications. *Journal of Management*, *37*(1), 352–388. doi:10.1177/0149206310383910

Hudson, R. (2014). The question of theoretical foundations for the spirituality at work movement. *Journal of Management, Spirituality & Religion*, *11*(1), 27–44. doi:10.1080/14766086.2013.801031

Jin, M. H., McDonald, B., & Park, J. (2018). Person–organization fit and turnover intention: Exploring the mediating role of employee followership and job satisfaction through conservation of resources theory. *Review of Public Personnel Administration*, *38*(2), 167–192. doi:10.1177/0734371X16658334

Kristof-Brown, A. L., Zimmerman, R. D., & Johnson, E. C. (2005). Consequences of individuals' fit at work: A meta-analysis of person-job, person-organization, person-group, and person-supervisor fit. *Personnel Psychology*, *58*(2), 281–342. doi:10.1111/j.1744-6570.2005.00672.x

Lauver, K. J., & Kristof-Brown, A. (2001). Distinguishing between employees' perceptions of person–job and person– organization fit. *Journal of Vocational Behavior*, *59*(3), 454–470. doi:10.1006/jvbe.2001.1807

Lee, T. R., Chen, S. Y., Wang, S. H., & Dadura, A. (2010). The relationship between spiritual management and determinants of turnover intention. *European Business Review*, *22*(1), 102–116. doi:10.1108/09555341011009034

Memon, M. A., Salleh, R., Nordin, S. M., Cheah, J. H., Ting, H., & Chuah, F. (2018). Person-organisation fit and turnover intention: The mediating role of work engagement. *Journal of Management Development*, *37*(3), 285–298. doi:10.1108/JMD-07-2017-0232

Milliman, J., Czaplewski, A. J., & Ferguson, J. (2003). Workplace spirituality and employee work attitudes: An exploratory empirical assessment. *Journal of Organizational Change Management*, *16*(4), 426–447. doi:10.1108/09534810310484172

Moynihan, D. P., & Pandey, S. K. (2007). The ties that bind: Social networks, person-organization value fit, and turnover intention. *Journal of Public Administration: Research and Theory*, *18*(2), 205–227. doi:10.1093/jopart/mum013

Nandram, S., & Bindlish, P. (2017). *Managing VUCA through integrative self-management.* Springer. https://link.springer. com/book/10.1007%2F978-3-319-52231-9

Narcıkara, E. (2017). *Spiritüel liderlik davranışının algılanan performans üzerine etkisi.* Yayınlanmış Doktora Tezi, Yıldız Teknik Üniversitesi.

Narcıkara, E. B. (2018). Spiritüelite (Ruhsallık) ve iş ortamında anlam arayışı. *Alanya Akademik Bakış, 2*(1), 11–25. doi:10.29023/alanyaakademik.337789

Narcıkara, E. B., & Zehir, C. (2016). Effect of Organizational Support in the Relationship between Spiritual Leadership and Performance. *International Journal of Humanities and Social Science, 6*(12), 29–42.

Peltokorpi, V., Allen, D. G., & Froese, F. (2015). Organizational embeddedness, turnover intentions, and voluntary turnover: The moderating effects of employee demographic characteristics and value orientations. *Journal of Organizational Behavior, 36*(2), 292–312. doi:10.1002/job.1981

Podsakoff, N. P., LePine, J. A., & LePine, M. A. (2007). Differential challenge stressor-hindrance stressor relationships with job attitudes, turnover intentions, turnover, and withdrawal behavior: A meta-analysis. *The Journal of Applied Psychology, 92*(2), 438–454. doi:10.1037/0021-9010.92.2.438 PMID:17371090

Puni, A., Agyemang, C. B., & Asamoah, E. S. (2016). Leadership styles, employee turnover intentions and counterproductive work behaviours. *International Journal of Innovative Research and Development, 5*(1), 1–7.

Rego, A., & Cunha, M. P. (2008). Workplace spirituality and organizational commitment: An empirical study. *Journal of Organizational Change Management, 21*(1), 53–75. doi:10.1108/09534810810847039

Saripudin, W., & Rosari, R. (2019). Does Spiritual Leadership Model Enhance Work Engagement? Empirical Evidence From an Islamic Hospital in Yogyakarta. *Journal of Leadership in Organizations, 1*(2). Advance online publication. doi:10.22146/jlo.45520

Schneider, B. (1987). The people make the place. *Personnel Psychology, 40*(3), 437–453. doi:10.1111/j.1744-6570.1987.tb00609.x

Sheep, M. L. (2004). Nailing Down Gossamer: A Valid Measure Of The Person-Organization Fit Of Workplace Sprituality. In Academy of Management Proceedings, Briarcliff Manor, Academy of Management. doi:10.5465/ambpp.2004.13862520

Sheikh, A. A., Inam, A., Rubab, A., Najam, U., Rana, N. A., & Awan, H. M. (2019). The Spiritual Role of a Leader in Sustaining Work Engagement: A Teacher-Perceived Paradigm. *SAGE Open, 9*(3), 2158244019863567. doi:10.1177/2158244019863567

Singhal, M., & Chatterjee, L. (2006). A person–organization fit-based approach for spirituality at work: Development of a conceptual framework. *Journal of Human Values, 12*(2), 161–178. doi:10.1177/097168580601200205

Tsui, K. T., Lee, J. C. K., Zhang, Z., & Wong, P. H. (2019). The Relationship Between Teachers' Perceived Spiritual Leadership and Organziational Commitment: A Multilevel Analysis in the Hong Kong Context. *Asian Journal of Social Sciences & Humanities*, *8*, 3.

Xiang, W., Chen, X., & Zhang, F. (2019). The Diffusion of Green Technology Innovation Based on Cloud Platform for Energy Saving. *Ekoloji Dergisi*, (107), 1641–1650.

Yusof, J. M., Zulkiffli, S. N. A., & Muda, M. S. (2016). The Influence Of Spiritual Leadership On Intention To Leave Of The Employees. *International Journal of Applied Business and Economic Research*, *14*(9), 113–9124.

Chapter 5
Existence of Therapeutic Techniques in Indian Psychology

S. Akila
Avinashilingam University, India

Benadict Savitha
Avinashilingam Institute for Home Science and Higher Education for Women, India

ABSTRACT

In the new millennium, therapies of Indian psychology have gained renewed interest as a distinct and holistic approach to understanding the mind and human behavior. The essence of psychotherapy existed in India since time immemorial submerged in social structures, religion, ancient scriptures, mystics, and alternate system of medicine including Ayurveda, Unani tradition, Siddha and Yoga, and so forth. The popularity of Indian psychology in the West has been driven by a growing interest in mindfulness, meditation, and other Eastern spiritual practices, which are increasingly being incorporated into Western therapy and wellness programs that focus on treating mental disorders and addressing individual problems. Numerous Western psychologists and therapists are beginning to incorporate Indian psychology techniques and principles into their practice. Indian psychology is one perspective in understanding mental health and is not a substitute for modern evidence-based approaches to mental health care.

INTRODUCTION

Healing is the goal of Indian psychological traditions. Cure is more or less external intervention and the treatment is relatively passive, whereas healing involves more caring and counselling. Healing is more active and the whole process is interactive and integral. In Indian wisdom tradition, cure and healing do not have such a distinction. In Ayurveda, svastyam, coming to self or being in self, could be compared to the concept of healing; and arogyam, balance of gunas or living according to one's prakrti, physical constitution, is similar to the concept of cure. (Menon, 2005).

DOI: 10.4018/978-1-6684-9778-4.ch005

From ancient times, our sages have endeavoured to comprehend the workings of the mind and various methods of controlling it. In India, psychology is essentially intertwined into the philosophical and religious traditions, as is widely believed. It combines cosmology, theology, mythology, and philosophy. Several psychological concepts, including mind, cognition, personality, emotions, and others, are thoroughly and sophisticatedly explained in ancient Indian texts. Indian methods to psychology, and more specifically counselling, do exist, as is demonstrated in classical literature. Many experts have recently drawn attention to this issue by showing the similarities between numerous psychological concepts from the west and the theories put forth in ancient Indian scriptures.

There are many psychological theories found in ancient Indian writings and scriptures that can be helpful for understanding counselling procedures. Additionally, India has used a range of culturally appropriate psychotherapy approaches all ages. The Vedas, Upanishads, Yoga, Buddhism, and its various schools may all have a strong influence on the average Indian. The Vedas and Upanishads are the main texts in India that provide knowledge on counselling procedures. The Upanishads explain ideas like perception, consciousness, cognition, and so forth. In particular, psychopathology and mental health issues are described in terms of the imbalance of the Tridoshas and Trigunas. (Kumar, 2023).

A unique and comprehensive approach to understanding the human mind and behavior is provided by Indian psychology. Indian psychology emphasises the connection between the individual and the collective consciousness while drawing on ancient philosophical and spiritual traditions. It also acknowledges the value of mindfulness, yoga, and meditation in fostering mental and emotional well-being. This emphasizes the importance of understanding the human psyche within the larger context of cultural, social, and spiritual factors. (Aakash, 2021). Indian psychology is becoming more and more popular in the West as a holistic and spiritual method of studying the mind and human behaviour, with mounting scientific data demonstrating the efficacy of its techniques. (Kumar, 2023).

A positive trait, enthusiastic parity, the ability to live a full, balanced, and creative life, and the flexibility to deal with life's inevitable challenges are all associated with mental wellness. The Indian society and theory are unique in how they encourage people to build their own autonomy. The system and belief that the human being has enormous potential hidden inside it are shared by Indian psychology study and philosophy. Indian Ancient Psychology studies also contains an endless display of methods for enhancing human awareness. Indian thought is filled with mental concepts that have not yet been fully explored by therapists or in other spheres of daily life. (Sedlmeier & Srinivas, 2016). Ancient Indian thought contains a wealth of mental information that is clear and unpretentious, elaborating on procedures and constructs such as psychological health, attention, feeling, emotions, perceptions, inspiration, self- and personality discernment, and psychopathology and its treatment.

CONTRIBUTION OF ANCIENT INDIA IN THE FIELD OF MENTAL HEALTH

Indian Psychology is a holistic approach to understand the mind and human behavior based on ancient Indian texts such as the Vedas and treating mental health issues includes addressing both the symptoms and the underlying causes. It emphasizes the integration of spiritual and psychological practices for overall well-being and differs from Western psychology, which focuses on treating mental disorders and addressing individual problems. Some key principles of Indian psychology that are relevant to mental health include

1. Atman
2. Karma
3. Dharma
4. Yoga and Meditation
5. Ayurveda

Atman

Atman originally meant "breath" and then came to be applied to whatever constitutes the essential part of man, his self or soul. The distinctive meaning of *Atman* is the inner self of man.

As per Indian Psychology the perception of Atman is to assist people to connect with their inner persons and to discover a sense of harmony.

Atman (the self) is the innermost individual being characterized by individual consciousness (*Chitta*). The essence of personality is something beyond body, life, mind and intellect. It is *Atman*, the self. Its chief attribute is consciousness. The self exists before, in and after the various states of consciousness: wakeful, dream and sleep. Denial of consciousness means denial of everything else. Hence, mind and self are not identical. The self is knower (*kshetrajna*), the seer (*drasta*), the witness (*sakshi*), and the immutable (*kutastha*). The composite whole of chit and achit (consciousness and matter), *kshetrajna* and *kshetra* (knower and known), *karta* and *karana* (doer and its instrument) is the total personality called *Jiva* and *Jivatman* – the embodied self.

Atman, according to the Upanishads, is *sat* (existence), *cit* (consciousness) and *anand* (bless). So, every form of happiness or pleasure, the Advaita maintains, should be derived from the *ananda* of *Atman*.

According to Nyayavaisesika, *Atman* has 14 qualities: *buddhi* (knowledge), *sukha* (pleasure), *dukha* (pain), *iccha* (desire), *dvesa* (hatred), *yatna* (striving), *sankhya* (number), *pramiti* (size), *prathaktva* (distinctness), *amyoga* (contact), *vibhya* (separation), *bhavana* (imagination), *dharma* (merit) and *adharma* (demerit) (Srivastava, 2010).

Karma

Varma emphasized the use of concepts of Karma in psychotherapy. (Varma, 1982). Karma is the belief that every action has consequences and that individuals are responsible for their actions and their effects on the world around them. Understanding Karma can help individuals understand how their actions impact their own mental and emotional well-being, as well as the well-being of others. When it comes to coping, adjusting, and adapting processes, the concept of karma is important in the Indian setting. It also affects how people approach their challenges.

Dharma

The belief that each individual has a unique purpose or role in the world and that living in alignment with one's Dharma can lead to greater satisfaction and fulfilment. Varma emphasized the use of concepts of Dharma in psychotherapy. (Varma, 1982).

Yoga and Meditation

Indian psychology emphasizes using yoga and meditation as tools for self-awareness and spiritual development. The Indian culture attaches huge importance to spiritual life which may not be synonymous with the mental health but it values inner mental life and experiences. (Wig, 1989). Detachment from material things and self-realization is the ultimate goal of life. This is the reason for yoga and meditation having a special place in Indian philosophy. Yoga originates from the word "*Yuj*" which in Sanskrit means "to unite." (Sood, Singh & Chadda, 2017). It has four divisions including *Mantra yoga, Hatha yoga, Laya yoga,* and *Raja Yoga*. (Pandurangi, et al., 2017).

The Yoga Sutras were compiled by Sage Patanjali who is also known as the father of Yoga. These Sutras form the basis of Raja Yoga which is considered the ultimate among the four divisions. (Pandurangi, et al., 2017). Raja Yoga contains the descriptions of the eight limbed path of yoga for overall personality development known as the "*Astanga Yoga"* which is the key to attain the ultimate spiritual goal of self-realization. (Khalsa, 2017). These eight levels are divided into preparatory phases, the internal and external aids to yoga. *Yama* (self-control) and *Niyama* (observation of rules) are the preparatory phases, and the two along with *Pranayama* (regulation of breath), *Asana* (assuming certain postures), and *Pratyahara* (restraint of senses) form the *Bahiranga sadhna* or external aids. *Antaranga sadhna* or internal aids consist of *Dhyana* (meditation), *Dharana* (steadying of mind), and *Samadhi* (contemplation of universal consciousness). (Pandurangi, et al., 2017). The cognitive apparatus, physical, psychological, and social self-interact with each other and remain in harmony according to Patanjali. The six foes including lust (*Kama*), anger (*Krodha*), pride (*Mada*), jealousy (*Matsar*), greed (*Lobha*), and desire (*Moha*) are comparable to Freudian Id and make the individual more vulnerable. (Abhyankar, 2015).

Ayurveda

Ayurveda, also known as the "Science of Life," is the most ancient formal Indian medical system. (Ravishankar, & Shukla, 2007). Its origin dates to the 6th century BCE. *Charaka Samhita* and *Sushruta Samhita* were the two important medical texts written during that period, with the former dealing with medical diagnosis and management, and the later dealing with surgical diagnosis and techniques. Descriptions of possession states can be found in *Charaka Samhita*. (Bhugra, 1992).

According to Ayurveda, the traditional concept of health in India was about maintaining balance between the five *bhutas* or elements which constitute the human body including earth, fire, air, sky, and water and three *doshas* or humors including wind (*vata*), bile (*pitta*), and phlegm (*kaph*). (Wig, 1989). To maintain the balance at physical, psychological, physiological, and spiritual level, the excretion and digestion must be unimpaired. The person must have clarity about mind, his senses, and soul, and must be blessed with tranquility. The ancient texts also mention a suprasensory organ, the *Manas* which regulates all other senses. *Manas* is equivalent to the concept of mind. There is also mention of an entity *Buddhi* (intelligence), ranked higher than *Manas* that refers to the judgmental capacity. (Wig, 1989). *Bhoot vidya* was one of the eight disciplines of Ashtanga Ayurveda which included the branch of psychiatry. (Abhyankar, 2015).

TRADITIONS OF INDIAN CULTURE IN THERAPY

Indian psychology is rooted in ancient Indian philosophy, many of its principles and practices can be adapted to modern Western psychology. The term "customary traditions" is used in Indian cultural traditions to refer to religious rites. Each one of them has been skilfully woven into the system to soften effect. The network of relationships contains the supportive or reassuring component of Indian psychological intervention. The most distinctive feature of Indian culture is the nurturing nature of relationships. The significant word in the therapy is "arise" (*uthishthe*). This arousal is from their areas of inactivity, from ignorance to knowledge, from apathy to a positive feeling and from inertia to purposeful activity.

Bhagavad Gita

The Gita shows what is absolutely important for a relationship between the teacher and the student. The counselling provided on the battlefield resembled a significant, brief crisis intervention. The conversation on the battlefield reveals the vast potential of human mental resources. These criteria suggest that Gita is a masterpiece of psychotherapy, addressing all facets of mental activity.

Nasto Mohan Smritit Labdha
tvatprasadhanmayacyuta
Sthitosrigatsamsehah
Karisyecacnamtava

"My delusion is destroyed. I have regained my memory through your grace Achyuta. I am firm. I am free from doubt. I shall act according to your word."

These psychotherapeutic traditions provided a global framework of physical psychological and spiritual health. The rescue from *teen jap-addhi, uyaadhi* and *upaadhi* was the goal of these traditions. (Srivastava, 2010).

The Bhagavad Gita offers insights into many distressing problems' therapeutic solutions. The three main techniques to comprehending and living a fruitful life are Jnana, Karma, and Bhakti. In the bhagavadgita, there are also other definitions of self that are important in understanding the Indian self-conception. In verse 7.4, self is defined as constituting of eight parts – earth, water, fire, air, space, manas, buddhi, and ahagkara. This is important because the concept of self is tied to the environment and could be divided into external and internal self. manas, buddhi, and ahagkara constitute the internal self, and together they are referred to as the antahkarana, or the interna instrument of mental, emotional, verbal, and physical activities. (Bhawuk, 2011).

The emphasis in Gita on the abandonment of materialistic pleasure and control over desires are among the differences in comparison to modern concepts. It may be argued that these concepts from Bhagavad Gita are traditional and there may be discrepancy while comparing and applying it to modern life. However, one should be aware that various Indian scholars like Vivekananda have found these teachings to be meaningful in modern society and have written about it. Even some Western writers have emphasized on their relevance and applicability for the Western culture. (Jeste & Vahia, 2008).

Wisdom, a multidimensional construct, has become another area of research in recent times. The concept could be of importance to modern psychiatry in the development of more individualistic and holistic psychotherapeutic interventions aiming at well-being in general and not just the reduction of psychiatric symptoms. The interest may be new, but the concept has been described in some of the ancient Indian texts. The Bhagavad Gita conceptualizes wisdom as having multiple domains. These include knowledge of life, control over desires, love of and faith in God, emotional regulation, duty and work, humility or insight, decisiveness, self-contentedness, yoga, and compassion/sacrifice. In Bhagavad Gita, the personality is compared to the chariot which is driven by horses. The intellect or *buddhi* is the charioteer, and the horses are comparable to our senses. Bhagavad Gita illustrates the principles of psychotherapy and crisis intervention and teaches the person to be his/her own master. (Abhyankar, 2015).

Ramayana and Mahabharata

Philosophical and religious concepts native to India can be utilized by therapists while dealing with patients as these are more acceptable. Surya and Jayaram included the legend of *Savitri* in their framework of psychotherapy. The mythological story of *Hanuman* (a character in the epic Ramayana), who was wise and brave but did not realize his potential to fly until *Jambavanta* (another character in the epic) reminded him of the same. This phenomenon is comparable to a patient who has lost his confidence and can be made to realize his potential which lies within him to change his life and was named as *Hanuman* complex by NN Wig. The concept has a great relevance in psychotherapy in India, especially in the background of depression, where the patient is reminded of his strengths. The traditional concept of Guru or teacher who is seen as a role model by the student was propounded by Neki as "*Guru-Chela*" paradigm in psychotherapy. The model is especially relevant in South Asia. (Chadda, & Deb, 2013).

Ramayana and Mahabharata also include descriptions of various psychiatric disorders. In Ramayana, a family history of unipolar depression can be found among different characters. King Dashratha dies in extreme grief, and in the end of the story, Lord Rama also goes into depression and kills himself by going into the Saryu river. Descriptions of other disorders such as impotence, alcoholism, and epilepsy can also be found in these ancient epics. (Bhugra, 1992).

Buddhism

The Buddhist culture offered a path to Nirvana. Nirvana was regarded by Psychology of Nirvana as the ideal state for mental health. Nirvana is obtained through transformation, which is a condition of emotional stability, inner peace, self-fulfillment, and accurate self-evaluation. Neki discusses the potential of Indian concepts including *nirvana*. (Neki, 1973). Verma viewed psychotherapy as, the 'interpersonal method of mitigating suffering' and found its roots in the communication of Buddha. (Varma, 1982).

Mindfulness

Mindfulness is a practice used in a various of religious and non religious traditions. Mindfulness was first described by Buddha as "Sati" 2500 years ago. It is documented as "Satipatthana Sutta" (Discourse on the Foundations/Establishment of Mindfulness) and subsequently as the "Mahasatipatthana Sutta" (The Great Discourse on the Foundations/ Establishment of Mindfulness in the Pali canon of Theravada Buddhism. (Iyer, 2022).

The four foundations of mindfulness as the Buddha described them are as follows:

- Related to the body and breathing,
- Related to the feelings aroused by perceptions from the various senses,
- Related to the mind,
- Related to the objects of the mind. (Hanh, 1991).

The Buddha described mindfulness as the method that may assist all people in overcoming suffering and achieve enlightenment. Practicing mindfulness can be understood as a way of relating to one's own experiences that helps in decreasing the pains associated with life's difficulties especially the self-imposed ones. It includes awareness, attention and remembering. Buddhism has long placed a strong emphasis on teaching mindfulness, and globally well-known practises like Vipassana mindfulness meditation. (Iyer, 2022).

Yoga

Yoga means union –union of the individual consciousness with cosmic consciousness. The ancient Indians set a high value on introspection and reflection. Through the meticulous study and practice of Yoga, they perfected their faculty of intuition, attained serenity of mind, and made very careful analyses of the constitution of the mind and the mental processes. (Srivatsava,K. 2010). The Buddha synthesized and integrated the main ideas of the Vedanta, Samkhya and Yoga schools, laying emphasis on the exercise of concentration, and developed the most comprehensive psychology of intuition, in which intuition was considered as a higher level/form of consciousness or *Bodhi*. (Bhattacharya, 1975).

Spirituality

Neki used the concept of Sahaja. Sahaja is an Indian ideal of mental and spiritual health. (Neki, J.S. 1975). Sahaja is both a process and a state characterized by spontaneity, bringing about harmony with oneself and culminating into illumination. He considers the healthy woman personality possessing - illumination, equipoise, spontaneity, freedom and harmony- a higher state of positive mental health as manifested through Sahaja. (Neki, 1977)

In his book on the history of spirituality, Eugene Taylor makes the prediction that Indian psychology will continue to have an increasing impact on global culture, particularly as a new epistemology, based on current tendencies. It will be appropriate to conclude that the core of Indian psychology is its spiritual understanding. Its real value will show itself when this spiritual knowledge is used not only for individual liberation, as it has done in the past, but also for a comprehensive, collective transformation of life, and this has future implications. The Indian philosophy and Indian psychology have a treasure house of practical and spiritual knowledge as its heritage. (Taylor, 1999).

Vedanta

It is based upon the Vedas and is primarily focused upon self knowledge and cosmic knowledge. There are four Vedas: Rig Veda, Yajur Veda, Sama Veda and Atharava Veda. These Vedas are laid down the basic framework of the traditional Indian medicine. (Sood, Singh & Chadda, 2017). Rig

Veda, one of the world's oldest scripture, includes the descriptions of surgical procedures. (Bhugra, 1992). The scripture also has details about prayers and methods to promote mental happiness, empower mind, and build up intelligence to aid in healing and the speed of mind. (Murthy, 2010). The Yajur Veda and the Rig Veda explain a variety of psychological concepts, such as the mind and mental illness. One of the most renowned counselling practice comes from Ayurveda, which is an Upa-Veda of Atharva Veda.

Vedic counselling emphasizes the concept of Dharma which includes the importance of right actions, right living and right awareness. Vedic counselling aim to enhance the self understanding of the person so as to uncover their true potential which would lead them towards a harmonious relationship with the universe as a whole. (Kumar, 2023).

Kosha

From an integrative viewpoint, a person is seen as an integration of their mind, body, and soul. In contrast to many western ideologies, this approach is centred on the interdependence of numerous aspects of a person's life. The Taittiriya Upanishad, which holds that a person has five dimensions, or five Koshas, gives rise to the integrative view to a person. These are Annamaya kosha, Pranamaya kosha, Manomaya kosha and Vijnanamaya kosha, Anandamaya kosha.

Based on the Kosha theory, the treatment approaches and intervention strategies will be separated into five separate categories. The true self is contained within the five koshas, or sheaths. Kornfeld writes, there are "five koshas, or layers of consciousness, in yoga: physical, energetic, mental-emotional, wisdom and bliss. Each kosha represents one aspect of our existence or consciousness and can potentially be open and accessible to the individual, or blocked" (para. 10). One must transcend each of the stages to be connected to his or her true self. This also allows one to gain and maintain balance in the gunas. The koshas include: Annamaya, Pranamaya, Manomaya, Vignanamaya, and Anandamaya.

These koshas can be transcended with the use of the eight different limbs of Patanjali's Yoga Sutra and with Ayurvedic treatment techniques. Patanjali's Yoga limbs include: yama, niyama, asanas, pranayama, pratyahara, dharana, dhyana, and samadhi (Anjali, 1994; Mohan, 1993). Ayurvedic techniques include: mantra vidya, ashvasan and upchar, dairya havan chikitsa, and prayaschittani. The koshas, yoga limbs and Ayurvedic treatment all work in tandem to help an individual. Other treatment modalities can also be utilized to assist in the transcendence of each kosha such as psychotherapy.

The ancient texts also mention three personality types or *trigunas*, one of which is present at the time of birth of an individual and determines his/her "*prakriti.*" These include the balanced type (*Satvika*), the emotional type (*Rajasik*), and the lustful (*Tamasik*). Psychosis is termed "*Unmad,*" a deluded state, and mental disorders are named after Gods and devils. Some endogenous disorders have loose correlation with the modern-day psychiatric disorders. These endogenous disorders are thought to be provoked by the three humors. *Vatonmad* is like schizophrenia, *Kaphonamad* is closer to depression, and *Pittonmad* is similar to mania. Causative factors as described include a lack of healthy habits and preoccupation with the six foes: nervous temperament, wrong diet, demonic possession, etc. (Abhyankar, 2015).

Four types of mental illnesses have been defined. These include illnesses caused due to exclusive involvement of emotions, due to exclusive involvement of the three humors, disorders of body mind involvement such as *unmada,* alcoholism, and disorders with mind–body involvement including psychosomatic illnesses. Treatment described included medications, psychotherapy, dietary modifications, and shock therapy. Exogenous disorders known as *bhutonmada* were treated using worships and psychotherapy.

(Bhugra D, 1992). Thus, there are many similarities in the descriptions of the mental illnesses as given in the ancient Indian literature with the modern psychiatry, though there are differences in approach to treatment. (Wig, 1989).

The knowledge pool related to psychiatry derived from our ancient texts has enriched international psychiatry. (Murthy, 2010). Classification and course of mental disorders, transcultural variations in clinical features and traditional methods of care such as yoga and meditation have been some of the important contributions of Indian psychiatrists to global psychiatry. (Murthy, 2010). The current concept of psychosomatic medicine has some parallel concepts in Ayurveda according to which multiple etiological factors contribute to the disease including various psychological factors. (Shamasundar, 2008).

ANCIENT THERAPEUTIC TECHNIQUES

Treating illness in the Indian tradition is prevention (Mishra, 2004). This can be attained by a dedicated practice of Ayurvedic principles such as diet, lifestyle, and positive interactions with others as well as participation in yoga practices such as Patanjali's yoga. Therapy in Indian psychology typically includes: living a healthy lifestyle, consciousness enhancing programs, psychotherapy, "nutritional programs, herbal medicines, hatha yoga, and other exercises, meditation, and detoxification and rejuvenation techniques" (Lad, 2002; Ninivaggi, 2008; Stiles, 2000; White, 2000, p. 674).

Types of Ancient Techniques

(I) **Atharva Veda & Psychotherapy:** dwells upon the ways of knowing individual psyche; deals with personality improvement & mental health.

Atharva Veda gives a description of possession by supernatural elements as leading to mental illness. Rig Veda and Yajur Veda describe mantras (rhymes), which help in development of noble thoughts that prevent mental pain (depression). (Avasthi, Grover, & Kate, 2013). Strong willpower and control over one's emotions can be made possible with the help of prayers and thus contributing to positive mental health. Yajur Veda and Atharva Veda conceptualize mind as the inner flame of knowledge, instrument of hypnotism, and a basis of consciousness. (Avasthi, Grover, & Kate, 2013).

Atharva Veda has 10 parts which include witchcraft, sorcery, hysteria, pathological fear, insanity, guilt, and jealousy. Mental illnesses were considered as occurring due to the curse of God. (Wig, 1989). Upanishads, described as synopsis of Vedas, have a more recent origin, and welcomed the new ideas marking a transition from the traditional Vedic ritualism, and include theories of consciousness, memory, thought, and perception. There are also descriptions of dreaming state, waking state, deep sleep state, and Samadhi.(Murthy, 2010).

The Psychotherapeutic Systems of Atharvaveda

1. **Samkalp or self determination:** building will power; positive suggestions repeated; similar to auto suggestion; associations with lions & elephant warriors to acquire energy & confidence
    i. Directive therapy by suggestion (Sadesh):

Therapist plays the role of a guide or teacher; symbolism, personification, similarity & contrast are used; re-educates & corrects thinking, feeling for sexual problems, increase energy in a weak person

ii. **Ritualistic Therapy:** Especially for the uneducated & children; rituals performed with suitable manthras; symbolization, dramatization & demonstration
iii. **Psychological defensive belief (Brahma Kavach):** applied for creating self- confidence & sense of control on the environment; helps to mobilise mental energy for the same by hymns & spiritual texts

2. **Cognitive change as therapeutic method (Ashvasan):** Therapist is dominant, directive; change the behavior patterns & ideas that are unhealthy;

Through encouragement, instilling hope & confidence modification of behavior on positive lines is made; methods used are persuasion & re-education.

3. **Prayaschittani:** Doing penance voluntarily with the aim of sublimating & purifying oneself; self - mortification by doing penance or tapas to overcome guilt; aims to improve super-ego & ego functions; to establish equilibrium of satvic, rajasic & tamasic qualities of a person.

Counseling in Bhagvad Gita

- Treatise to guide, resolve conflict, get clarification, assurance (based on Karma Yoga) & enlightening the individual to achieve adequate ego strength.
- Form of crisis intervention; instant therapy
- Techniques of clarification, assurance, faith, enlightenment, surrender from spiritual perspective.
- Arjuna complex: -goes through crisis in view of ground realities & typical stress reactions; dealt with by Krishna by clarification, assurance & emphasizing the importance of duties & responsibilities; may be used effectively in suitable cases
- Hanuman complex:- used to bring out the inner potentials that are dormant, e.g. in cases of inferiority complex, lack of social skills; also with depressives
- For e.g. the student is simply asked to find out who is he? Body (Annamaya) Sensation (Pranayama), thought (Manomaya), Consciousness (Vynanamaya) or something unexplainable (Anandmaya)?
- When the student understands that he is none of these, he understands the real nature of 'Self'.

Ayurvedic Psychotherapy (Medico Religious Therapy)

Philosophical principles were joined together with biological & psychological principles & systematized as science of life.

- **Causes of mental illness:**

    (i) endogeneous (nija)
    (ii) Exogeneous (Aguntaja) and
    (iii) Psychological (manas)

Broad ranged therapy suggested; Charaka classifies them into 3 categories:-

- **Faith healing:** incantation (mantara); herbs (aushadi), wearing precious gems (mani) etc.
- **Rational therapy (Yukti Vyapasraya):** consists of 5 karmas- i) cleaning nasal passage (nasya) ii) Vomitting (Vaman); iii) Purgation (Virichan) iv) Enema (nirodha) & v)
- **Nutrition;** single drugs and faith healing also suggested Sattvavajaya (psychotherapy): drugless measures for restraining the mind from impulses & unwholesome objects;

Applied aspects of Sattvavajya are summarized under 8 headings:-

A- assurance; B- replacement of emotions; C- regulation of thought processes; D- reframing of ideas; E- Channeling of presumptions; F- Correction of objectives & ideals; G- proper guidance & advice for taking right decisions & H- proper control of patience

Ritualistic or Action Oriented Psychotherapy

- Vedic rites & rituals systematized for personal & social hygiene in Post vedic religious text called "Dharmashastras"
- Therapeutic value depends upon & encourages:-
  (a) Righteous action (dharma)
  (b) Conscious satisfaction of material pleasure (Artha)
  (c) Conscious & righteous satisfaction of biological instincts (karma)
  (d) Achievement of Summum bonum (Moksha)
    - Prescribes a mode of conduct of life that can prevent psychological disturbances
    - Tools for therapy: adoration to gods through repeating their names (japa or bibliotherapy) & various sacrificial rituals were developed.

Yoga

The yoga philosophical tradition reports that health is gained when the sattva guna is in dominance. This literature contends that if one has sattva guna dominance then he or she is in good psychological health and able to easily overcome any short comings that may be present.

Yoga is helpful for both psychological and physical illnesses, such as back pain, unease, and sadness. Yoga therapy provides resources to those who are facing weakening emotional instability and long-term reliance on the healthcare system to assist them overcome their innate limitations.

Types of Yoga

Hatha Yoga: It is one of the earliest types of yoga and consists of the asanas (postures) and pranayama (breathing exercises) that calm the mind and body and assist the body be ready for meditation and other more in-depth spiritual practises. Hatha-Yogic techniques are being used as adjunct to the other psychotherapeutic system as a part of psychosomatic rehabilitation and relaxation training. (Tripathi, K.M., 2021)

Vinyasa Yoga: In the late 1980s, a vigorous and athletic style of yoga was developed from the conventional ashtanga technique. It basically refers to forceful movement that is in time with the breath and is based on the quick flow of the sun salutation. It also describes the smooth transition between postures.

Ashtanga Yoga: Ashtanga is a style of yoga that Sr.K.Pattabhi Jois introduced to the contemporary world. This type of yoga consists of six series, each of which is a predetermined order of asanas. Usually, it moves quickly, vigorously, and is physically demanding.

Power Yoga: Power yoga is the name given to intense vinyasa-style yoga. Today, power yoga is done and taught all over the world.

Bikram Yoga: The practise includes 26 postures in total, and there are 2 breathing exercises. This type of yoga enables participants to go more fully into postures, flush out toxins, and control their body weight.

Jivamukti Yoga: In 1984, this particular form of yoga was developed. This type of yoga includes chanting, meditation, readings, and affirmations.

Iyengar Yoga: To allow one to pay closer attention to the particular musculoskeletal alignment inside each asana, poses are held for a great deal longer in this particular form of yoga. The use of props, such as blocks, belts, bolsters, chairs, and blankets, to accommodate injuries, tightness, or structural imbalances as well as teach the student how to move appropriately into a posture, is another distinctive characteristic of iyengar yoga.

Anusara Yoga: The anusara style is a completely novel school of hatha yoga that emphasises elegance and following your heart while providing a set of fundamental concepts of alignment that underpin all yoga poses. It is capable of being roughly divided into the three categories of attitude, alignment, and action, or the "three A's."

Sivananda Yoga: Savasana (also known as the relaxation position), kapalabhati, and anuloma viloma typically take place first, then several repetitions of surya namaskara. Then it performs each one of Sivananda's twelve asanas, which work together in order to render the spine more flexible and strong. It might additionally involve meditation and chanting.

Viniyoga: Viniyoga was an approach of practising yoga that tailors every practitioner's practise to their particular requirements, interests, and conditions. This type of yoga aids in growing as an individual and self-discovery.

Kundalini Yoga: Multiple movements or exercises, dynamic methods of breathing, chanting, meditation, and mantras have all been included in kundalini. A specific kundalini exercise, or kriya, is a movement that is frequently carried out and synchronised to the breath. In order to direct energy upward through each of the seven chakras, this practise is aimed at waking up the energy at the base of the spine.

Yin Yoga: Yin yoga is a slow-paced technique that places are held for a minimum of five minutes. Although being passive, yin yoga can turn out to be extremely challenging due to the extended holds, particularly when your body is not accustomed to them. In order to enhance flexibility and increase the supply of blood to the joints, moderate stress is imposed on the connective tissue, which includes the tendons, fascia, and ligaments.

Vipasana

The word "Vipassana" can also be provided as "understanding," which refers to being in touch with the three characteristics of presence that are constant throughout time and space: change, intolerability, and pitifulness. The concept of "Insight Meditation" is derived from the Pali name for this form of practise, Vipassana Bhavana, and this signifies the growth of knowledge.

Meditation

Meditation has born in India (East) and 'Therapies' have been developed in the West. Meditation can help a person to come out of depression, anxiety and sufferings. 'Meditation (Dhyana) is a multidimensional state of awareness where not a single iota of thought exists.' For being in a state of meditation a person has to purify his or her body, thought and emotion; and become aware of his body, thought and emotion, then one can be in a state of witnessing (sakshi) which is a core feature of meditation. (Choudhary, Maitreya, Kumar, & Richa, 2021).

Meditation helps the people to improve their general sense of wellbeing and blissfulness in persons by growing multidimensional awareness (sakshi); enhancing and rejuvenating: great silence, peace, sensitivity, compassion, love and intelligence. Broadly speaking, there are many different types of contemplation for the many psychiatric problems, just as there are many different treatments for the various physical illnesses.

Osho has developed 'Meditative Therapies' for purification of body, thought and emotion of the participants, so that they should become ready to be in a state of meditation. These therapies dissolve tensions of the participants. Participants are also able to cathart out all the repressed emotions. These therapies are easy and are very useful, interaction among the meditators are very less. The energy which is created during therapy session, help them to go very deep in meditation. These therapies are: **'The Mystic Rose Therapy'**, **'No-mind Therapy'**, **'Born Again Therapy'**, **'Dynamic Meditation'** etc. These meditative therapies have been used to treat many patients suffering from psychogenic headache, anxiety, depression, psychosexual dysfunctions and OCD etc. (Choudhary, Maitreya, Kumar, & Richa, 2021).

Reiki

The word "reiki" is derived from the Japanese terms "rei," which means "universal," and "ki," which refers to the vital life force energy that permeates all living things.

Reiki is a form of energy healing that draws on the inherent universal energy that each human possesses. A practitioner of reiki who has completed the required training will use it as a sort of physical therapy to stimulate the human body's chakras and aura. The recipient of the primary energy healing receives it. A person's hormonal shifts and secretary defects are balanced as a result of energy healing, and disease exacerbation is regulated. Following protocol, the practitioner administers the necessary healing energy to the patient. Effective physical therapy can minimise diseases that cause death and has produced some remarkable results. Reiki's primary goal is to promote overall health—mental, physical, and spiritual. Some Reiki techniques:

1. Centering.
2. Clearing.
3. Beaming.
4. Extracting harmful energies infusing.
5. Smoothing and raking the aura

EXISTENCE OF THERAPEUTIC TECHNIQUES IN INDIAN PSYCHOLOGY IN TREATING MENTAL DISORDERS

Yoga

Using therapeutic yoga techniques like breath work, asanas, and attention to the present moment, those who struggle with emotional problems may learn to see their mood swings of stress and despair as passing rather than permanent conditions of awareness.

Some of these concepts of yoga and meditation have been prevalent in India for centuries and used for the treatment of anxiety and psychosomatic disorders. They help in developing control over the voluntary and involuntary nervous functions. (Vahia, Vinekar & Doongaji, 1966). The therapeutic adequacy and validity of these practices have been reported by the Indian researchers for more than 50 years. (Vahia, Vinekar, & Doongaji, 1966). A meta-analysis conducted in 2011 indicated the statistically significant role of yoga therapy as an adjunctive treatment of depression and anxiety disorders. Yogic principles may be useful as complementary treatment options for mental illnesses and have the privilege of having fewer side effects and contraindications. (Cabral, Meyer & Ames, 2011). Yoga and meditation are increasingly recognized for their potential benefits in treating many mental health conditions, including anxiety, depression, and stress. (Kumar, 2023).

Some studies have tried to look for the neurobiological basis of action of yoga. Practice of Sudarshan Kriya Yoga decreases the adrenocorticotropic hormone and serum cortisol levels and increases P300 amplitude. These changes correlate with improvement in psychiatric symptoms. (Varambally & Gangadhar, 2012). Gamma-aminobutyric acid (GABA) levels tend to decrease in anxiety and depressive disorders, and yoga sessions increase GABA levels. Deactivation of the limbic region has been seen on functional MRI while chanting *Om* during Yoga sessions, and this could possibly lead to the regulation of emotions. (Varambally & Gangadhar, 2012). Some studies have also highlighted similarities between the trance state in Patanjali yoga sutras and trance in hypnosis. (Chowdhary & Gopinath, 2013). The similarities are in the fields of induction and deepening techniques, and the phenomena described during the trance states.

The teachings of Bhagavad Gita also held relevance in dealing with the COVID-19 pandemic and recently, some authors have revisited these teachings. The three paths of yoga emphasized in Gita may hold relevance in reliance-focused psychotherapy while dealing with the burden of the pandemic. First is the path of knowledge (*jnana yoga*) which helps in shifting our focus from "I" to "we," thus helping in self-awareness so that we can focus on dealing with the pandemic in a collective manner. Second is the path of action (*karma yoga*) which is applicable to all front-line workers for working selflessly. The guiding principle for the health-care workers is *karma* or duty. Third is the path of meditation (*raja yoga*) which may help in developing resilience and reducing stress by adopting a healthy lifestyle. (Keshavan M., 2020).

Meditation

The great benefit of meditating can be seen with depressed clients because meditation reduces the tendency to ruminate and worry about the future. The practice of mindfulness meditation has several variations where an individual can focus on objects, use the five senses, use the breath, or even engage in mantra chanting (Iqbal et al., 2015).

Ayurveda

Ayurveda not only treats the symptoms but also recognizes the root cause of mental illness is biological as well as psychosocial factors. Ayurvedic treatment of the mentally ill prescribes changes to biopsychosocial factors through various modalities, such as diet change, meditation, or yoga (S. Kumar & Nathani, 2014).

Mindfulness

It is a technique which involves focusing on the present moment without judgement. Mindfulness assists the persons become more aware of their thoughts, emotions, and bodily sensations.

Naturopathy

Nathuropathic practice is based on the premise that the body has the capacity to heal from within (Ahmad et al., 2015). In rural areas of India, traditional medicine is more popular than allopathic medicine (Samal, 2014). At present, less than 30% of households use traditional healing systems (Ahmad et al., 2015). In rural areas, where people cannot afford allopathic medicines, the use of naturopathy is more popular because of its lower costs as well as the belief in the healing properties of natural prescriptions (Samal, 2014).

Music Therapy

Research has demonstrated that music profoundly affects your body and mind (Scott, 2011).

Music therapy has a great influence on mental health. It helps in alleviating both physical and mental pain and also acts as a medium through which negative emotions such as anger and hostility can be released more acceptably. It also plays a key role in improving anxiety and stress by reducing stress hormones such as cortisol. Moreover, it helps people suffering from other disorders such as addiction, personality disorders, PTSD, and many more. (Verma, 2021).

Sattva Enhancement Therapy

Indian-psychology based psychotherapy approach called as Sattva Enhancement Therapy with a client. Thematic analysis of core yoga texts, i.e., Yoga Vasishta, Bhagavadgita, and Patanjali Yogasutra, led to the development of a heuristic model of therapeutic approach, with six interlinked themes as the primary focus of intervention. This approach was success- fully utilised with a 68 years old man presenting with complaints of sadness, anger, bitterness and guilt. (Agrawal, 2021)

In India throughout the 19th century, a traditional healing method called reiki was employed to assist people in keeping their physical, mental, emotional, and spiritual balances.

Pranic Healing

Pranic Healing is an ancient science and art of healing using vital energy or 'Prana'. This Prana keeps the body alive and function healthy in a proper manner. The term "Pranic" originated from the Sanskrit word "Prana", which denotes Pranic healing is a simple, yet powerful and effective no-touch, no drug healing therapy that uses only prana or energy to heal a person with respect to, psychological disorders, physical illness, improved health and stamina, reduced stress, greater self-esteem, and better interpersonal skills. To heal the mental health of an individual, Pranic heal therapy plays a vital role in Indian context (Sharma, 1998). It was observed that Pranic Healing is an excellent resource for mental and emotional health (Clark, 1998). The study findings reveal that pranic healing therapy has a significant effect on mental health. (Sharma, 1998).

INDIAN PSYCHOLOGY IN MODERN PSYCHOTHERAPY

In the new millennium, therapies of Indian psychology have gained renewed interest as a distinct and holistic approach to understanding the mind and human behavior. It is based on the ancient Indian texts known as the Vedas and emphasizes the integration of spiritual and psychological practices for overall well-being. This approach differs from Western psychology, which focuses on treating mental disorders and addressing individual problems. The popularity of Indian psychology in the West has been driven by a growing interest in mindfulness, meditation, and other Eastern spiritual practices, which are increasingly being incorporated into Western therapy and wellness programs that focus on treating mental disorders and addressing individual problems. Numerous Western psychologists and therapists are beginning to incorporate Indian psychology techniques and principles into their practice.

The essence of psychotherapy existed in India since time immemorial submerged in social structures, religion, ancient scriptures, mystics and alternate system of medicine including Ayurveda, Unani tradition, Siddha and Yoga and so forth. Girindrasekar Bose who brought modern psychoanalysis to India, made original contributions on the theory of mental life and on the gunas (temperament).

He drew substantially on the cultural, religious and psychological ethos of India, as he worked on concepts related to repression, defiance, ambivalence, free association and opposite wishes (Bose, 1931).

Similarities between psychodynamic theories of drives and psychic structures, and the concept of three gunas have been elucidated (Reddy 2008; Bhatia et al. 2013). Krishna's analytic (therapeutic) function was not interpretative per se, but more an object that facilitated the development and maturation of Arjuna's ego (psychic). Specifically, it is Krishna's allowing Arjuna to use him as a transformational object from a psychoanalytic viewpoint. The cardinal techniques of abstinence, anonymity, and neutrality were both observed and violated by Krishna.

The pivotal and transformative violation of anonymity, by Krishna's self-disclosure promoted the therapeutic regression and psychic reorganization that lead to Arjuna's existential transformation. Arjuna under duress exhibited elements of distorted thinking. Lord Krishna help remedied this through a process akin to Cognitive Behavioral Therapy (CBT) (Balodhi & Keshavan, 2011). Hence Gita lends ways of dealing with issues from psychodynamic as well as cognitive approaches.

One of the highly acclaimed citations is in Bhagavad Gita where Lord Krishna works out for a change of behaviour through verbal communication with the hesitant Arjuna at the battle field of Kurukshethra. (Janetius, 2017)

There are similarities in the teachings of the Bhagwad Gita and psychotherapy in modern times (Bhatia et al., 2013). Some commonalities include the use of a conversational style, the therapist as a guide, the inclusion of psychoeducation, and modifying behavior. Cognitive behavioral therapy (CBT) works toward resolving the cognitive distortions that impair functioning. CBT also focuses on how the views of the self, others, and the world can affect functioning. (Kalra, 2020).

Dialectical behavior therapy (DBT) is a cognitive behavioral treatment. The therapy is developed to treat chronically suicidal individuals who diagnosed with borderline personality disorder (BPD) and it is now recognized as the gold standard psychological treatment for this population. In addition, research has shown that it is effective in treating a wide range of other disorders such as substance dependence, depression, post-traumatic stress disorder (PTSD), and eating disorders. As such, DBT is a transdiagnostic modular treatment.

Eye Movement Desensitization and Reprocessing (EMDR) is an integrative psychotherapy approach that has been extensively researched and proven effective for the treatment of trauma. EMDR is a set of standardized protocols that incorporates elements from many different treatment approaches. (Bhattacharya, 1975).

Transactional Analysis was developed by Berne in 1957. He suggested three “ego states”, the Parent (P), Adult (A) and Child [C] go states, which were largely shaped through childhood experiences. It is used primarily as a therapeutic tool though it also has relevance for facilitating a deeper understanding of behaviours which affect relationships in a wide range of settings. The use of transactional analysis enables patients to modify their immature and unsuitable interpersonal communication styles.

In the past 25 years, yoga and meditation have gained popularity as treatment programmes for psychological distress. Yoga is an ancient Indian technique detailed in the Ashtanga Yoga of Patanjali’s Yoga Sutras. Yoga as it is commonly called today either refers to only the asanas or body posture component or to breathing practices or pranayama, or to a combination of the two.

Meditation refers to the practice of focusing attention on breath or on an object or thought or a mantra. Here attention is focused. In Vipasana meditation, also known as mindfulness based meditation, there is no fixed object or thought to hold the attention. The person passively observes the various bodily sensations and thoughts that are passing through in her or his awareness.

The rapid breathing techniques to induce hyperventilation as in Sudarshana Kriya Yoga (SKY) is found to be a beneficial, low-risk, low-cost adjunct to the treatment of stress, anxiety, post-traumatic stress disorder (PTSD), depression, stress-related medical illnesses, substance abuse, and rehabilitation of criminal offenders. SKY has been used as a public health intervention technique to alleviate PTSD in survivors of mass disasters. Yoga techniques enhance well-being, mood, attention, mental focus, and stress tolerance. Proper training by a skilled teacher and a 30-minute practice every day will maximise the benefits. Research conducted at the National Institute of Mental Health and Neurosciences (NIMHANS), India, has shown that SKY reduces depression. Further, alcoholic patients who practice SKY have reduced depression and stress levels. Insomnia is treated with yoga. Yoga reduces the time to go to sleep and improves the quality of sleep. Kundalini Yoga taught in the USA has been found to be effective in treatment of mental disorders. The Institute for Nonlinear Science, University of California, San Diego, USA has found that Kundalini Yoga is effective in the treatment of obsessive-compulsive disorder. Kundalini Yoga combines pranayama or breathing techniques with chanting of mantras. Prevention of repeated episodes of depression may be helped by mindfulness-based meditation or Vipasana. This meditation would help the patients to process emotional stimuli better and hence prevent biases in the processing of these stimuli. (NCERT, 2021).

Mindfulness-based Stress Reduction (MBSR) founded by Jon Kabat Zinn in 1982 and Mindfulness-based Cognitive Therapy (MBCT) described by Segal, ZV, Williams, and Teasdale in 2002. Together these are described as Mindfulness-based Interventions (MBIs) and there is an extensive body of literature describing the use of these techniques in a wide variety of disorders including anxiety, depression, and posttraumatic stress. Mindfulness has also been used in healthy people in their workplace including healthcare professionals working in high-stress environments like intensive care units (ICUs) with high rates of burnout. Adaptations of MBIs include therapies that use mindfulness skills like acceptance and commitment therapy (ACT), dialectical behavior therapy (DBT), shorter retreats and residential programs (typically 3 days), brief mindfulness interventions (2–3 weeks), lab-based mindfulness training (3–4 days), and Internet and smartphone-based applications. (Iyer, 2022).

CONCLUSION

Indian psychology emphasises the connection between the individual and the communal consciousness and acknowledges the value of mindfulness, Sativk enhancement therapy, Ayurveda, Music therapy, yoga, and meditation in fostering mental and emotional well-being. It does this by drawing on old philosophical and spiritual traditions. In India the traditional Psychology based on religio-philosophical concepts need to be incorporated into theories of human behaviour and life so that current life and behaviour of the people could be explained correctly and accurately for a better therapy outcome. Some mental health professionals have begun incorporating these principles into their treatment approaches for certain conditions. It is important to note that Indian psychology is one perspective in understanding mental health and is not a substitute for modern evidence-based approaches to mental health care. Indian psychologists can significantly contribute to the cause of bettering everyone's mental and emotional health. However, it can be a useful complement to Western-style therapy and medication.

REFERENCES

Aakash. (2021). *Introduction to the Indian Psychology concept.* Mantracare. https://mantracare.org/therapy/therapy-types/indian-psychology

Ahmad, A., Khan, M. U., Kumar, B. D., Kumar, G. S., Rodriguez, S. P., & Patel, I. (2015). Beliefs, attitudes and selfuse of Ayurveda, Yoga and Naturopathy, Unani, Siddha, and Homeopathy medicines among senior pharmacy students: An exploratory insight from Andhra Pradesh, India. *Pharmacognosy Research, 7*(4). PMID:26692742

Akthar, S. E. (2005). *Freud along the Ganges psychoanalytical reflections on the people and culture of India.* Rave Media.

Avasthi, A., Grover, S., & Kate, N. (2013). Indianization of psychiatry utilizing Indian mental concepts. [PUBMED]. *Indian Journal of Psychiatry, 55*(6), 136–144. doi:10.4103/0019-5545.105508 PMID:23858244

Balkrishna, V., Sanghvi, L. D., Rana, K., Doongaji, D. R., & Vahia, N. S. (1977). The comparison of psychophysiological therapy with drug therapy. *Indian Journal of Psychiatry, 19*, 87–89.

Bhatia, S. C., Madabushi, J., Kolli, V., Bhatia, S. K., & Madaan, V. (2013). The Bhagavad Gita and contemporary psychotherapies. *Indian Journal of Psychiatry, 55*(2), 315–321. doi:10.4103/0019-5545.105557 PMID:23858274

Bhattacharya, H. (1975). Yoga Psychology, Nature of Mind and Its Activities. *Indian Psychology*.. The Ramakrishna Mission Institute of Culture.

Bhugra, D. (1992). Psychiatry in ancient Indian texts: A review. *History of Psychiatry, 3*(10), 167–186. doi:10.1177/0957154X9200301002 PMID:11623029

Bose, G. (1931). A new technique of psychoanalysis. *The International Journal of Psycho-Analysis, 12*, 387–388.

Cabral, P., Meyer, H. B., & Ames, D. (2011). *Effectiveness of yoga therapy as a complementary treatment for major psychiatric disorders: A meta-analysis*. Prim Care Companion CNS Disorder.

Chadda, R. K., & Deb, K. S. (2013). Indian family systems, collectivistic society and psychotherapy. *Indian Journal of Psychiatry, 55*(6, Suppl 2), S299–S309. doi:10.4103/0019-5545.105555 PMID:23858272

Chadda, R.K. & Rajhans, P. (2021). Learnings from Ancient India: Relevance to Contemporary Psychiatry. *Perspective/Viewpoint, 3*(150-153)

Choudhary, K., Maitreya, Kumar, K., & Richa. (2021). Meditative Therapies in Clinical Psychology. *Indian Journal of Clinical Psychology, 48*(1).

Chowdhary, S., & Gopinath, J. K. (2013). Clinical hypnosis and Patanjali yoga sutras. *Indian Journal of Psychiatry, 55*(6, Suppl 2), S157–S164. doi:10.4103/0019-5545.105516 PMID:23858248

Debroy, B., & Debroy, D. (2006). *The Holy Vedas: Rig Veda, Yajur Veda Sama Veda and Atharva Veda* (13th ed.). BR Publishing Corporation.

Hanh, T. N. (1991). *Old path, white clouds: walking in the footsteps of the Buddha*. Parallax Press.

Iqbal, N., Singh, A., & Aleem, S. (2015). Effect of dynamic meditation on mental health. *Journal of Religion and Health, 55*(1), 241–254. doi:10.100710943-015-0082-x PMID:26179581

Iyer, S. (2022). Mindfulness-based Interventions: Can They Improve Self-care and Psychological Well-being? [Google Scholar]. *Indian Journal of Critical Care Medicine : Peer-Reviewed, Official Publication of Indian Society of Critical Care Medicine, 26*(4), 407–408. doi:10.5005/jp-journals-10071-24194 PMID:35656051

Janetius, S. T. (2011). *Indigenous therapeutic counselling in the Indian context*. Research gate.

Jeste, D., & Vahia, I. (2008). Comparison of the conceptualization of wisdom in ancient Indian literature with modern views: Focus on the Bhagavad Gita. *Psychiatry, 71*(3), 197–209. doi:10.1521/psyc.2008.71.3.197 PMID:18834271

Kalra, V. (2020). *Psychotherapy Model for the Training Counsellors in India*. National Louis University. https://digitalcommons.nl.edu/cgi/viewcontent.cgi? article= 1443&context=diss

Keshavan, M. (2020). Building resilience in the COVID-19 era: Three paths in the Bhagavad Gita. *Indian Journal of Psychiatry, 62*(5), 459–461. doi:10.4103/psychiatry.IndianJPsychiatry_829_20 PMID:33678824

Khalsa, S. (2017). A perspective on yoga research: Past to present. *Yoga Mimamsa.*, *49*(1), 1–2. doi:10.4103/ym.ym_10_17

Kumar, M. (2023). *Psychotherapy and Indian thought.* Tutorials Point. https://www. tutorialspoint.com/psychotherapy-and-indian-thought.

Kumar, M. (2023). *Indian Psychology in the New Millennium*. Tutorials Point. https://www.tutorialspoint.com/indian-psychology-in-the-new-millennium

Kumar, M. (2023). *Indian Psychology: Implications and Applications*. Tutorials Point. https://www.tutorialspoint.com/indian-psychology-implications-and-applications

Kumar, S., & Nathani, N. (2014). Preventative and therapeutic measures of Ayurveda for mental health care. *Pharma Science Monitor*, *5*(1), 176–183.

Manickam, L. S. S., & Sahya. (2004). The concept in Indian philosophical psychology and its contemporary relevance. In: Joshi K. & Cornelissen M. (eds.), *Yoga and Indian approaches to psychology*. New-Delhi: Centre for the Study of Civilizations.

Menon,S.(2005). What is Indian psychology: Transcendence in and while thinking. *The Journal of Transpersonal Psychology, 37*(2), 83-98.

Murthy, S. (2010). From local to global contributions of Indian psychiatry to international psychiatry. [PUBMED]. *Indian Journal of Psychiatry*, *52*(7), 30–37. doi:10.4103/0019-5545.69202 PMID:21836699

Neki, J. S. (1973). Guru-Chela relationship: The possibility of therapeutic paradigm. *The American Journal of Orthopsychiatry*, *43*(5), 755–766. doi:10.1111/j.1939-0025.1973.tb00847.x PMID:4742816

Neki, J. S. (1977). Psychotherapy in India. *Indian Journal of Psychiatry*, *19*, 1–10.

Pandurangi, A., Keshavan, M., Ganapathy, V., & Gangadhar, B. (2017). Yoga: Past and present. *The American Journal of Psychiatry*, *174*(1), 16–17. doi:10.1176/appi.ajp.2016.16080853 PMID:28040996

Ravishankar, B., & Shukla, V. J. (2007). Indian systems of medicine: A brief profile. *African Journal of Traditional, Complementary, and Alternative Medicines*, *4*(3), 319–337. doi:10.4314/ajtcam.v4i3.31226 PMID:20161896

Sachin, K. S. & Pranati, C.R., (2020). Reiki: Old Indian therapy as new methodology. International Journal of creative research thoughts, 8, 694- 703.

Samal, J. (2014). Indian public health standards for Ayurveda, Yoga and Naturopathy, Unani, Siddha and Homoeopathy facilities: An assessment. [Google Scholar]. *International Journal of Medicine and Public Health*, *4*(4), 331. doi:10.4103/2230-8598.144058

Sedlmeier, P., & Srinivas, K. (2016). How Do Theories of Cognition and Consciousness in Ancient Indian Thought Systems Relate to Current Western Theorizing and Research? *Frontiers in Psychology*, *7*, 343. doi:10.3389/fpsyg.2016.00343 PMID:27014150

Shamasundar, C. (2008). Relevance of ancient Indian wisdom to modern mental health a few examples. [PUBMED]. *Indian Journal of Psychiatry*, *50*(2), 138–143. doi:10.4103/0019-5545.42404 PMID:19742213

Sharma, S. (1998). Life force as a unique Divine greatness (2nd ed.). Akhand Jyoti Institution, Mathura.

Sood, M., Singh, S., & Chadda, R. (2017). Relevance of traditional Indian medical concepts in psychosomatic medicine. [India]. *Annals of the National Academy of Medical Sciences (India), 53*(3), 148–155. doi:10.1055-0040-1712757

Srivastava, K. (2010). Human nature: Indian perspective revisited. [Google Scholar]. *Industrial Psychiatry Journal, 19*(2), 77–81. doi:10.4103/0972-6748.90335 PMID:22174527

Srivastava, S., Patel, A., Tiwari, S. K., & Gupta, K. (2019). Effectiveness of Pranic Healing on Mental Health. *Journal of Psychosomatic Research, 14*(1), 163–168.

Taylor, E. (1999). *Shadow culture: Psychology and spirituality in America*. Counterpoint. [Google Scholar]

Thapar, A. (2002). *The Penguin History of Early India: From the Origins to AD 1300*. Penguin Books.

Therapuetic Approaches. (2021). *National Council of Educational Research and Training*. NCERT. https://ncert.nic.in

Vahia, N., Vinekar, S., & Doongaji, D. (1966). Some ancient Indian concepts in the treatment of psychiatric disorders. *The British Journal of Psychiatry, 112*(492), 1089–1096. doi:10.1192/bjp.112.492.1089 PMID:5971528

Vahia, N. S., Jeste, D. V., Kapoor, S. N., Ardhapurkar, I., & Nath, R. S. (1973). Further experience with the therapy based upon concepts of Patanjali in the treatment of psychiatric disorders. *Indian Journal of Psychiatry, 15*, 32–37.

Varambally, S., & Gangadhar, B. (2012). Yoga: A spiritual practice with therapeutic value in psychiatry. *Asian Journal of Psychiatry, 5*(2), 186–189. doi:10.1016/j.ajp.2012.05.003 PMID:22813667

Varma, V. K. (1982). Present state of psychotherapy in India. *Indian Journal of Psychiatry, 24*, 209–226. PMID:21965915

Wig, N. (1989). Indian concepts of mental health and their impact on care of the mentally ill. *International Journal of Mental Health, 18*(3), 71–80. doi:10.1080/00207411.1989.11449136

Wig, N. (2004). Hanuman complex and its resolution: An illustration of psychotherapy from Indian mythology. *Indian Journal of Psychiatry, 46*, 25–28. PMID:21206772

Chapter 6
From Ancient Wisdom to Modern Science:
Indian Psychology for the Modern Age

C. Vijayabanu
https://orcid.org/0000-0002-0125-4534
School of Management, SASTRA University, India

Madhu Midha
School of Management, SASTRA University, India

Siddharth Ram
School of Management, SASTRA University, India

ABSTRACT

In India, psychology, yoga, and Ayurveda have deep-rooted traditional importance that spans centuries. These disciplines have contributed to the holistic well-being of individuals by addressing physical, mental, and spiritual aspects of life. In contemporary times, the traditional importance of psychology, yoga, and Ayurveda in India continues to thrive. They have gained global recognition for their holistic approach to well-being. Many people worldwide now practice yoga, engage in Ayurvedic treatments, and study Indian philosophical concepts to enhance their mental, physical, and spiritual health. This chapter helps us understand the psychological problems humans face and remedies for such illnesses through various practices of yoga and Ayurveda. This chapter helps us to gain wisdom on psychology, yoga, and Ayurveda. This chapter will provide visions to students, corporate professionals, practitioners, scholars, researchers, etc.

INTRODUCTION

Ancient Wisdom to Modern Science" explores and integrates traditional knowledge into various practices, modern scientific advancements, and technologies. The insights from traditional knowledge are

DOI: 10.4018/978-1-6684-9778-4.ch006

more valuable and embedded in multiple cultural and conventional methods that are still relevant and useful to the contemporary world. The Indian culture and traditional knowledge comprise accumulated information over thousands of years through trial & error methods, experience, cultural beliefs, assumptions, and deep connection with nature and the environment. The traditional knowledge of India comprehends a wide assortment of disciplines, such as Ayurveda, Yoga, astrology, and spiritual practices. The conventional wisdom in India is a cherished and valuable resource several generations have passed down.

It is also equally acceptable that India's rich heritage and traditional knowledge dating thousands of years back has lots of evidence from the Vedas, Upanishad, and epics with thoughtful psychological perspectives and profound insights into mindfulness, human consciousness, emotions, and well-being.

BACKGROUND OF THE STUDY

Traditional knowledge systems in India focus on and study a comprehensive overview of Ayurveda Yoga, examine the concept of spirituality based on Vedantic literature, and propose that spirituality is a climatic construct that encompasses concern for both the social and natural environment at a macro level. This holistic understanding of spirituality highlights its connection to the overall well-being of individuals and communities. Moreover, Parasmani, Sharma, and Bindles (2014) developed an consolidative structure of working environment spirituality that incorporates aspects from Indian spiritual traditions. Spirituality is an consciousness of a being or force that exceeds life's material concerns and imparts a profound sense of the universe's unity or interconnectedness. (Myers & Williard,2003). The current chapter explores the implications of traditional knowledge systems towards Yoga, ayurvedic Practices, and the role of spirituality towards the well being

Moreover, these practices have inspired scientific research and have influenced modern psychology and medicine. Mindfulness-based therapies, for instance, have roots in ancient Indian contemplative practices and are now widely used in psychological treatments for stress, depression, and anxiety. This chapter also focuses on the emotions of humans in this corporate world. Yoga and Ayurveda are very cost-effective for treating mental illness that acts as a barrier for humans. India is the home for most yoga practitioners; around 80% of people in India and Nepal practice Ayurveda. India has announced several schemes for yoga and Ayurveda like Ayush Medicines/Aid for community/Primary Health Centers, Promotion of Public Health Activities, Ayush Village, Starting Yoga Wellness, etc., to promote yoga and Ayurveda among the public to improve their psychological well-being

AYURVEDA-INDIAN PRACTICES

History of Ayurveda

Ayurveda began in the 2nd Century BC. Ayurveda was started from the earliest Hindu philosophical traditions renowned as Vaisheshika and the academy of logic was named Nyaya. It is the background of Samkhya, and it was introduced in the same era during the introduction of the schools Nyaya and Vaisheshika.

The Vaisheshika school has addressed the implications and insights gained about a patient's compulsive ailment for treatment. On the other hand, the school Nyaya proliferated its lessns based that one must have in-depth data of the patient's condition. The institute of Vaisheshika categorizes the characteristics of the article into six types: Matter, Meticulousness, Activity, Generalization, Inherence, and Superiority, which are commonly known as Dravya, Vishesha, Karma, Samanya, Samaveda, and Guna, respectively, in Sanskrit. Later, the schools Vaisheshika and Nyaya combined and initiated the Nay–Vaishesika school. In later periods, the Nay–Vaishesika school brought grandeur to the ancient wisdom and helped in circulating the wisdom of Ayurveda. Even before the schools were founded and even today, the origin of Ayurveda was regarded as deific, from the Hindu God, Brahma, who is known as the inventor of the world. Lord Brahma passed the holistic healing wisdom to the sages for their humanity.

Again, from sages, the wisdom was passed onto the followers and then to the public through literatures and verbalized narrations. The knowledge regarding the therapeutic properties of the herbs was detailed in poetries called "Shlokas." Sages are commonly used to define how to use medicinal herbs. The Hindu structure is thought to be based on four renowned accumulations of acquaintance (Vedas) called Yajur Veda, Rig Veda, Sama Veda, and Atharva Veda. The most difficult and most cult values have been described in the Rig Veda, consisting of 67 plants and 1028 shlokas. At the same time, the Atharva Veda and Yajur Veda comprise 293 and 81 herbs information.

The preparation of Ayurveda is basically from the wisdom expanded from these Vedas. The sculptures and works in Rig Veda and Atharva Veda are accredited to "Atreya," who gained knowledge about Ayurveda from Lord Indra, who originally acknowledged it from Lord Brahma. Agnivesh gathered the expertise or information from the Vedas, and Charaka and some other renowned scholars rewrote it, and currently, it is known as "Charaka Samhita." Charaka Samhita defines all the characteristics of Ayurvedic medicine, and Sushruta Samhita describes the science and surgery. Many physicians of traditional medicine still use these two legendary compilations. These antique writings are accessible in several transformations and lingos like Tibetan, Greek, Chinese, Arabic, and Persian. Still, Charaka Samhita is considered the most honored of them all.

Traditional Medicine for Mental Illness-Herbal Psychopharmacology

Traditional medicine is commonly used as a cure for mental disorders by using different methods. Psychological illnesses like sadness, nervousness and sleeplessness are often discovered in an individual and they have a similar nervous basis, the process for curing these kinds of sicknesses conceivably entangled with each other, when aspects turn on a particular aim, a commotion can be seen in another target which may affect the treatment for other associated mental disorders

Herbal Anti-Depressants and Depression

According to practitioners, depression is considered a usual psychological illness with great costs to human capability. Furthermost, synthetic anti-depressants have severe side effects such as a slight gamut of anti-depressants, hostile responses, high medication prices and easy reappearance exist. Most persons are slowly revolving in the direction of traditional medicine to discover the various targets of anti-depressants with a minimal poisonousness. The development of sadness is complex, and it is discovered that various types of psychological disorders have similar genetic changes. Nevertheless, the minute system were not the only reason for gloomy sicknesses; the main reason for depression is due to the act of neuroendocrinological irregularities and also stress; fluctuations in cytokine, steroids and dysregulation of improper sleeping. The persistent plant known as Rhodiola rosea extract (considered as stonecrop family of Rhoiola genus) comprises 96 types in the world with the most in China. This plant has additional 40 different varieties of chemical mixtures and can be used to reduce the signs of tension, anoxia and exhaustion to recover immune function and shield the vital nervous system along with the cardiovascular system. Ayurvedic medicines like Saffron (stigmas of Crocus sativus l.) have remained used for remedial purposes around millenniums. The two main constituents of Saffron are Safranal and Crocin. They are revealed as anti-depressant

Herbal Anxiolytics and Anxiety

Anxiety is categorized into comprehensive anxiety, panic, post-traumatic anxiety, OCD, and anxious disorders. Anxiety is considered the primary symptom of various psychological disorders. The function of nervousness illnesses is still unknown. In the opinion of these trials, various drugs are regarded as beneficial to fight anxiety disorders—however, continuous usage of these medications results in many unavoidable lateral effects or acceptance. However the use of natural extracts and plant preparations have been considered as the best remedy for fighting anxiety disorders. The remedies for menopausal psychotic syndromes are gardenia fructus, and the Kampo formula Kamishoyosan could be used.

Many herbal substances have been used to achieve anxiolytic effects by increasing central GABA (Gamma-Aminobutyric Acid) levels. The most potent inhibitor of GABA-T was determined to be an liquid abstract of Melissa officinalis (lemon balm) . The fruit of Marinda centifolia, a traditional medicine used for several healthiness aids, including anti-inflammatory, antioxidant, detoxifier, cell-rejuvenator properties, has hydrophilic components that exert a GABA-A receptor agonistic activity. Similar to benzodiazepine medications, valerian and its principal active ingredient, valerianic acid, has sedative and anxiolytic effects that are primarily mediated by GABA-ergic processes.

Asian countries have utilized Zizyphus jujuba Millvar. Spinosa (Rhamnaceae) Zizyphi Spinosi Semen (ZSS), the dried seed, to cure anxiety and insomnia. Sanjoinine, one of the main alkaloid chemicals in ZSS, is thought to have anxiolytic-like effects through activating the Cl-Channel and GABA-benzodiazepine receptors. Sun ginseng (ginseng heated at a higher temperature), Along with the previously listed herbal anxiolytics, coumarins from Angelica archangelical Linn., root bark extract from Rauwolfia vomitoria, lavender oil, Stachys tabetic Vatke, and Magnolia officinalis are also accountable for the minor tranquilizer activity.

Natural Sedatives and Insomnia

Insomnia, the most common sleep disorder, is routinely ignored. Long-term sleep and wakefulness issues affect around one-third of the general population, according to estimates. Numerous medicinal plants and complex formulas are routinely used to treat sleeplessness. The GABA receptor, cortisol levels, cytokines, circadian rhythm (melatonin secretion, adenosine receptors), and excitatory amino acids (glutamate and aspartate) are just a few of the pathways that might be abnormal, leading to sleep issues.

Patients' symptoms of sleeping problems and other diseases, especially those in the elderly, may be improved by L. sativa seed oil. The commonly used saffron, which is the stigma of the stemless perennial herb Crocus sativus L (a member of the Iridaceae family), has been shown to have various effects on the central nervous system. Safranin has neuropharmacological properties, as was shown in a study that examined the effects of saffron water extracts and its constituent parts on mice. According to the literature review, a number of additional herbal treatments, such as Passiflora incanata (passionflower), Eschscholzia californica (California poppy), P. methectic and Scutellarin later ifera (scullcap), also seemed to have potential advantages for treating insomnia.

YOGA AND SPIRITUALITY OF WELL-BEING

While most individuals practice Yoga for their physical advantages, Yoga can help us in numerous ways. Yoga has strong spiritual roots, and numerous postures have deeper purposes beyond strengthening and stretching muscles. Yoga's comprehensive effect enables interpreters to enhance their physical stamina, inflexibility, feelings, intelligence, and focus. The spiritual outlook of Yoga helps yogis to improve their blending of the inner being as well as the ultimate supreme consciousness within oneself. It begins with the body and the asanas, otherwise known as postures.

Yoga's Impacts on Depression and Quality of Life

Research has found that Yoga is thought to be the most successful kind of exercise for enhancing both physical and mental health, including stress, quality of life, mood swings, heart rate variability, respiratory functions, etc. Based on numerous independent research, it is clear that toxicity and weight gain are the most frequent adverse consequences of a variety of treatments. In order to counteract these dangers, yoga may be a useful and less toxic adjunctive therapy for the majority of mental health issues.. Yoga helped to understand that prisoners' health and mental illness, such as subjective well-being, executive functioning and so on, have been improved. Also, Yoga improved pregnant women's quality of life and interactive relationships. Over the decades, Studies have demonstrated that yoga can aid with breast cancer treatment by enhancing psychological well-being, and yoga has also been used as a monotherapy to treat MDD (Mild to Moderate).

Also there has been strong evidence that Yoga has been used as an adjunctive therapy. Several studies have indicated:

a) Yoga is considered a better treatment than improving MDD
b) Yoga is viewed as an equal to tricyclic anti-depressants (TCAs) in severe MDD
c) Combined with anti-depressants, Yoga is considered the most effective treatment for depressive symptoms.

Patients who do Yoga have their experience of connectedness with others and everything. When someone goes into a depressed state, they feel alone and tired of coping with stress, and cogitations help them to feel good compared to before Yoga. They started to concentrate on optimism instead of the wrongs they had done in the past, to come out of regret or the feeling of being unable to do anything. Yoga helps them motivate and try things they were afraid to do before.

How Does Yoga Work?

Yoga has a proven track record for excellent health promotion, disease prevention, patient management, therapy, and intrusion mitigation. According to several researches, yoga alters gene expression, the cardiac system, and the nervous system in a positive way. Pneumogastric nerve stimulation causes the autonomic nervous system's parasympathetic activity to increase, which in turn amplifies GABA's (a neurotransmitter) effect inside brain.

Parallel to other types of corporeal activity, conscious and movement have a optimistic impression on cardiac well-being. The breath connects the mind and the body in yoga. Slow and deep breath is important to maintain peace of mind. Performing Yoga aids to develop psychological steadiness, serenity, and peace in the first place because of breathing.

Practitioners can link mobility and hush. Physicians can connect within through this immobility and hush. Practically, all yoga practices, such as asana (postures), pranayama (Breathing practices), dhyana (meditation), boost softness and concentration within oneself. Yoga helps a person to develops endurance, merciful, less likely to become angry and sorrowful. Moreover, Yoga helps physicians to get back to their natural selves. Most asanas are formed by imitating different animal and plant poses like trees, dogs, snakes, and cats. The end or final part of Yoga is the relaxation known as savasana (corpse pose) where individuals lie on the floor and open their hands and forelegs. Ayurvedic practitioners suggest savasana to most patients as the best treatment for modern existing.

Savasana links profound breathing through organized slackening of each part of the body. While few people may go to sleep while performing savasana, the intention of this asana is to maintain consciousness with resting our body. In India, the savasana as a dead body pose is built partially on the concept that the cadaver is the final piece of a living being. Additionally, Yoga motivates physicians to understand the meaning of an open heart. Many yogic practitioners have said that, Yoga helps to connect our hearts in a metaphorical way. To go deep, Yoga helps activate the chakra system used to awaken the seven chakras. To activate these chakras, particular asanas are to be performed to activate each chakra. The Arda chakras Ana (back bend), kapotas (pigeon pose) and ustrina (camel pose) help to widen the centre of the chest where Anahita chakra is located, the yogic heart centre. Therapies and pranayama are also considered as a tool for open-heartedness.

Spirituality and Well-Being

Nations all across the world are transitioning from an agro-based economy to an industrial economy and then to a post-industrial economy. The current concern is the extent to which the quickening socio-economic, political, and demographic changes have been put up to benefit society and the subjective well-being of people. Life satisfaction and spiritualistic happiness are two different types of subjective happiness. Happiness comes in many different ways that are directly related to humankind's aspiration. Additionally, there are disparities in how people define happiness on a cultural and conceptual level.

Buddhism believes that by forgoing all sensuous and materialistic pleasures (verkakte) and cultivating the wisdom of respect and sympathy for all beings, one might achieve ultimate bliss. The Hindu philosophy of the Vedas, on the other hand, focuses on continuous endeavors towards achieving greater types of bliss, from material to mental to spiritual happiness. Lord Krishna tells Arjuna in the Hindu mythical book Bhagavad Gita to carry out his duties without worrying about the consequences (Nishka karma). The complete absence of all cravings (moksha) is the single condition necessary to attain the highest level of contentment.

HISTORY OF PSYCHOLOGY

Although psychology has only recently emerged as a field of study from a scientific perspective, it has long been recognized as a topic of human inquiry. Some psychological ideas and theories are shared across all countries. They are described using a variety of terms, including "inexperienced psychology," "common sense psychology," "ethnopsychology," "everyday psychology," and "the psychology of the populace". The outline of modern scientific psychology is to change from inexperienced and common-sense notions to a globally applicable set of theories and, principles, theories and philosophies. Psychology is an indigenous knowledge system which is present in many cultures and societies, gives rise to a variety of perspectives on reality, cause, competence, innate traits, self-assertive qualities, admired traits, behavior consequences, moral principles, Human versus nonhuman, life against death, joy versus sorrow, normal versus abnormal, family structure and function, social status, justice, ethnicity, labor and play, and numerous more issues (Thomas, 2001).

INDIAN PSYCHOLOGY

Implications of Global Psychology

The two techniques mentioned above show that we are able to classify gaps in the works that signify hypothetical, procedural, and applied shortcomings by starting with Western or cross-cultural psychological models and ideas. To close these gaps, the global psychology creates indigenous or emic models and compares them to cross-cultural or Western models.. As an alternative, the etic views could be used to fill in the gaps in the literature and advance global psychology.

These theoretical advancements or methodological breakthroughs, particularly those involving the creation of measurement scales, don't appear to significantly advance native psychologies or viewpoints Bond et al.,2004). (Bhawuk, 1999, 2003a; Hwang, 2004; Yang, 1997), The indigenous model-building technique frequently broadens the choice of philosophy and technique for development, accentuates gaps in the literature, and raises new concerns. We must thus support the two methods since they appear to improve distinct types of value to our knowledge of global psychology. Cultural and cross-cultural scholars should concentrate more on the second research paradigm because the first one predominates. As indicated in the conversations, the studies on insinuation conduct and headship, there is a lot of potential for the synthesis of homegrown thoughts in administrative psychology in India. I advise psychologists to forbid conducting pseudoetic research in Indian organizations as a result. Organizational commitment is a prime illustration of how organizational research, in general, highlights the risks of mindlessly adopting Western culture.

It was provided in a research summary of group and team effectiveness. They came to the conclusion that team performance is influenced by organizational structure, context, or environmental factors., as well as through work. Team effectiveness is influenced by the personalities of its members as well as by its internal and external processes. In addition, a meta-analysis showed a significant negative association between interactions and challenging tasks, team productivity, and member satisfaction. However, it is not clear that these results apply to different cultural contexts.

From the standpoint of cross-cultural studies, theories of individualism and collectivism can be utilized to assess popular Western conceptions of group development. Open issues are addressed and cultural change at various stages of group growth is investigated based on her four key concepts of individualism and collectivism. This strategy shows a desire to begin with cross-cultural theory.

The 1980s have been dubbed the decade of individualism and collectivism by academics due to the tremendous influence individualism and collectivism have had on psychological study. Triandis summarizes the material and suggests that individualism has four universal qualities that set it apart from collectivism:

Self-independence and inter-reliant are defined as, group goals independent of group compatibility goals, emphasize attitudes relative to the norm and the relationship's rationality. According to Schwartz (1990), the study of individualism and collectivism could be better if the terms were broken down into more precise dimensions.

EMOTIONS FROM THE INDIAN PERSPECTIVE

According to Indian psychology, philosophical texts and scriptures, a clear picture of emotion has not been defined as a separate concept. They are portrayed as a trait, personality, or character of a living being that arises due to contact of ego (Ahamkara). This is because "emotions are considered as something that has been transcended to achieve the eventual goal of life". Emotions are considered as ego (Ahamkara) and one's true self (Atman). It establishes the relationship between ego and the outside world. Indians believe that, emotions are viewed that they come from what are their needs and wants. There has been a strong belief that pleasure and pain (Sukha and Dukkha) are distinctive from each other. Emotions are related to mind and have effect on both food and air. Emotions and their touching experiences are inclined by mind.

Every emotion arise from desires and desire is triggered by a sense of faultiness, incompleteness or disappointment that has been felt within oneself. If the desire is stronger, it creates a stronger emotional experience. When a need or want is not fulfilled or dissatisfied it creates anger (Krodha), jealousy (Asuya), unhappiness (Dukkha) and suffering and if desire has been met it has the positive impacts within one self like happiness (Sukha) and enjoyment. Often these desires are carried out by a by a single emotion called greed (Lodha). If one need or want is met, a person desires more and more to live his life as his wants and need are never ending. This is because of the enjoyment one feels within. When these are accepted, one may develop arrogance (Made) and envy (Mansaray). Also, there is one emotion that is most vital and it is known as fear (Bhabya) of losing. One's mind and mental disturbance cause all these emotions. Although, not all emotions are viewed as harmful. In simple words, emotions are considered the asset, but when it interferes with one's decision, it creates a sense of weakness.

Although there are occasional objections to such a understanding (e.g., Ranganathan, 2008), the two classifications of Samkhya and Yoga are frequently considered as tightly connected and they are habitually studied together. The Samkhya structure is attributed to one legendary Kapila, but the most primitive works from the 2nd century appears to be lost, and the Samkhya Karika of Ishvaraskrishna (circa 200 CE, e.g., Dasgupta, 1997, p. 212) is believed to be the trustworthy text that express the essence of Samkhya philosophy (Raju, 1985, p. Flood (2004) from the ages of the fifth century BC.

We indicated Samkhya-Yoga as it possess emormous psychological theories which is perhaps one of the most vital systems of India and it encompasses theoretical components that is widespread beyond the Western Psychology compared to Indian Systems. The reputation of Samkhya-Yoga is demonstrated by the fact that the recommendations to it can be route in throughout the most dominant works, including the previous Upanishads, the Bhagavad-Gita, and other chapters of the Mahabharata (Puligandla, 1997, p. 119). Samkhya-Yoga is strongly inter-connected with ancient Indian writings known as Veda (knowledge). However, there are only grim chances of extracting the theories of psychology straight from Vedas since they contain significant servings devoted to rites, in addition they are frequently inscribed in a elegiac and clear way. As a result, we relied on a methodically developed methodology that includes well acknowledged scholarly explanations of the Vedas.

Cognition From an Indian Perspective

A person, according to Yoga and Samkhya, is made up of two "mechanisms," one is made into materialistic while the other was not (for more information, see Dasgupta, 1930; Chatterjee and Datta, 1984; Puligandla, 1997; Jha, 2008; Rao and Paranjpe, 2008). Prakriti (largely translated as "nature") which is comprised of three "qualities," or gunas: sattva (purity), rajas (energy), and tamas (inertia). Prakriti, in the form of the three gunas, is the essence of the universe as well as the foundation for a person's individuality. The unique character and stuff which includes the mind too and they are regarded as result of a "mixture" of the three gunas.

People who possess high level of sattva are supposed to have a optimistic view of the world, a well-intentioned boldness toward others, to be well-organized, peaceful, and tranquil, to have tolerance towards the stress, to live a hale and hearty lifestyle. On the other hand, people with a high rajas level have difficulty relaxing and favor acts that provide them with interim desire or comfort but they are eventually hazardous in the long-run. Furthermore, people lead an unwholesome routine and waste their liveliness. Lastly, people with large tamas personality are unhappy in their life and more inclined for neglect in their health. Yet, the combination of these energies are not viewed as inherently stable: Growing sattva is widely regarded as a necessary goal, also when sattva is bulging in a person, that individual can reach exceptional spiritual goals.

Purusha is the non-material element of a person and also of the world, often decoded as truthful person or true-self, but then it is often condensed as untainted realization. Prakriti and purusha form the obvious world for the person in its entirety. The mind contains a wide range of dispositions and memories. It is divided into three practical aspects: sense of mind, ego mind, and intellectual mind or intellect.

For example, how discernment function in this method? Through peripheral logic organs, the sense of mind selects an exterior body. The ego consciousness subsequently seizes this item, which associates it with the situation. The intelligence then denotes the body (represents an item) later forms decision or else makes a judgment about likely activities. The thought, that is unconscious by essence (part of prakriti), it becomes mindful (and reasonings become possible) as it comes into connection with purusha. To be specific, cognition would be impossible without the operation of purusha. However, communication among purusha and intelligence operates in one way for amateurish people. Purusha "practices" the mind, whereas the intellect "practices" purusha. Without "seeing" pure consciousness in its pure form, it just reflects it. This reflection, on the other hand, gives us uncomfortableness and our particular perception about the world. The evidence thet mind uses doesn't rely solely from the senses. They could have alsox be derived from implications, verbal sources, or recollection. Furthermore, it covers instinctive leanings acquired through the consequences of historical deeds and prior incarnations, which have an impact on the contemporary existence. The intelligence includes remembrance insides from previous understandings (previous lifetimes).

Let us use an example to demonstrate the operation of the mind. Suppose the senses are presented with a banana, for example. In that case, the sense of mind gathers each and every available perceptions of hue, form, palate, etc., and merges them and distinguishes entire unified item constructed in a way different from other matters. The ego-mind then claims ownership of the thing, as in "I see a banana." The thing in query (e.g., a banana) is a thing of one's knowledge but they are not viewed as an thing of the unbiased world at this level of perception. The intellect creates such an item by making an assertion or judgment that results in roughly like "this is a banana" as the result of the decision process.

Furthermore, it accumulates various characteristics of banana, (the banana tree), how its eaten, its worth, vitamins, etc., and it associates these with the seeming banana in collaboration with the other areas of the mind. This encounter is also remembered. Nevertheless, entire course is solitarily possible with assistance of untainted mindfulness, which is "mirrored" in the mind and senses.

All section of the mind are believed to have bodily form, although their subtlety varies, with the intellectual, being the greatest delicate and sensory concentration being the minimum. However, every components are thought that thay are made in a far more delicate material than the body (that includes brain) and the minds. It is worth noting that, in Samkhya-Yoga, the mind, while material, is extraterritorial; it doesn't have to be located in the brain (e.g., Rao, 2005). Furthermost crucially, and obviously contrary to popular belief, the mind alone cannot work solely: Cognizant cognition requires a linking between the intellect and the basic module of the Yoga scheme: untainted mindfulness.

ETHICAL IMPLICATIONS OF USING INDIAN PSYCHOLOGY IN THE MODERN AGE

Ethical Difficulties In the following situations, psychological well-being physicians employed with aged clients will expect to meet moral dilemmas.

1. When opposing ethical principles exist.
2. When moral, lawful, and/or structural standards conflict.
3. When confronted with a comparatively new area of medical exercise, moral norms or laws fail to deliver enough direction.
4. The physicians must depend on his or her decision.

In the framework of finishing evaluations, implementing interpositions, offering sessions in sickbays or hospitals, and doing investigate, senior mental health physicians frequently face moral problems. We offer a few situations from our clinical experience of providing psychological therapies to the mature people affected with dementia that emphasize moral issues.

Example One: Contribution in Mental Interventions is the First challenge

Mr M was identified with late-onset mild Alzheimer's illness and advised to be present group CST sittings. However, he consented to go and engage in the CST sittings advised by the clinic, he remained resistive once he began appearing. His primary caregiver, his spouse, mentioned that he protested regarding the extended drive to the epicenter and he was hesitant to get dressed for attending the sittings. His spouse convinced him, arranged conveyance and made him to the sittings. He requested to leave the center shortly after arriving for the first few sessions. He seemed to be more anxious and uneasy. Convincing him to come and not to go away from the sittings, by presenting a new process or a novel group associate remained frequently met with annoyance and hostility. Due to his cognitive limitations, he was unable to explain the source of his uneasiness, discomfort, and rage. After speaking with his wife, we concluded that these symptoms were most likely caused by the new atmosphere and the existence of unfamiliar person. We requested him if he wanted to cease appearing the sittings since he stood unwilling to participate. When ewas all set to, his spouse remarked that he wasn't friendly to unfamiliar person and new surroundings, and she requested him to attend few more sittings, with the understanding that if he remained hesitant. She even stated thet he appeared to be more curious and conversational after attending the sittings. Mr M was ahead from the CST sittings, despite his reluctance to participate. He physician asked the spouse not to force him to attend but to softly boost him to attend the sittings. Mr M appeared calmer throughout the sessions during the next two weeks, and his partner commented that he was very anxious about the sittings. Over time, he became over active in the sittings. The obligation to reconcile the patients' independence along with their well-being (generosity) is a recurring ethical challenge in the medical exercise of geriatric psychological practitioners. While physicians wanted to promote their patients' right to make self-governing choices about health, when victims are incapacitated and the judgments are inconsistent about well-being, physicians often discover it difficult to care their conclusions. In this case, understanding the victims' standards and desires will result in conflict resolution.

Example Two: Bottomless Collection of Mental Interventions is the Second Challenge

Mrs N, a retired headteacher who has vascular dementia. She is found to be self-sufficient and determined. She often dominated and contemptuously of other participants while engaging in CST groups. She was more emotional in her voice and deeds, creating nasty remarks on the mistakes other CST group members made, and she was often dominating and disrespectful of other participants. She was also acknowledged to be a more uninhibited participant in making and concerning their appearances. Mrs N sustained to interrupt the group despite the efforts of the facilitators. Her family members said, she seemed to advantage from the sittings because she tend to be better-off at home and beheld onward to them during each week. Though, other members became less engaged with her and began grouchy on her conduct. Though her conduct may have been influenced by emotion caused by the neurodegenerative procedures inherent in vascular dementia, the right test for geriatric psychological well-being physicians have to strike a balance between her "autonomy," the "generosity" of getting the involvement, and the code of "not to harm patients" towards other participants. Mrs N was offered individual CST sessions following a chat with her and her family, she was transferred to Individual CST in a distinct chamber.

Example Three: Discontinuing Interventions is the Third Challenge

Mrs S is an older lady suffering from late-onset Alzheimer's disease dementia. She went through one round of CST. She attended the facility regularly once in a week for about two or more years. Her mental functions and everyday active tasks remained deteriorating over time. She could not significantly withstand to participate in group programs. This seemed to have a detrimental effect on other members of the group, as the organizers spent huge time assisting Mrs S, making other members feel unheeded. On the other hand, her relatives noted that she seemed to like being out of the house. On the days when she went to therapy, she seemed to be happier after the sessions. While the facilitators of the group were conscious about the uselessness of Mrs S's maintenance CST, they also thought that socialising will help her emotionally. It was approved by the CST, but for maintenance it may not be the ideal option simply to stretch sociability. Following, a conversation between her and her family, she was moved to another group that met once a calendar week solely meant for socialising. She seemed to adore this new cluster and regularly attended the sittings. In particular, for psychological well-being physicians who work with elder persons, the moral principles of "uselessness of treatment" and "non-abandonment" has become crucial in their daily practice. Specific interventions may become ineffective as dementia progresses or conditions change. As soon as their victims no longer profits from therapies, the psychotherapist must acknowledge "uselessness of treatment" and attempt for change or terminate them. The term "non-abandonment" denotes to the psychotherapist's duty to guarantee that the patient receives proper care which is both positive and non damaging to them. In Mrs. S's siuation, continuing maintenance CST was pointless, and that appearing for a "socialization group" remained most appropriate and consistent with the belief of "non-abandonment."

CONCLUSION

The practice of Yoga, Ayurveda and the positive psychology of the Indian perspective display a promise for endorsing improved people mental health. It is agreeable, reachable, lucrative and ambitious. Yoga is the sole well-being encouraging exercise that can be perfromed neither in large number nor reinforced by people. Performing Yoga in group, in workrooms, institutes and further surroundings, displayed a positivity in population in mental health. Yoga promotes a sense of inner peace from the mental illness. It encounters the three-way aim of developing well-being, attention and reduction price. Yoga interventions and assorted study populations, Yoga naturally improves complete sign of anxiety and depression. Yoga and spiritual health are inter-related. When it comes to the use of Ayurveda, it uses several principles like Dincharya, Raticharya, Ritucharya, Achara Rayasana, Aahara, Sadvrutta and regularly performing Yoga like Asanas, Pranayama and Meditation have a large part in betterment of mental health. These practices galvanize the mind for mental work, improve physical and mental balance, develop concentration and calm the mind which results in good mental health. There are two sources of knowledge: collated syntheses of descriptions of retrieval from mental illness and pragmatic proof about well-being from the academic discipline of optimistic psychology. These two are highly harmonizing and provide a counter-balance to the old focus of mental health services of discrepancy improvement. Assessment and action of the individual need to be changed if the aim is to promote well-being rather than treating the illness. There are also wider trials for mental health professionals who have become more outward looking in the context of their corresponding role and to build their job as more than working with individuals. A view on developing social inclusion, becoming social activists who contest stigma, judge and encourage societal well-being may have to become the model otherwise being an exception for mental health practitioners in the 21st century. The chapter will facilitate the learning and rich knowledge source in the Indian traditional knowledge management discipline. It also provides insights to economists, academicians, researchers, practitioners and other learned audiences.

REFERENCES

Al-Farabi, A. N. (1995). *Tahsil Al-Sa'ada* [Attainment of Happiness]. Ja'far Al Yasin.

Bhawuk, D. (2011). *Spirituality and Indian psychology: lessons from the Bhagavad-Gita*. Springer Science & Business Media. doi:10.1007/978-1-4419-8110-3

Biswas, S. K., & Debnath, M. (2017). *Yoga and Ayurveda: Concomitant preventive therapeutics for some important lifestyle disorders*.

Bond, M. H., Leung, K., Au, A., Tong, K. K., De Carrasquel, S. R., Murakami, F., Yamaguchi, S., Bierbrauer, G., Singelis, T. M., Broer, M., Boen, F., Lambert, S. M., Ferreira, M. C., Noels, K. A., van Bavel, J., Safdar, S., Zhang, J., Chen, L., Solcova, I., & Lewis, J. R. (2004). Culture-level dimensions of social axioms and their correlates across 41 cultures. *Journal of Cross-Cultural Psychology*, *35*(5), 548–570. doi:10.1177/0022022104268388

Brown, J. L. C., Eubanks, C., & Keating, A. (2017). Yoga, quality of life, anxiety, and trauma in low-income adults with mental illness: A mixed-methods study. *Social Work in Mental Health*, *15*(3), 308–330. doi:10.1080/15332985.2016.1220441

Chaudhry, N., Bhandari, R. B., & Gaur, V. (2023). Yoga perspective on personal excellence and well-being. *Journal of Ayurveda and Integrative Medicine*, *14*(3), 100717. doi:10.1016/j.jaim.2023.100717 PMID:37224682

Contrada, R., & Baum, A. (Eds.). (2010). *The handbook of stress science: Biology, psychology, and health*. Springer Publishing Company.

Cornelissen, M. (2011). *Foundations of Indian Psychology Volume 2: Practical Applications*. Pearson Education India.

Daaleman, T. P., Cobb, A. K., & Frey, B. B. (2001). Spirituality and well-being: An exploratory study of the patient perspective. *Social Science & Medicine*, *53*(11), 1503–1511. doi:10.1016/S0277-9536(00)00439-1 PMID:11710425

Fallot, R. D. (2001). Spirituality and religion in psychiatric rehabilitation and recovery from mental illness. *International Review of Psychiatry (Abingdon, England)*, *13*(2), 110–116. doi:10.1080/09540260120037344

Gergen, K. J., Gulerce, A., Lock, A., & Misra, G. (1996). Psychological science in cultural context. *The American Psychologist*, *51*(5), 496–503. doi:10.1037/0003-066X.51.5.496

Gerhard, W. A. (1964). Heimann," Facets of Indian Thought"(Book Review). *The Journal of Asian Studies*, *24*(1), 182. doi:10.2307/2050470

Hodge, D. R. (2004). Spirituality and people with mental illness: Developing spiritual competency in assessment and intervention. *Families in Society*, *85*(1), 36–44. doi:10.1606/1044-3894.257

Jaiswal, Y. S., & Williams, L. L. (2017). A glimpse of Ayurveda–The forgotten history and principles of Indian traditional medicine. *Journal of Traditional and Complementary Medicine*, *7*(1), 50–53. doi:10.1016/j.jtcme.2016.02.002 PMID:28053888

Kamradt, J. M. (2017). Integrating yoga into psychotherapy: The ethics of moving from the mind to the mat. *Complementary Therapies in Clinical Practice*, *27*, 27–30. doi:10.1016/j.ctcp.2017.01.003 PMID:28438276

Kim, U., Yang, G., & Hwang, K. K. (Eds.). (2006). *Indigenous and cultural psychology: Understanding people in context*. Springer. doi:10.1007/0-387-28662-4

Kumar, S. K. (2008). Indian thought and tradition: A psycho-historical perspective. Handbook of Indian psychology, (pp. 19-52). Cambridge Press.

Mishra, L. C., Singh, B. B., & Dagenais, S. (2001). Ayurveda: A historical perspective and principles of the traditional healthcare system in India. *Alternative Therapies in Health and Medicine*, *7*(2), 36–43. PMID:11253415

Myers, J. E., & Williard, K. (2003). Integrating spirituality into counselor preparation: A developmental, wellness approach. *Counseling and Values*, *47*(2), 142–155. doi:10.1002/j.2161-007X.2003.tb00231.x

Nagendra, H. R. (2013). Integrated yoga therapy for mental illness. *Indian Journal of Psychiatry*, *55*(7, Suppl 3), S337. doi:10.4103/0019-5545.116299 PMID:24049195

Obeyesekere, G. (1970). Ayurveda and mental illness. *Comparative Studies in Society and History*, *12*(3), 292–296. doi:10.1017/S0010417500005867 PMID:11614363

Pandey, A., Gupta, V., & Gupta, R. K. (2019). Spirituality and innovative behaviour in teams: Examining the mediating role of team learning. *IIMB Management Review*, *31*(2), 116–126. doi:10.1016/j.iimb.2019.03.013

Pardasani, R., Sharma, R. R., & Bindlish, P. (2014). Facilitating workplace spirituality: Lessons from Indian spiritual traditions. *Journal of Management Development*, *33*(8/9), 847–859. doi:10.1108/JMD-07-2013-0096

Park, C. L., Finkelstein-Fox, L., Sacco, S. J., Braun, T. D., & Lazar, S.C. L. (2021). How does yoga reduce stress? A clinical trial testing psychological mechanisms. *Stress and Health*, *37*(1), 116–126. doi:10.1002mi.2977 PMID:32797683

Ramaprasad, D. (2013). Emotions: An Indian perspective. *Indian Journal of Psychiatry*, *55*(6, Suppl 2), S153. doi:10.4103/0019-5545.105514 PMID:23858247

Rao, K. R., & Paranjpe, A. C. (2016). *Psychology in the Indian tradition*. Springer India. doi:10.1007/978-81-322-2440-2

Reat, N. R. (1990). *The origins of Indian psychology*. Jain Publishing Company.

Rieber, R. W., & Robinson, D. K. (Eds.). (2001). *Wilhelm Wundt in history: The making of a scientific psychology*. Springer Science & Business Media. doi:10.1007/978-1-4615-0665-2

Sedlmeier, P., & Srinivas, K. (2016). How do theories of cognition and consciousness in ancient Indian thought systems relate to current Western theorizing and research? *Frontiers in Psychology*, *7*, 343. doi:10.3389/fpsyg.2016.00343 PMID:27014150

Shilpa, S., & Murthy, C. V. (2011). Understanding personality from Ayurvedic perspective for psychological assessment: A case. *Ayu, 32*(1), 12. doi:10.4103/0974-8520.85716 PMID:22131752

Shroff, F. M., Asgarpour, M., & Fm, S. (2017). Yoga and mental health: A review. *Physiother Rehabil, 2*(132), 2573–0312.

Shukla, R. (2013). Indian perspective of spiritual well-being. *Indian Journal of Positive Psychology, 4*(1), 114–116.

Shukla, S. (2020). Spirituality in Ayurveda. *Spirituality in Clinical Practice, 7*(2), 103–113. doi:10.1037cp0000181

Singh, K., Raina, M., & Sahni, P. (2017). The concept and measure of Sukha–Dukha: An Indian perspective on well-being. *Journal of Spirituality in Mental Health, 19*(2), 116–132. doi:10.1080/19349637.2016.1231604

Slade, M. (2010). Mental illness and well-being: The central importance of positive psychology and recovery approaches. *BMC Health Services Research, 10*(1), 1–14. doi:10.1186/1472-6963-10-26 PMID:20102609

Starnino, V. R. (2016). When trauma, spirituality, and mental illness intersect: A qualitative case study. *Psychological Trauma: Theory, Research, Practice, and Policy, 8*(3), 375–383. doi:10.1037/tra0000105 PMID:26783761

Subudhi, C. (2014). Culture and mental illness. *Social Work Practice in Mental Health: Cross-Cultural Perspectives, 141*, 132–140.

Thomas, R. (2001). *Folk psychologies across cultures*. Sage Publications, Inc. doi:10.4135/9781452233901

Vijayabanu, C., Therasa, C., & Daisy, S. A. (2019). Impression Management Tactics as a psychological booster for the communication of IT employees–SMART PLS Approach. *Revista de Psicología, 37*(2), 683–707. doi:10.18800/psico.201902.012

Chapter 7
Holistic Approach as a Strategy for Special Education in India

Reena Ryall
Brindavan Education Trust, India

ABSTRACT

Overcoming socio-cultural pressures in India with reference to special education will render intervention and remedial practices effective especially with a holistic approach which includes regional adaptations and multidisciplinary approaches to create a suitable framework within the Indian context for successful special education assessment with particular concern for hidden disabilities like learning disabilities which require and benefit from a holistic approach. Tracing a path through analysis of the Indian philosophical perspectives in education to possible current applications in educational practice this chapter provides a sound basis for adopting the holistic approach in education at a macro level and bringing about change in assessment practices at the micro level.

INTRODUCTION

In India, a host of circumstances surround every situation. When a child is found to be lagging in multiple skill areas, a process of denial, protecting the child from society as well as declining appropriate professional help to the child creates a trickle-down effect through the years resulting in uneven development in the child. The Rights of Persons with Disabilities Act (2016) aims to provide inclusive education in all schools, macro-level cultural factors like language barriers and economic barriers have affected the efficacy of this aim and at a micro level pedagogical practices within classrooms, remain resistant to change, again due to cultural specificities. Special education at the heart of its intention seeks to ease the child through the process of inclusion to a life within a normal environment as opposed to segregating and grouping children. Much has been accomplished in the last two decades in India, but hidden disabilities like learning disabilities are yet to see the light of day in terms of adequate awareness, early diagnosis, and early intervention. The scenario is additionally complicated by economic disadvantages and cultural pressures. The multilingual Indian context further exacerbates the situation. Hidden disabilities like Specific Learning Disability (SLD), comprise a

DOI: 10.4018/978-1-6684-9778-4.ch007

heterogeneous group of disorders with the main impairment being cognitive processing, which leads to challenges in academic performance and has psychosocial implications. Impairment should be present in history, school reports, and psychological assessment and persistence for at least six months as per Diagnostic and Statistical Manual 5th version (DSM-5) criteria by American Psychiatric Association (2013). From research by Chacko &Vidhukumar (2020), it is known that the prevalence of learning disabilities among primary school children in India is 11.2% for dyslexia, 12.5% for dysgraphia, and 10.5% for dyscalculia. In the current scenario, the approach of schools is to refer only children who are noticeably struggling with formal assessment which would be at the high school level, and extend available provisions like exemption of second language. The children struggling at the primary level are left languishing till their difficulties are so great that the delayed intervention they receive is often too little too late and they end up dropping out of school and shifting to special schools. A major goal of inclusive education led to the development of an early warning identification system by UNICEF (2017) which looks at the environmental circle as well as behavioral patterns of the child within a wider social context. Today, inclusion has thus been added to the preschool curriculum at Anganwadi centers in the hope of promoting early identification and providing holistic development. All along there have been recommendations to adopt a holistic approach in early childhood development. A holistic approach has been described as taking into consideration all facets of the development of a child including physical, emotional, economic, and intellectual. It allows the child to develop uniquely, focusing on individual strengths without the constraints of the traditional classroom which is norm based and competitive. It is relevant to consider the holistic approach as a valuable approach toward inclusion. Both keep the child s interests at its core. In special education, the holistic approach is relevant from two aspects, assessment as well as intervention. Holistic education aims to equip children to face challenges in life in a healthy manner.

INDIAN PHILOSOPHY AND EDUCATION

The holistic approach to education is rooted in Indian philosophy. Rabindranath Tagore's ideals for education were based on the individual's innate capabilities (Andrews, 1938). He believed children should feel free to be inventive so their creativity could develop (Tagore, 1931). His worldwide travel on educational missions contributed greatly to educational reforms in India (Lal, 1984). His ideas on education encompassed learning amidst nature, aligning one's skills in harmony with one's surroundings and thus bringing out the best in each child. Roy (2021) has shown the benefits of holistic teaching and learning as seen among children educated according to the principles laid out by Tagore in Shantiniketan. His was a combination of East and West keeping the good of the child as of utmost importance, inculcating education as well as nurturing the goodness within. The essence of his approach was that nature and arts could put one in harmony with the universe. He felt freedom in the mind facilitated the exercise of mental faculties, he viewed education as a vehicle to appreciate others' cultural differences (O'Connell, 2010). If children were rooted firmly in their cultural identity, they would find it easy to relate to other cultures. Similarly, if they were confident in themselves, they would blossom in their creativity and individual strengths. His main ideology was that education should aim to develop harmony within one's self as well as with the outer world. It was a journey of self-realization (Goswamee & Saikia, 2017). His idea of consolidation of cultures is particularly relevant in present times with regard to the Right to Education Act, of 2009 which makes education a right for every child and requires private schools to reserve 25% of seats based on economic, caste, and other reservation basis. The global village which Tagore envisioned is now a classroom reality, however, educational reforms are a work in progress and the time is ripe to contemplate changes in approaches such as a focus on holistic education. The profile of the child with learning disabilities beckons a deeper understanding of individual strengths, talents, and need for freedom from the rigid classroom environment, and promoting of an inner sense of self-worth, self-acceptance, and inner harmony which in turn would reflect in outer ability to follow true paths of potential and thereby lead to a life of satisfaction. Tagore s concept of spiritualism in education which encompassed values of caring and acceptance of others sits well with the special education environment where every individual is different yet can coexist in harmony with others. His firm position on teaching in the mother tongue is central to the holistic approach as he believed that true self-expression was possible only through the mother tongue as it was the basis for generating ideas (Mishra, 2014). This is appropriate for children who find English as a medium of instruction akin to a second language hence their difficulties constitute what is referred to as English as Second Language learners or ESL. If taught in their mother tongue, their language proficiency increases (Suntharesan, 2012). All in all Tagore's ideology of education remains relevant, for neurodiverse children as well as neurotypical children.

LEARNING DISABILITIES PROFILE IN THE INDIAN CONTEXT

The profile of the child with learning disabilities warrants a symptomatic overview to understand how the holistic approach would fit well for observational purposes, screening and assessment as well as teaching. Unlike other disabilities which are obvious to the eye, such as motor handicaps or visual impairments, learning disabilities are hidden and as such cause much turmoil for the child as often related areas give rise to secondary factors like socio-emotional disturbance and behavioral issues. A child with learning disabilities is one with a developmental disorder of scholastic skills (World Health Organization, 1993) where the child has difficulties with reading, writing, or math, observable in academic settings like the classroom, hence difficult to identify in early years. Such children are good potential however they seem to lack attention or fail to pick up some cognitive skills unless they are provided with intervention. The traditional classroom environment places demands on them that are beyond their coping which presents a case of lack of attention, incomplete notes, and a feeling of inadequacy. When taken for professional intervention they are placed in a secure environment where they are encouraged to be creative, spontaneous, unique, and confident. However, in school and at home they feel the weight of expectation on them. The main difficulties faced by children with learning disorders are errors in reading like reversals, omissions, substitutions, errors in spelling like reversals, inversions, phonetically consistent spelling for irregular words, errors in writing like poor spacing, inconsistency in size and pencil pressure, inability to form sentences, etc. Math errors usually manifest as digit reversal or rotation, confusion between computation signs, difficulty to maintain rows and columns, and difficulty with numerical relations and spatial relations. An exhaustive study by Ramaa. S (2000) brings to light the additional issue of multiple languages in India as well as the need for Indian language assessment instruments. An interesting study explored the spelling ability of children in their mother tongue Kannada and the medium of instruction English, it found that though Kannada was a transparent script, children committed errors possibly due to the complexity of the script and cognitive difficulty of spelling acquisition (Silva & Padakannaya, 2009). There is no treatment for learning disabilities however early identification and remedial intervention can reduce the gap children experience between potential and performance. This places the needs of the child squarely in the educator's hands. If the classroom environment provided the freedom to the child to move about, pursue that activity that is of interest to the child, and allowed creativity in learning all of which Tagore recommended, the child would experience those benefits that Tagore firmly believed led to confidence and ability to face challenges of life.

A BLEND OF WEST AND EAST THROUGH TAGORE

The starting point should well begin with observation and screening. This process is facilitated through a multidisciplinary team consisting of parents, teachers, special educators, psychologists, speech therapists, and all those who are involved in the progress of the child. This multidisciplinary approach leads to a comprehensive evaluation (Silver, 1986). It bears a striking parallel to the holistic approach where the child is seen as a whole and all aspects of the child s development are taken into consideration. In special education in particular the holistic approach will abundantly point the care-givers in the right direction. Through careful consideration of physical health, academic difficulties, individual talents, aptitudes, and strengths, socio-emotional and behavioral concerns a truly individualized educational program can be developed holistically. Burnette (2000) gives comprehensive multidisciplinary guidelines for culturally and linguistically diverse child screening where the focus is on determining whether the difficulties are arising from cultural or linguistic factors among other factors and deciding which language the child will be assessed in as well as compiling information from all aspects of the child's environment. This falls in line with Tagore's philosophy that the child should be the center of the education process.

Some of the valid aspects of the holistic approach are experiential learning and learning in one's language rather than a new language. This is especially true of children with learning disabilities who characteristically have difficulties acquiring a second language much less study in it or think in it. When it is suspected that a child is having difficulty learning, an important criterion when screening and assessing is to check if the child is comfortable in the mother tongue or language spoken at home before concluding that the child does indeed have a learning disability as per formal guidelines. It is well-researched that students suffer from a lag in academics due to English being a second language and efforts are necessary to make the learning an integrated experience accommodating a multilingual environment, motivating the student, creating a safe feeling, small class size, and many other steps which would increase second language acquisition as well as factors like family background (Raja & Selvi, 2011).

THE HOLISTIC APPROACH OF NEP FROM AUROBINDO

Aurobindo Ghosh philosopher of the twentieth century, well known for his principles of education has given a rich holistic approach to teaching the child. He wanted education to be child-centered according to his aptitude and capability. An analysis by Rani (2017) clearly summarizes the importance he stressed on teaching through discovery, the importance of cultivating observation, teaching as well as learning in the mother tongue and he expounded that if the child were encouraged to pursue individual interests it would lead to mental as well as spiritual development. He believed that the child was at the center of the education process while the teacher was the guide, not imposing upon the child but rather leading the child through the process of learning. His writings inspire the teacher to bring out the best in the child so that there will be holistic development. His ideas of integralism in education (Choudhary, 1953) focus on seeing the child in wholeness. This approach if looked at in the field of special education will greatly reduce the present divide between education and practical living. A child who is trained to do math in class but who cannot use money in practical daily living is suffering from a lack of all aspects of development being integrated. In his approach spiritual development was important in child development and he gave equal importance to knowledge and wisdom, love and compassion as well as action. Shirazi (2011) has presented an account of the principles originally given according to the philosophy of Aurobindo Ghosh expounded by Choudhary which explains the need for integral or holistic education as a responsibility of teachers to develop a curriculum that includes physical, cognitive-pragmatic-vocational, instinctual-emotional, socio-ethical and religious-mystical-humanistic aspects of development in a child. When viewed from a special education angle it can be understood that intervention as part of the therapeutic or healing process needs to draw out from the child an individual latent talent and thereby live in harmony as an integral being according to each one's environment rather than be a product of the world. When this philosophy is applied to each child, the child with learning disorders is accepted and nurtured according to individual strengths and aptitudes. The pressures of a rigid educational system can be replaced with a system of assessment that is criterion based rather than norm-based with the teacher being a helper and guide not a taskmaster. In recognizing the value of Aurobindo Ghosh's philosophy the latest reforms in education in India have been formulated to incorporate multimodality in learning, which is beneficial not just for children with learning difficulties but for every child as a unique human being. These reforms have culminated in the New Education Policy (2020) which aims at the development of knowledge, skills, creativity, moral values, character, and many other aspects which contribute to holistic development. Intervention includes hands-on learning, skill-based learning, opportunity to learn in the mother tongue, flexibility and range of subjects, freedom to teachers to bring out the best in the students, and many more solutions for the benefit of every child (Kumar, Prakash & Singh, 2020). The NEP 2020 with its basis in the philosophy of Aurobindo Ghosh has hope and value for children with special needs. Children who are differently abled or who have learning disorders and who are recognized as neurodiverse face the following challenges in the traditional classroom:

- lack of experiential learning
- lack of individuality
- one size fits all approach in a mixed-ability class or lack of differentiated teaching
- ignoring children with learning handicaps and other handicaps

Zaki (2022) has presented the relevance of Aurobindho's philosophy to NEP 2022 in a concise manner extolling the links, benefits, and applications of his philosophy to education. The study highlights the focus on an India-centric education by giving importance to the medium of instruction as to the child's mother tongue and regional language to build imagination, use of biographies and interesting books to inspire children from true events, and enabling life skills from experiential learning. His philosophy covers all areas of development to which the NEP 2022 aspires. In special education approach the implementation of the NEP 2022 would apply in the following ways:

- substituting rigid curriculum with flexible curriculum according to strengths and needs of the learner. It aims at an inclusive classroom where all children benefit.
- viewing diversity holistically rather than as a deficit.
- barrier-free access to all children with disabilities implies not just ramps and Braille books but also language-appropriate teaching materials, technology, and assistive equipment appropriate to the child's needs.
- teachers will be trained to identify learning disabilities.

ANALYSIS OF THE NEP FRAMEWORK

While the educational system has remained unchanged for too long and rest of the world has taken huge strides, finally India has emerged with a seemingly comprehensive educational policy that is holistic in nature. If one looks at the new framework from a bird's eye view it is apparent that the pros are many. Some of the benefits are:

- Choice of subjects in high school allows for specialization in areas of interest and aptitude.
- Option of vocational training based subjects recognizes creative talents and multiple intelligences.
- Reduction in volume of curriculum and emphasis on core knowledge.
- Child can opt for mother tongue as medium of instruction.
- Multidisciplinary flexibility allows for broad based education.
- Inclusive education provision has been highlighted.
- Development is aimed at intellectual, creative and social and life skills which is a holistic approach.
- Teacher training will now shift focus from only teaching and imparting knowledge, to tracking true student learning.

Overall it appears that the new framework does not rely on rote learning but rather on individual interests, experiential learning and socio-emotional development. There are a few drawbacks which deserve to be mentioned. They are:

- It is theoretically strong however clarity is needed on implementation at the policy, pedagogical and managerial level.
- Specifics like who will be considered qualified to teach vocational based subjects, in what way will teacher training improve and how can assessments be done in a holistic manner are a concern.

Banerjee et al (2021) have provided an insightful analysis highlighting identification of educational stages in a child's life, the power of language through multilinguism and pedagogical issues like focus on discussion, presentation, debate and multidisciplinary thinking. Kumar & Singh (2022) also bring to the fore some concerns as well as support systems to be incorporated for NEP related to special needs to be successful. They bring attention to the lack of guidelines as to how the curriculum will be modified to include all, the link between disability and poverty, the lack of financial resources allocated by the government, and the social as well as emotional aspects that have to be considered in the case of special needs children and many other related important aspects that should be dwelt on before implementing it. Some of the recommendations are:

- Scribes for children with learning disabilities
- Counselors to support students
- Remedial teaching for children with learning disabilities

All in all at the heart of the intent is the holistic development of the child, not just the child with special needs but every child. There are linked concerns such as the sociopolitical aspects of the family and community from which arise discrimination, bias, and superstition. India being a country that attaches deep value to society and its support either through familial or community recognition places the family with a special needs child in a difficult spot. Whatever the factor at blame whether it is belief, superstition, or pride, at the end of the day all this has to be kept aside and the focus has to be on going forward and keeping the progress of the child as the goal. This is easier said than done. Very often though teachers or special educators alert a parent on certain lags in the child, parents prefer to turn a blind eye for as long as possible, many times till it is too late, past the crucial window of learning age for specific skills. It is important to understand the basis for this before choosing a workable interventional approach. Many socio-cultural factors affect the efficiency of screening and providing intervention such as language, religion, status, etc. as well as demographic factors like gender, age, region, culture, etc. Amidst an educational scenario of diversity in ethnicity, linguistically, culturally as well as socioeconomically it is challenging to appeal to the parent to lay aside these social and psychological pressures to plan the appropriate development for the child by focusing on the learning diversity or neurodiverse elements within the child. There are many obstacles to be overcome before inclusive education can become a reality and one of them is the social obstacle, where the support of the family is the starting point. A detailed paper by Singhal (2009) helps to understand the scenario with clarity. There is low enrolment of children with disabilities in education, and a combination of structural factors like caste, gender, and poverty when intersecting with a disability is overwhelming, though many efforts have been made progress is slow, diversity or difference being seen as undesirable leading to stigma and thereby marginalization from the mainstream. The case of India being steeped in social pressures particularly reflects in its effects on the child with disabilities. Taking the case of children with learning disabilities it is seen that parents know there is a problem but delay seeking help, withdraw from societal interaction, and experience anxiety about the future.

There is a tendency to view people with disabilities negatively. One of the biggest challenges people with disabilities face is social prejudice. Negative attitudes develop in a social context reflecting the hard and heartless face of society, where children with disabilities, as well as their parents, experience either subtly or openly both in school as well as in the community. Over a period of time, children with disabilities internalize this negativity and experience a lack of confidence due to low self-esteem. If attitudes are learned responses then there is hope that attitudes can be changed, however long it may take. The socio-religious attitudes in India are rooted in myths, legends, and folklore causing a greater challenge than the environmental challenges faced by the differently abled. Children with disabilities experience rejection at young ages; they also sense shame and dejection in their parents and segregation from the larger society. Several studies have documented the prevalence of negative attitudes, stigma, and discrimination against those with disabilities. Norwicki & Sandieson (2002) found that children preferred children without disabilities; Paterson (2000) found attitudes to be negative towards those with a visual impairment, Mathias et al (2018) found the prevalence of social distance and Siperstein et al (2004) concluded that inclusion in India is hampered by attitudinal barriers. In moving towards change Dalal (2006) explains clearly how the focus needs to be on an attention shift from disabilities to abilities, changing societal mindset is possible through community-based rehabilitation projects where role reversal such as children with disabilities are involved in helping collect funds for flood victims, breaking mental barriers that disability is related to destiny by identifying strengths to make them economically independent and opening of integrated schools to help break prejudices and provide a community forum. The outcomes indicated positive change.

Another consequence of social stigma is the reluctance to seek help. Parents are often ashamed to ask for help lest their families hear of it. They hesitate to shift the child to a special school where the child would truly learn and would rather the child remain in a classroom that is not suited in terms of skill level and readiness level.

Apart from societal mindset, there are some psychological co-morbidities that children with learning disabilities experience which further strengthen the case for a holistic approach. In addition to remedial teaching, such children need their emotional and behavioral needs addressed. Sahoo et al (2015) gives a detailed study of this. The concern is that 30% of children with learning disabilities suffer from behavioral and emotional problems like attention deficit hyperactivity disorder, and anxiety; they are victims of bullying and suffer from depression. The recommendations are for a comprehensive holistic approach to treatment. The conclusion is that including mental health in general health care as well as networking between all those involved with the child i.e. parent, doctor, teacher, and other service providers like speech therapist is essential.

NEP, 2020 holds hope in addressing the socio-emotional needs of every child. It recognizes the social and educational barriers children face. It has created a representation of those who have been hitherto unrepresented under the grouping of SEDG (Socio Economically Disadvantaged Groups) thereby moving from exclusion to inclusion. It aims to train teachers in learning disabilities, conscious steps to include students in community participation, and develop values through learning about Indian culture.

CULTURAL CONTEXTUAL RELEVANCE OF GANDHIAN PHILOSOPHY

If the holistic approach is considered it will provide a framework to understand the odds a child with special needs faces. Currently, only academic performance is analyzed and suitable remedial teaching is recommended while talents, aptitude, inhibitions, trauma, and language barriers are ignored. The school system is rigid requiring competitive levels of written work and preventing alternate methods of testing like oral tests or the assistance of a scribe. There is a lack of awareness of the socio-behavioral impact of learning disorders and a tendency to reject, ostracize and bully such children as well as a poor understanding of behavioral management within the classroom. Without a school pass certificate job opportunities are bleak and skill development opportunity is low. It is like a vicious cycle that the child is unable to break out of. Only if society changes its approach and starts analyzing what the child can do instead of what all the child cannot do will a new viewing lead to tapping the strengths of the child rather than only rectifying the weakness. This approach was explained by Gandhi who provided a model of education that is suited for the modern world. He had a vision of integration between child and community such that all school learning would serve a higher purpose of serving society. His philosophy is that the purpose of education is for the upliftment of society and education is an all-around development of a person. Education should not only cater to economic needs but should also cultivate values. He believed in vocational training and the dignity of labor. He valued handicrafts and viewed it as a productive work that resulted in intellectual development. His final aim was harmony between mind, body, and spirit.

To him, education was not just literacy but also character-building. The main focus of his educational philosophy was free and compulsory basic education which would alleviate gender, poverty, caste, and language barriers. He also emphasized handicraft education to develop the value of productive work, the dignity of labor, self-sufficiency, etc.

His philosophy and application have been summarized by Mahakul (2020) as a correlation between environment, craft, and other subjects. By bringing out the talents of the child, various dimensions like psychological, sociological, and economic will develop a personality in totality.

Bala (2005) has linked the Gandhian concept of education to the need of present-day challenges, studying various committee and commission reports based on his philosophy that recommend vocational education to quell youth unrest due to unemployment.

Gandhian philosophy of education tackles ground realities in the present age. The main difficulty faced by neurodiverse children is that they are not recognized as individuals with unique brain functioning. Often their behavioral challenges are negatively labeled and pose further risks of stigma and isolation. A holistic view of the child through early screening would quickly identify children at risk for learning disabilities, enable special educators to intervene and this would pave the way to inculcate vocational and life skills in a timely manner. Some of the challenges faced by children with learning disabilities are:

- these children are intelligent and creative, they are not able to learn in a typical way, however, they do not receive any accommodations in the classroom like step-by-step instructions or reduced homework load.
- they exhibit behavioral and emotional adjustment problems due to frustration, low academic performance, and low self-concept.
- traditionally the common classroom is time pressured and syllabus driven leaving the child with learning difficulties trailing behind with incomplete notes and unable to catch up.
- their other nonacademic skills are often not recognized. They are not exposed to vocational skills and are unprepared for life after school.

The heterogeneous nature of learning disorders serves as a basis for taking into account all aspects of each child in a holistic manner to truly help them. The benefits of early and holistic intervention could prevent later deep learning difficulties. There is adequate research to support early phonemic awareness building, it has demonstrated effectiveness in identifying children when they are very young, developing reading skills as well as enhancing cognitive and metacognitive skills (Ehri et al, 2001). Metacognitive skills like directing oneself to learn or applying strategies that suit one's style of learning are low in children with learning difficulties, often they are unable to know how to improve their memory or adjust their speed to fit a particular quantity of work. It is here that a supportive environment can bring to their attention ways to be more self-aware and regulate their cognitive processes more efficiently.

Gandhian philosophy of education steps in here to provide scaffolding through the child's inner circle of parents and teachers, who impart not fragmented knowledge, but true learning by building self-awareness in the child through works that are in harmony with the child's level of development and learning ability. Knowledge was supposed to come from experimentation, experience, and gradual growth in complex thinking. His idea of a craft-centered education focuses on the child's true aptitude, skills, and level of knowledge which suits the child with learning problems in particular as they have unique talents that are not tapped into at school.

With a balanced view it is good to keep in mind some contemporary philosophies that are relevant in the educational system such as Montessori method which is a child-focused approach given by Maria Montessori of Italy who believed in fostering self-motivated learning and learning should revolve around the child's natural interests (Gutek, 2004). A contemporary philosophy gaining ground is the Science of Living or Jeevan Vigyan ("Values education," 2023) which emphasizes a combination of health, values, emotional and spiritual education to create balanced individuals who remain in touch with their inner being.

TAKING THEORY TO PRACTICE

The theoretical framework allows for the creating or aligning of thought with action. When looking at the three greats of Indian philosophy in education Tagore, Gandhi, and Aurobindo what emerges in common are sensitivity to diversity, equality, and harmony. Tagore aspired for self-realization through education while Gandhi emphasized the complete development of the child through noncasteism in society. Both Tagore and Gandhi believed that school should be an environment rich in experience and creativity, learning and thinking are best in the mother tongue and self-discipline was preferred to harsh imposed discipline. Tagore emphasized nature while Gandhi emphasized craft. Both loved Indian culture however Tagore had a wide view of bringing harmony between East and West by appreciation of all cultures while Gandhi emphasized the role and importance of community in the development of the child. Aurobindo aimed at developing consciousness within the child through imparting holistic teaching which included both body and mind and a universal culture to inculcate values.

Overall the role of Indian educational philosophy is reflected in the psychological principles of self-realization as personality development, acceptance of diversity as extending to neurotypical children as well as neurodiverse children, the naturalism of learning by doing supports experiential learning and differentiated teaching, teacher as guide upholds curriculum modification and curriculum adaptation to suit each child and skill-based, craft-based learning forms the basis for vocational training and acquiring knowledge through the senses gives weightage to the multisensory method of teaching.

Applying these psychological methods through a holistic window changes the view and presents different goals, curricula, and evaluation priorities. For the child with learning difficulties, the focus shifts from academic performance to overall development. The idea of implementing or choosing holistic education is currently rapidly gaining ground. Fullan (2015) has over the recent years been analyzing at length the need, possibility, and changes for a holistic overall view of the educational system through decision-making at the local school community level to the state level and national level. Recently there has been an attempt to introduce new elements to the educational system in Delhi aiming at holistic development through the Happiness Curriculum and many positive changes were observed through mindfulness, critical thinking, and socio-emotional building (Khanna & Peterson, 2023).

There is a convincing need for learning to overlap with other constructs like cognitive, social, emotional, and linked developments. The main dimensions of the holistic approach are:

- Intellectual
- Emotional

- Social
- Physical
- Cultural
- Moral Spiritual

For the child with learning needs each dimension further develops into further related issues.

Intellectual: To teach effectively and ensure intellectual development the instructional component has to meet the comprehension and communication needs of the child. This calls for curriculum modification which enables parts of a chapter or syllabus to be altered in terms of length, complexity, and presentation. It also entails curriculum adaptation which refers to how the lesson needs to be suited to the child's learning ability or style. This requires freedom for the teacher to decide how to rework the chapter content.

Emotional: When viewed through the holistic perspective the emotional dimension includes establishing emotional stability and building emotional intelligence. For the child with learning difficulties emotional wellbeing is yet another area of challenge and requires encouraging of self -awareness and building of confidence through a supportive environment. Some of the signs that a child is struggling with emotionally could be avoidance behavior like wanting to go out of the class on some pretext or the other, anxiety symptoms like fidgeting with hair or bed wetting, physical symptoms like headaches, stomach aches, as well as low self-esteem and low resilience from being constantly misunderstood.

Physical: The physical dimension places importance on outdoor activities to enhance physical well-being like sports and other recreational activities amidst nature so that children can experience freedom of space, explore, play creatively, learn team spirit, and improve focus and coordination among many other valuable learning.

Cultural: In India the cultural scenario is the background of every child. If used positively to share and build cultural acceptance this could be a rather than a barrier in the educational setup. Every child comes embedded with a social system that is unique in terms of language, regional, traditional, and socioeconomic experiences. When this is taken into consideration rather than being shut out of the curriculum, it places the child in a comfort zone that will support learning.

Moral Spiritual: With the ideals of holistic development comes the issue of building morality in children. Through the school, it is possible to build conscience and increase consciousness thereby leading to values like compassion, honesty, and sincere work which create a foundation so that the child can face challenges as the child grows. Self-realization and metacognitive understanding contribute to well-being in a person who is not seen as only an individual but rather a member of society that aims to live in harmony. For the child with learning difficulties, the moral sphere is complex wherein they are judged as lazy and dull though often they put in double the time and effort to achieve what comes easily to others. However if established with the aim of holism then morality is seamlessly connected to all other areas enabling the child to value self, and others to value the child with a disability. Morality leads to spirituality and in India, this is a part of the ethos and way of life.

PRACTICAL APPLICATION OF SPECIAL EDUCATION TECHNIQUES

The holistic resource room where children with learning disabilities are trained is an environment rich in visuals, teaching aids, teacher prepared worksheets, student specific individualized worksheets, word walls and other language rich exposures. The whole process needs to be carefully understood at the practical level. It is a process of moving from conscious learning to unconscious learning. Knowledge, experience and comprehension go hand in hand in the learning process. The teacher is a facilitator providing the stimulus and allowing the student to spontaneously respond. The teacher's supporting role extends to nudging the thought processes to a higher level, gradually building vocabulary, gently assisting the student in sentence formation and leading the student to a level of confidence. The resource teacher has drawn up a professional individualized educational plan which forms the basis for the lesson plan of the day. Several goals may be accomplished without the student or any observer realizing it. For example through showing a picture, goals of expressive language like naming, giving the function of an object, identifying verbs, forming a phrase or sentence, building visual memory, visual association and countless other goals can be accomplished. The atmosphere is usually light, the special educator is calm, joyful, enthusiastic, affectionate and encouraging. Children look forward to these learning sessions, they know it is a space where they are accepted, they realize their potential is being tapped and often through feedback they understand and recognize their progress. The underlying approach is to establish a web of mindmaps where concepts, applications, subjects and fluidity of understanding begins to form. This prevents gaps in knowledge. Holistic approach provides for integration and linking of constructs rather than a rigid subject based division of knowledge. Goal setting in holistic education involves linking a goal to multiple areas. A simple example could be that of spelling development which is traditionally seen as the responsibility of the English teacher or the language teacher, but in the holistic approach the teachers assist the student in learning spelling whatever be the subject. Therefore the teacher discussing science concepts would also help the student identify difficult words in the chapter, guide the student through specific spelling techniques and keep spelling improvement as one of the goals, wherein the content or material are science based words. This may be unheard of in traditional learning systems, however for holistic approach in the seamless merging of knowledge lies true learning.

It is relevant to take into consideration the pragmatic aspects of holistic approach one of which is teacher preparedness. In India most teachers are not trained in special education as it has hitherto been a specialized area of education. A study by Das, Kuyini & Desai (2023) found nearly 70% of the regular school teachers in Delhi had neither received special education training as well as lacked experience with such children, 87% of the teachers lacked support systems in their classrooms and finally the primary school teachers felt inadequate to cope with students who might have disabilities. It is of paramount importance to train the trainer as teacher preparedness is vital. This has a direct effect on the progression of learning in each child. Apart from teacher preparedness other practical aspects relate to infrastructure like mandatory equipment, teacher-student ratio, safety and security issues, identification and provisions for gifted children and a host of other practicalities that will emerge as and when the steps begin to be implemented.

CURRENT IMPLEMENTATION

Currently in India there is a scheme of Integrated Education for Disabled Children (IEDC) implemented by the Ministry of Human Resource Development's department of Secondary and Higher Education. The objective is to retain special needs children in the school system as well as to integrate children from special schools back into mainstream education. A three-member assessment team consisting of a doctor, psychologist and special educator recommend if a child is eligible to be enrolled in school through this scheme. This holistic approach is beneficial to the child's progress. Another successful endeavor that is holistic in approach is the National Institute of Open Schooling (NIOS) an autonomous institution under ministry of education, Government of India, which offers schooling, as well as vocational courses allowing a choice from a range of subjects, including programs for individuals with disabilities. It is holistic in nature as it provides a choice for students to choose subjects of their strength, allows students to go at their pace and permits multiple attempts (Andrade, 2008). It recommends techniques like task analysis, peer teaching, cooperative learning, learning corners and multisensory approach. It has no age limit for enrolling.

In India most special schools follow the holistic approach. Education World, a publication which ranks schools, regularly presents rankings of special schools, which can serve as a guide for parents. These special schools and schools with resource rooms are currently implementing holistic approach as the aim of the remedial program is not just academic training but all round development. In special education the following plan process could be considered:

All of the above would be a balance between academics, remedial training as well as socio-emotional and behavioural modification, thereby ensuring cognitive skills like problem solving and thinking are systematically established alongside with other brain functions like attention, sitting tolerance, emotional self -regulation, creativity, speech and communication etc.

Figure 1. Flowchart of specific implementation plan process

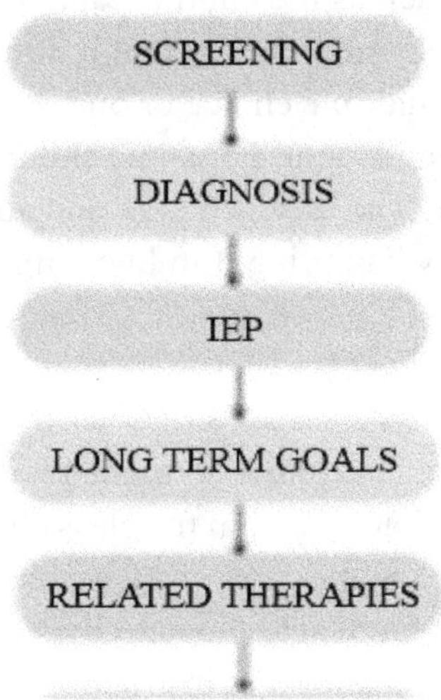

SCREENING AND ASSESSMENT ADAPTATIONS

The purpose of examining the holistic narrative is to identify crucial areas where new perspectives can be considered. Some questions to ponder over are:

Can screening tools be developed for Indian children that are suitable in terms of cultural and experiential context?

In present times westernized tools are yielding results that are limited in terms of being inclusive of understanding holistic aspects of the child such as family background, socioeconomic background, and many other dimensions such as medium of instruction being a challenge and content of testing material culturally unfamiliar. If the flexibility to alter the content is permissible then words that are familiar to the child can be substituted for words that are unfamiliar such as mud instead of snow, pot instead of mug, cap instead of hat etc.

Can teachers be trained in special education as part of regular teacher training?

It is difficult to fathom why teacher education excludes basics of child development like developmental milestones, at-risk factors, early identification, the prevalence of handicaps, common developmental issues, screening at kindergarten, etc. If every teacher were familiar with the alarm bells children would receive help early and thereby save severe handicaps like not picking up reading or language. Referring a silent or stammering child to a speech therapist for example can reduce the symptoms as well as avoid escalation of the condition.

Can teachers be given flexibility in altering the lesson in terms of quantity or complexity depending on the capability of the child?

Often the lesson is designed for a child of full capacity who can compete with others and maximize self-potential. Most often the lesson is not considered in light of children who cannot keep up with the high achievers. If the lesson could be designed to contain at least three levels, then the teacher can allow flexibility for the child to do as much as the child is capable of whatever the level. Those who are struggling can stop at the simplest level where the content is summarized and only direct questions are framed. Also, the questions will be of multiple choice or one-word answers to ascertain if the child has picked up the basics of the concept being taught. For some children, the middle level may suit while for the rest the complete lesson is possible. The idea is that lesson adaptation and modification will reduce the pressure of quantity and complexity and bring it in line with the comfort level of the child.

Can classroom instruction be differentiated?

This implies that children within a class cannot be treated with a one size fits all approach. Though the content is planned for each grade suitably, within the class children learn differently, in other words, differentiated teaching will benefit all. Some areas which children with learning disabilities require differential teaching is the method used to teach, the activities done to learn and the personal requirements of the child such as extra time or repetition of instructions and environment in the classroom such as allowing a child to walk about and learn if the child cannot sit still for long periods. Differentiated teaching requires grouping of children according to ability so that they are comfortable in their group in terms of the pace of work, level of work, etc. A child's learning can be assessed through differentiated application of the content in order to ascertain mastery of it.

Can teaching be multimodal?

Multimodal refers to the use of all the senses. When a lesson is taught it should be presented visually, accompanied by an auditory explanation and some kind of related activity that would allow for the use of tactile and kinesthetic senses or even olfactory senses. When multiple modes are used to deliver content the learning experience is more effective. This is particularly relevant to children with learning disorders as they tend to be stronger in one sense more than the other senses, for example, a visual learner will struggle to grasp a verbal explanation given by the teacher and an auditory learner will get lost in the notes given visually. A multi-sensorial approach to teaching holds great scope. The advantage is that it benefits children who are identified as well as those who are not identified. It supports diverse learning needs and through this method the rigor of the lesson can be broken down and made manageable for every child. When children are offered choice of modality, learning conditions are more suited to individual needs. Thus a visual learner is offered graphics, an auditory learner needs to hear the content, and the kinesthetic learner gets an opportunity to learn in a hands-on manner. This requires supplementing the curricula with a variety of activities that target different modalities.

Can assessment instruments be developed in regional languages?

This is a glaring gap that is present in India as far as the assessment of children is concerned. Usage of Western material has been the practice and though it gives a fairly clear diagnosis and prognosis, the ease of the child has not been taken into consideration and the results would be fully valid if conducted in the language choice of the child. Often the child cannot follow the instruction or the task may be unfamiliar like rhyming words. It could lead to a complicated picture where the child is learning spelling by rote and unable to read the same words or children were proficient in skills taught in class such as letter naming but low in knowledge of phonological awareness for reading and spelling of new words. (Silva &Padakannaya, 2009). Two excellent Indian assessment tools NIMHANS Index for Specific Learning Disability (Kapur et al, 1991) and Grade Level Assessment Device (Narayan, 1997) are currently serving an excellent purpose however they are in English and based on Western tests. The Sarva Shiksha Abhiyan (2011) program aims at the universalization of primary education through improved curriculum, educational planning, and management. It provides classroom teachers with informal screening checklists that have been of great help to the teachers. When assessment as well as teaching is done in regional languages, using regional vocabulary will reinforce learning that is comprehension-based.

PSYCHOLOGICAL INTERVENTIONS

Four major models have guided interventions in learning disabilities, the medical approach which traces the etiology of learning disorders, the developmental model which focuses on stages of development in childhood and maturation, the educational model gives importance to diagnosis and remediation and the behavioral model looks into environmental adaptations to alleviate symptoms. However they do not come together or converge as a complete approach, as each has its own approach and limitations. Kirk and Kirk (1971) have given three approaches to remediation which on closer look go well with the holistic approach. They are training of deficient areas, using areas of strength and use of multisensory methods. Practically this translates into utilizing strengths to compensate for weak skills as well as to gradually build up weak areas. Use of multisensory approaches refers to enabling a child who is visually highly perceptive to learning through the visual mode such as presenting teaching aids that are colorful and high in clarity of text or presenting information verbally to a child who prefers auditory mode of learning. Similarly a child who cannot write letters could be taught through tracing in a sand tray so that the tactile stimulation of the sequence of movements is neurologically impressed upon the memory through the brain. These are some of the interesting and fascinating psychological interventions that can be used in the holistic approach.

CONCLUSION

After due analysis of the historical wisdom of educating a child holistically and the current scenario of challenges under the present methods, keeping in mind, especially the child with learning disorders, it is evident that combining all aspects of holistic education will surely benefit the growing child. When the spiritual moral element is brought into focus it will contribute to improvement in metacognitive skills and metamemory skills like gathering relevant information, knowing how much is understood, realizing what has not been comprehended, and devising strategies to support the brain in improving itself. The

Figure 2. Multimodal team

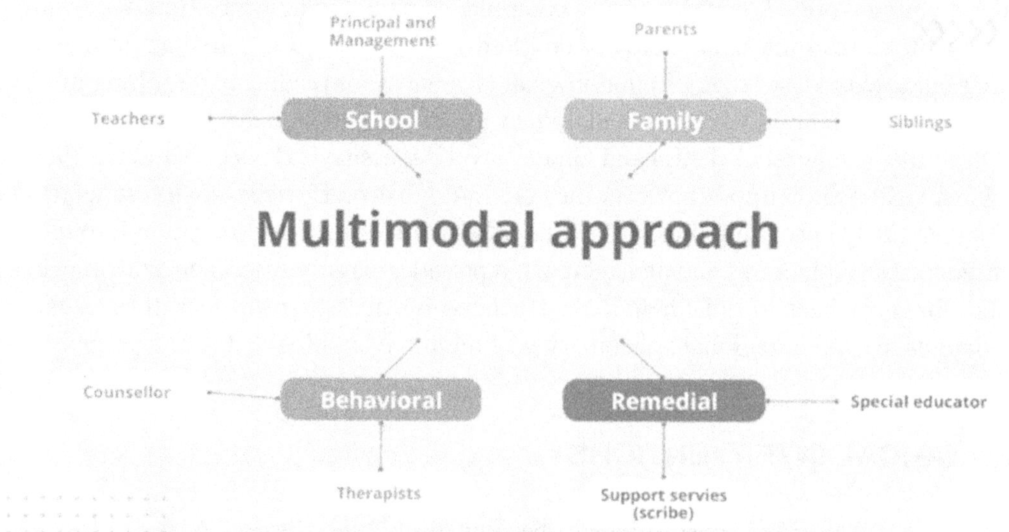

Gandhian approach of Basic Education centered on holistic understanding and development of the child as a member of the community. This approach is aligned with the special educational goal of inclusion. Aurobindo's goals of nurturing latent potential in harmony with the environment or being an integral human being again point in the direction of holistic development. Tagore aspired for inner freedom and inner enlightenment which was through developing moral and spiritual aspects in the child. The Indian philosophy of education revolves around the acceptance of all. This value resonates in special education as seen in the report by UNESCO (2020) which states that inclusive education is justified not just from an educational point and economic point but there is also a social justification that will result in changed attitudes and non-discriminatory society. It also identifies the crucial role of teachers and recognizes that inclusive practices will lead to improved teaching, quality curriculum, ongoing assessments, and flexibility in teaching because of learners' needs.

Intervention to be Multimodal and Multispecialty

A multimodal approach to teaching engages multiple senses to promote a greater understanding of the concept. Using visual, aural, kinesthetic, and tactile senses allows each child to perceive and store information in their brain the way it works best for them. This promotes a positive learning environment and prevents children from feeling overwhelmed because learning is in only one mode and that mode may not suit them. Different learning formats keep students interest activated. This approach is in line with the Indian philosophy of nurturing the child in a stimulating environment and allowing the child to pursue and develop talents that require multiple usages of senses. This supports the holistic perspective which prepares a child with life skills and vocational skills.

When speaking of multimodal, multispecialty goes hand in hand. An individualized educational program (United States, 2011) is a document that guides the long term development of a child with special needs. It is written by a team that ideally should consist of specialists from all the fields related to the child's development. It should include the teacher, educational administrator, special educator, parent, speech/occupational therapist, counselor, pediatrician, and any other service provider to the child. The goals for the child's progress are planned such that a consensus criterion for the management of the child is established. Regional adaptations like training in the mother tongue are recommended to best achieve maximum potential which the holistic approach advocates.

Through the holistic process of school as a community, experiential learning, self-awareness, and self-guided learning integrated support can be extended to every child. The interdisciplinary value of holistic education will contribute to overall cognitive growth. At the macro level, this chapter aims at fostering awareness for change at the policy level whereby inclusion in schools will truly bring out the holistic fullness including spiritual harmony as well as other latent potentials in every child within the Indian context. At the micro level, it is hoped that understanding that the child's daily challenges can be understood and met through holistic assessment, intervention, holistic pedagogical practices, and utilizing special education interventions in the educational community for the best educational outcome.

REFERENCES

American Psychiatric Association. (2013). *Diagnostic and Statistical Manual of Mental Disorders* (5th ed.). American Psychiatric Association Publishing., DSM-5.

Andrade, C. (2008). The National Institute of Open Schooling. *Indian Journal of Psychiatry, 50*(3), 227–228. doi:10.4103/0019-5545.43618 PMID:19742229

Andrews, C. F. (1938). An open-air school. *Visva-Bharati News. Bulletin*, 1930.

Bala, S. (2005). Gandhian conception of education – It's relevance in present times. *Indian Journal of Poultry Science, 66*(3), 531–548.

Banerjee, N., Das, A., & Ghosh, M. S. (2021). National Educational Policy (2020): A critical analysis. *Towards Excellence*, 13(3).

Burnette, J. (2000). *Assessment of culturally and linguistically diverse students for special education eligibility* (Report No. EDO-EC-00–13). Arlington, VA: ERIC Clearinghouse on Disabilities and Gifted Education. (ERIC Document Reproduction Service No. ED449637)

Chacko, D., & Vidhukumar, K. (2020). The Prevalence of Specific Learning Disorder among School-going Children in Ernakulam District, Kerala, India: Ernakulam Learning Disorder (ELD) Study. *Indian Journal of Psychological Medicine, 42*(3), 250–255. doi:10.4103/IJPSYM.IJPSYM_199_19 PMID:32612329

Chaudhuri, H. (1953). The Integralism of Sri Aurobindo. *Philosophy East & West, 3*(2), 131–136. doi:10.2307/1397259

Dalal, A. K. (2006). Social interventions to moderate discriminatory attitudes: The case of the physically challenged in India. *Psychology Health and Medicine, 11*(3), 374–382. doi:10.1080/13548500600595392 PMID:17130074

Das, Ajay, & Kuyini, Ahmed Bawa & Desai. (2013). Inclusive Education in India: Are the Teachers Prepared? *International Journal of Special Education*, 28.

Ehri, L. C., Nunes, S. R., Willows, D. M., Schuster, B. V., Yaghoub-Zadeh, Z., & Shanahan, T. (2001). Phonemic awareness instruction helps children learn to read: Evidence from the National Reading Panel's meta-analysis. *Reading Research Quarterly, 36*(3), 250–287. doi:10.1598/RRQ.36.3.2

Fullan, M. (2015). The new meaning of educational change. Teachers college press.

Goswamee, G., & Saikia, R. (2017). A study on the educational philosophy of Rabindranath Tagore and its influence on elementary education with special reference to Assam. *The Clarion- International Multidisciplinary Journal, 6*, 71-74.

Gutek, G. (2004). *The Montessori Method: The Origins of an Educational Innovation: Including an Abridged and Annotated Edition of Maria Montessori's The Montessori Method.* Rowman & Littlefield Publishers, Inc.

India's most respected special schools 2022-2023. (2022, October). Education World. https://www.educationworld.in/indias-most-respected-special-needs-schools-2022-2023/

Kapur, M., John, A., Rozario, J., & Oommen, A. (1991) NIMHANS Index for Specific Learning Disabilities. Department of Clinical Psychology, NIMHANS Publication, Bangalore.

Khanna, D., & Peterson, A. (2023). *State-led education reform in Delhi, India, A case study of the Happiness Curriculum*. Brookings Institution. https://policycommons.net/artifacts/4139426/state-led-education-reform-in-delhi-india-a-case-study-of-the-happiness-curriculum/4948375/

Kirk, S. A., & Kirk, W. D. (1971). *Psycholinguistic learning disabilities: Diagnosis and remediation*. University of Illinois Press.

Kumar, D., & Singh, D. (2022). India's New Education Policy (NEP) 2020 Creating Children with Disability. *International Journal of Advanced Research in Science. Tongxin Jishu*, •••, 70–74.

Kumar, K., Prakash, A., & Singh, K. (2020). How National Education Policy 2020 can be a lodestar to transform future generation in India. *Journal of Public Affairs*, *21*(3), e2500. Advance online publication. doi:10.1002/pa.2500

Lal, S. (1984). Rabindranāth Tagore's Ideals of Aesthetic Education. *Journal of Aesthetic Education*, *18*(2), 31–39. doi:10.2307/3332497

Mahakul, B. K. (2020). Mahatma Gandhi's vision on education: its relevance in the 21st century. *International Journal of Creative Research Thoughts (IJCRT)*, *8*(2,).

Mathias, K., Kermode, M., Goicolea, I., Seefeldt, L., Shidhaye, R., & San Sebastian, M. (2018). Social Distance and Community Attitudes Towards People with Psycho-Social Disabilities in Uttarakhand, India. *Community Mental Health Journal*, *54*(3), 343–353. doi:10.100710597-017-0211-y PMID:29143156

Mishra, Sreetama. (2014). Some Reflections on Pedagogy: In the Light of Paulo Freire and Rabindranath Tagore. *Indian Journal of Applied Research*, *4*(1).

Narayan J. (1997). *Grade Level Assessment Device for Children with Learning Problems in Schools (GLAD)*. Secunderabad: National Institute for the Mentally Handicapped (NIMH).

National Education Policy. (2020) *NEP Final*. NEP. https://www.education.gov.in/sites/upload_files/mhrd/files/NEP_Final_English_0.pdf

Nowicki, E. A., & Sandieson, R. (2002). A meta-analysis of school-age children's attitudes towards persons with physical or intellectual disabilities. *International Journal of Disability Development and Education*, *49*(3), 243–265. doi:10.1080/1034912022000007270

O'Connell, K. M. (2010) Tagore and Education: Creativity, Mutuality and Survival. *Asiatic: IIUM Journal of English Language and Literature*, *4*(1), 65–76. https://journals.iium.edu.my/asiatic/index.php/ajell/article/view/518

Paterson, J. (2000). Workers of south India their attitudes and their education. *Asia Pacific Disability Rehabilitation Journal*, *10*(1), 1–16.

Raja, B., Dharma, & K, Selvi. (2011). Causes of Problems in Learning English as A Second Language as Perceived by Higher Secondary Students. *i-manager's Journal on English Language Teaching*, *1*, 40-45. . doi:10.26634/jelt.1.4.1604

Ramaa, S. (2000). Two decades of research on learning disabilities in India. *Dyslexia (Chichester, England)*, *6*(4), 268–283. doi:10.1002/1099-0909(200010/12)6:4<268::AID-DYS177>3.0.CO;2-A PMID:11129452

Rani, A. (2016). Sri Aurobindo Ghosh's Philosophy of Education. *International Education and Research Journal*, 157–157.

Rani C (2017). A Study of Educational Vision of Aurobindo Ghosh. *International Journal of Indian Psychology*, *5*(1). doi:10.25215/0501.125

Roy, A. G. (2021) Reflection of Tagore's educational thought on his dream school Patha Bhavana, Santiniketan. *International Journal of creative research thoughts-IJCRT*.

Sahoo, M. K., Biswas, H., & Padhy, S. K. (2015). Psychological Co-morbidity in Children with Specific Learning Disorders. *Journal of Family Medicine and Primary Care*, *4*(1), 21–25. doi:10.4103/2249-4863.152243 PMID:25810984

Shirazi, B. A. K. (2011). Integral education: Founding vision and principles. *Integral Review*, *7*(1), 4–10.

Silva, Reena & Padakannaya, P. (2009). Spelling homophonic words in Kannada and English: A cross-linguistic study. *Journal of Psychosomatic Research*, *4*, 183–191.

Silva, R. & Padakannaya, P. (2007). An Analysis of Early Literacy Skills among Indian Children at Lower Kindergarten. *Indian Journal of Applied Linguistics*, *33*(2) p129-140

Silver, L. B. (1986). Learning disabilities. The primary care role in multidisciplinary management. *Postgraduate Medicine*, *79*(8), 285–296. doi:10.1080/00325481.1986.11699438 PMID:3714591

Singal, N. (2009). Education of Children with Disabilities in India. *Postgraduate Medicine*, *79*(8), 285–296. doi:10.1080/00325481.1986.11699438

Siperstein, G. N. Sugumaran, K., Bardon, J., Norins & Parker, R. C. (2004). *Attitudes of the Public in India towards People with Intellectual Disabilities.* University of Massachusetts Boston. https://media.specialolympics.org/soi/files/healthy- athletes/ResearchStudies/India_FullReport.pdf

Suntharesan, V. (2012). Role of Mother Tongue in Teaching English as a Second Language to Tamil Students (Special Reference to Undergraduates of the University of Jaffna, Sri Lanka). *Language in India*, *12*(12).

Tagore, R. (1931). *My Educational Mission*. The Modern Review.

UNESCO. (2020). *Towards inclusion in education: status, trends and challenges: the UNESCO Salamanca Statement 25 years on*. UNESCO.

UNICEF. (2017). Improving Education Participation. Policy and Practice Pointers for Enrolling All Children and Adolescents in School and Preventing Dropout. UNICEF.

World Health Organization. (1993). *The ICD-10 classification of mental and behavioural disorders: Diagnostic criteria for research*. WHO.

Zaki, S. (2022). Relevance of Sri Aurobindo's philosophy of education to national education policy 2020. *International Journal of Health Sciences*, *6*(S3), 9601–9608. doi:10.53730/ijhs.v6nS3.8288

KEY TERMS AND DEFINITIONS

Holistic: All-inclusive support to an individual as a whole for all round development.

Learning Disabilities: Difficulties involving development of academic skills of reading, spelling, writing and math.

Multimodal: Use of varied modes through multiple senses, for learning.

Chapter 8
Interconnections of Yogic Practices With Mental Health

Vaishnavi Agarwal
Christ University, India

Aditi Rastogi
Christ University, India

Anika Tyagi
Christ University, India

K. Sreenath
https://orcid.org/0000-0002-9028-6174
Christ University, India

Ashi Bansal
Patanjali, India

ABSTRACT

Yoga, an ancient practise of humankind, attempts to promote a lifestyle that is free of maliciousness with emphasis on inculcating qualities that would aid the individual in living a life that is truly actualizing. Practise of yoga is not limited to holding specific asanas but various components of yoga such as pranayama, pratyahara, etc.; all attempt to enhance an individual's wellbeing. The chapter has contextualized yoga therapy including pranayama, mudras, and chakras to biopsychosocial models, and attempted to identify yogic practises that bring holistic enhancement. Yoga, being cost-effective, and having no side effects, unlike pharmacological treatments, can be used as an adjunctive therapeutic agent in improving symptoms or improving mood and reducing stress. However, it is important to note the feasibility and limitations of yoga interventions, like proper trained professionals to minimize any ill effects. The chapter attempted to promote the practise of yoga as an adjunctive form of treatment which would thereby aid in improving biopsychosocial wellbeing.

DOI: 10.4018/978-1-6684-9778-4.ch008

INTRODUCTION

Sutra II of Yogic philosophy involves obstructing the patterns that arise within all aspects of consciousness. It goes beyond simply disconnecting from daily external experiences but also requires putting aside the vision experienced during deep meditation and elevated states of Samadhi. As one surpasses the expressions of individual awareness on various planes, the state of yoga emerges. This represents the sequential progression and evolution of one's consciousness.

The literal roots of term "yoga " originates from Sanskrit literature signifying "to join" (Shroff & Asgarpour, 2017). The fundamental concept of this South Asian discipline is the unity of mind and body, as well as the integration of individual and collective identities. All forms of life, according to the philosophy of yoga, are interwoven and unified. Therefore, the existence of Yoga in the world is attributed to the interconnectedness of all the various domains effecting human existence. (Shroff & Asgarpour, 2017).

Yoga, rooted in the Indian tradition, aims to bring joy, freedom from sorrow, mental balance, and peace. Throughout history, seekers of self-realisation, known as rishis or yogis, have utilised yogic practises to restore mind-body equilibrium and enable spiritual realisation (Singh, 2017). Various terms, such as 'Nirvana,' 'Moksha,' and 'Atmasakshaatkar,' describe the ultimate states of human mental health development, converging on the concept of liberation from suffering. In the present era, Yoga is increasingly being embraced as a "healing system" that promotes physical and mental well-being in modern society (Capon et al., 2019). Its popularity is rising in Western countries, with a growing number of people participating in yoga practises. Capon (2019) highlighted that conventional treatments for mental health involve medication and psychotherapy, like cognitive behaviour therapy (CBT). While effective for many, a significant minority struggles to engage with these treatments. Antidepressant efficacy varies, with only half reporting positive experiences. Over half of those with mental health challenges do not seek treatment. As a result, there is growing interest in exploring the potential of Yoga for common mental health disorders. Evidence suggests that Yoga can alleviate symptoms of anxiety, depression, and PTSD through various mechanisms. However, uncertainty remains, and healthcare professionals hesitate to recommend Yoga as a supplementary treatment.

History of Yoga

Yoga, originally practised as a form of healing, is one of the oldest physical and spiritual disciplines in the world (Varambally & Gangadhar, 2016). In India, the science of Yoga originated thousands of years ago, even before the whole belief system was born. The sculptures discovered in the Indus Valley at Harappa and Mohenjo-Daro show deities resembling Lord Shiva and Shakti practising asanas and meditation (Mooventhan, 2020). Mythical beliefs attribute the foundation of Yoga to Shiva, with Parvati serving as his initial student.

The Vedas, the ancient and revered texts of Hinduism, describe the earliest form of Yoga as a reflective practise centred on rituals of sacrifice. Scholars believe that Sanskrit-speaking individuals who settled in the Indus Valley between 1800 and 1500 BCE composed the Vedas (Raghuwanshi, 2011). The Vedas served as guides for performing rituals and sacrifices to enhance various aspects of life.

With the emergence of the Upanishads between 600 and 550 BCE, yogic philosophy underwent a radical transformation. Unlike the instructional nature of the Vedas, the Upanishads delved into profound existential inquiries. They invited students to sit near enlightened teachers and learn their profound wisdom. The Upanishads laid the groundwork for the development of Yoga as we know it today and became the fundamental wisdom of various yoga traditions.

Concurrently, the sage Patanjali compiled the Yoga Sutras, concise statements encapsulating yogic knowledge, which formed the basis of Classical Yoga. The Sutra was open to interpretation, leading to extensive commentary and analysis throughout history.

Hence, Yoga encompasses a wide range of practises; it is recognised as a therapeutic method for the mind and body, serving as an alternative treatment within the holistic approach of modern medicine (Raghuwanshi, 2011). Its application yields positive effects and complements other forms of therapy and natural healing.

The Eight Limbs of Yoga

Yoga helps us achieve a balance between our inner and outer worlds. Ashtanga yoga or "eight-limbed yoga" is how Patanjali (200 BCE) typically refers to yoga (Patanjali, 1978). The eight limbs consist of a set of ethical guidelines that guide individuals towards leading a purposeful and significant existence. They serve as a code of conduct and self-control, offering guidance for moral behaviour while also emphasising the importance of physical well-being and recognising the spiritual dimensions of human nature (Maehle, 2011). Patanjali's eight limbs have given rise to a plethora of yogic disciplines, each with its own distinct approach to disease prevention and treatment (Woodyard, 2011).

The first four limbs are associated with the external world and the physical response to external actions. Under the outside world's influence, one begins to regulate and explore the higher limbs of Ashtanga yoga. These higher limbs employ various meditational states that aid in reflecting on one's inner self and accepting one's presence. These eight steps, or limbs, help establish a connection between the physical and mental spaces by completing this gradual process.

Yama

The initial aspect of yoga involves the practise of restraining desires (Yama). It encompasses five moral values that guide our interactions with others and the world (Kirk et al., 2005). These virtues serve as ethical guidelines and principles that govern our actions, speech, and thoughts within ourselves and in relation to others. Swami Adgadanand Ji (2010) provides the following description of five yams:

Ahinsa (non-violence), Satya (Truthfulness), Asteya (Abstinence from stealing the possession of others), Brahmacharya (Observance of Celibacy), and Aparigraha (Abstinence from possessing unwanted things) are the five principles that fall under the category of Yam. Ahinsa refers to the practise of treating oneself with kindness and compassion. Satya represents the sincere and unwavering pursuit of spiritual truth. Asteya involves approaching one's chosen deity with a pure and open heart. Brahmacharya entails directing all senses and energies towards the ultimate reality, Brahman. Aparigraha serves as a means of safeguarding oneself from accumulating diverse impressions and experiences.

Niyams

The second limb emphasises the importance of staying engaged and accountable in life while staying true to personal objectives (Kirk et al., 2005). It involves five principles of self-awareness regarding our physical presence, behaviours, speech, and thoughts, which govern our relationship with ourselves.

Varambally and Gangadhar (2016) asserted in their review article that the objectives associated with yama and niyama are intrinsic to the individual. Yogic purists emphasis on the importance of practicing yoga as a holistic discipline, encompassing more than just physical postures and breathing techniques. They stress on aspects like 'Yama' and 'Niyama' that hold significant value as guiding ethical principles for one's lifestyle (Varambally & Gangadhar, 2016). In scientific terms, this means that yoga should be approached comprehensively, incorporating not only the physical aspects but also the moral and ethical dimensions represented by 'Yama' and 'Niyama.'

Asana

These postures aim to enhance physical strength, cognitive stability, and positive emotional states (Kirk et al., 2005). Yoga is the most widely recognised form of physical practise in Western cultures. Initially, these postures were developed as seated positions that promote a healthy environment for meditation. In modern times, asana practise has evolved into a physical discipline with the goal of promoting and facilitating mindful awareness and internal psychological processes (Brems et al., 2016).

Pranayama

A set of breathing techniques developed to aid practitioners in mastering the vital life force is referred to as pranayama. It involves the regulation and expansion of prana, which can be defined as the conscious control of breath (Brems et al., 2016). Today, pranayama Is understood as breathing practises that establish a connection between the mind and body, bridging the realms of consciousness and the subconscious.

Pratyahara

The process of withdrawing the senses, mind and consciousness from external stimuli to redirect attention towards oneself is known as pratyahara.

Dharna

Intense and concentrated mental focus is achieved in the sixth limb of yoga. It is accomplished once the body has been strengthened via asanas, the mind polished through pranayama, and the senses tamed by pratyahara. (Kirk et al., 2005). At this stage, the student experiences a heightened state of concentration and attention.

Dhyana

Meditation or Dhyana involves the act of redirecting one's consciousness inward, towards the essence of the soul (Kirk et al., 2005). It is a practise of withdrawing awareness from external distractions and turning it towards the depths of one's inner being.

Samadhi

Ecstasy is the state of merging with the divine and attaining self-realisation (Kirk et al., 2005). It is an experience where one becomes fully immersed in consciousness, truth, and indescribable joy. Maslow's concept of self-actualization is generally contrasted with attainment of Samadhi in ancient literature.

YOGIC PRACTISES AFFECTING ONE'S MENTAL WELL BEING

In 2022, the World Health Organisation published a report defining positive mental health as a condition in which every person realises their own abilities, can deal with typical stressors, can work effectively and efficiently, and can make contributions that are beneficial to their community. (WHO, 2022).

The first sutra of the Yogic Shastra opens by explaining what Yoga is, which is defined as the stillness of activities in one's mind, which is achieved by strenuous efforts of restraining operations in the mind. The status thus achieved help the self to get established in its real form. Yogic philosophies suggest that the self is always entangled with cognitive operations, thus causing distress. The following section will expand on some practises laid down by the disciple to achieve a sense of self.

However, before starting with the specificities of each practise, it is important to understand two critical components, as explained in the yogic literature, that play an important role in extracting benefits from yogic practises. These are named Faith and *Sadhana.* Lord Krishna in the Bhagwat Geeta endorses the importance of faith for any spiritual devotee. The idea has been preserved in Yogic literature; faith is necessary for intelligently pursuing the ultimate goal of Yoga step by step. After faith, the second requirement is a steady mind, or sadhana. A devotee should always keep the goal in view with an essence of eternal vigilance.

Yogic Asana (Hatha Yoga)

Yogic asanas are considered a conscious effort to examine Sadhana. Sitting in a comfortable, immovable position means asana. For mastering the art of asanas, physical capabilities are necessary; however, an absorbed mind characterised by Yam, Niyam, Tap, and Svadhyaya are central features. This was studied by revered Gurudev, who had crooked legs and could not even think of the postures of asanas, but they came out to be the best Mahapurush of their age.

Maharishi Patanjali suggests that as soon as Asana is mastered, the duels or conflicts of the mind subside. The pairs like *Raag-Dwesh,* that is, attachment and hatred, that throw the mind into a dilemma are softened, leading towards a path of mental satisfaction and pleasure. Using brain imaging techniques such as EEG, scientists have determined that practising yoga poses enhances neural activity in the grey matter as well as the performance of the amygdala and prefrontal cortex.

Yogic Breathing

The idea propelled by yogic breathing is that the repeated act of expelling the air out stabilizes the mind by taking out the "polluted air" from one's body and mind. The Yog Darshan of Patanjali provides a coherent picture of pranayama, diverting from the traditional idea of it being considered a breathing exercise. Breathing is a biological, life-sustaining process that provides very little room for modification.

While breathing, good and bad thoughts are intermingled in one's mind, but the capability to discard both kinds of thoughts is called pranayama. The applicability of yogic breathing can be contemplated with John Locke's idea of Tabula Rasa. Yogic breathing, which guides the practitioners to reach a state similar to tabula rasa helps them refocus their inner strength to freedom of self. An individual is subjected to achieve a 'blank state' and clear their head from the rushing automatic thoughts. It gives them a break and a chance for a rebirth of a fresh mindset (Petryszak, 1981).

Bhramari Pranayama, a breathing exercise with a humming sound like a black bee exhaling, has been used as an intervention during the COVID-19 breakout by Jagadeesan et al., in 2022. The 15-day online participation of 42 voluntary participants was conducted for a 20-minute Bhramari Pranayama session. There was a significant reduction in the scores on the Depression, Anxiety, and Stress Scale-21. The participants reported an improvement in the quality of sleep, as also reported on the Pittsburgh Sleep Quality Index (PSQI). A significant difference in scores at baseline and post-intervention was also noted on the WHO Quality of Life scale (Jagadeesan et al., 2022).

Yogic Diet

The association between diet and mental health has been intensively studied, and although the mechanism remains obscure, numerous investigators have concluded that there is a bidirectional relationship between food consumption and various physical and psychiatric disorders. Diet impacts mental health through its direct influence on mood, whereas the development of psychiatric disorders can contribute to dietary changes. (Bremner et al., 2020). While food is considered an essential component for the effective functioning of the physical body, eating right also has an impact on one's energy, mind, intelligence, emotions, and spirit (Suresh et al., 2020). The Upanishad philosophers propagated the notion that the food we consume transforms into three distinct forms: the heaviest portion is transformed into excrement, the medium density portion into flesh, and the tiniest particles go up to form the mind. (Sivananda, 1986).

Philosophies of yoga talk about different types of diet, namely the Sattvic diet, which calms the mind; the Rajasic diet, which excites the mind; and the Tamasic diet, which sedates the mind. The Sattvic diet nourishes the body and keeps it calm. It helps purify the body, which eventually enhances one's awareness and directs them towards positive actions (Shankar et al., 2017). Cereals, nuts, seeds, and honey are some ingredients of the Sattvic diet. Rajasic foods are stimulants. They tend to disturb the mind-body balance, leaving the mind restless. Stimulants like tea, coffee, and spicy foods are included in the Rajasic diet. The Tamasic diet has been found to produce no benefit to the mind or body. Yogic philosophers argue that such a diet reduces one's resistance to diseases and fills them with emotions like anger and greed. However, such food is helpful during times of physical and/or psychological pain (Suresh et al., 2020).

Chakras

The word Chakra literally means "wheel" or "disc." The physical body, according to a yogi, is a manifestation of psychic and psychosomatic energy within. The energy system is divided into seven primary chakra vortices that align along a core energy channel, or *nadi*, that extends between the base of the spine to the highest point of the head. The basic purpose of chakra yoga is to awaken the dormant kundalini energy at the base of the spine so that it can reach the crown of the head in its active state. The flow of energy by activating chakras has been studied by Sakthivel et al., 2023 while studying the effects of chakra yoga on psychopathologies namely, DID and PTSD. The process starts by chanting Bija Mantra as a part of chakra therapy which causes an activation of associated glands in one's body leading to activation and improved functionality of various parts of the nervous system (Sakthivel et al., 2023).

Yogic literature has identified approximately 7200 nadis of energy on an individual's body, out of which three are primary. The central sushmana, the ida, and the pinghala The ida is the left-side channel that controls an individual's features, such as being soft, sensitive, and reflective. On the other hand, the right side channel, which is the pinghala, corresponds with strength, heat, and activity. Each chakra has a specific physical location that is in tune with its physical, emotional, and energetic characteristics. For example, the manipura chakra along the waist line is also referred to as the "band of self-esteem."

Bandhas

Bandhas are described as a series of energy gates that have the responsibility of regulating the flow of psychosomatic energy. The analogy can be made with the valves of one's heart, which are responsible for regulating and pumping blood in one direction. Yoga practitioners learn a set of tones and rhythms that give them the ability to lock and desirably regulate the subtle energy channels. Three major bandhas are *Mulabandha, Uddiyana Bandha,* and *Jalandhara Bandha*, which, when performed together, help mobilize psychic and psychosomatic energy and clear blockages from the central energy pathway. Bandha entails a profound comprehension of our inner beings, which serves to invigorate the vital force known as Prana, and activate the energy centers.

These were some of the many practices that have been proposed by the discipline of Yoga enhancing the overall functioning of an individual. All of these practices have been emerged by the knowledge of Yogic philosophers and as presented have been empirically tested by researchers across the world. However these practices also bring with themselves some complications and scrutiny. Yogic practices like asanas have limitations for people with disability and has also been identified as a cause for physical injuries especially when practiced by under trained participants. Therefore it can be concluded that yoga is not a point of blind trust and require careful analysis before adapting any practise for oneself. The following sections will cover these aspects in greater details. However, before jumping into those it is important to understand what all areas of one's functionality are affected by Yoga and related practices.

A BIO-PSYCHO-SOCIAL PERSPECTIVE ON ANALYSING THE BENEFITS OF YOGA

In 1977, George Engel published "The Need for a New Medical Model: A Challenge for Biomedicine," proposing an evolution from the 'one-dimensional biomedical model to comprehend the ill-health of people (Santos et al., 2018). The book titled European Psychiatric/Mental Health Nursing in the 21st Century highlights essential features of the BioPsychoSocial (BPS) model:

- The model highlights a holistic view of any person's health, including several domains like physical, emotional, social, economic, and spiritual.
- It is based upon General Systems theory, which helps to understand the 'relationships' that various domains and systems contain within themselves.
- It gives an ecological perspective on health, which paves the way towards understanding interpersonal, community, and public policy issues.
- It helps in Person-Centred Health care, which disapproves of traditional notions of patients being passive recipients of care and rather posits that they are equal participants in any form of treatment.

Understanding Yoga and related practices in light of the BPS model will help to gain a better and more comprehensive insight into the benefits that the practices have on an individual's health and overall functioning. The following section will look at Yogic practices as an asset for multidimensional refinement of one's physical and mental health. The three segments, namely biological, psychological and social have been presented in the chapter, independently for in depth understanding of each. However, Engel's model proposes a harmonious convergence of the three perspectives to offer a holistic approach (refer to Figure 1).

Biological Aids With Respect to Yogic Practises

The scientific evidence of the benefits of yoga on one's mind and body has been significantly increasing, as assessed by MRI, fMRI, and SPECT. Randomised control trials have found a positive association between yoga practise and improvement in diabetes, cardiovascular function, and musculoskeletal conditions. Neuroanatomical evidence suggests that regular yoga practise benefits the functioning of the hippocampus, amygdala, and prefrontal cortex (PFC).(Gothe et al., 2019). Gothe et al. (2018) conducted an experiment to determine the effects of yoga on working memory by evaluating yoga practitioners on the Sternberg working memory task. An MRI scan revealed that the yoga practitioners' left hippocampus contained more grey matter than the controls. Further examination revealed that experienced yoga practitioners demonstrated decreased stimulation in the left dorsolateral prefrontal cortex (PFC), the region responsible for the encoding of information as perceived by the senses, indicating improved working memory performance.

GABA is one of the primary inhibitory neurotransmitters found in the brain which works to reduce neural activity. A 27% increase in GABA levels in the yoga practitioners was found as compared to the control subjects who indulged in reading sessions. Conclusively, yoga can be used as an intervention practise for the treatment of disorders like generalised anxiety disorder (Streeter et al., 2007). Empirical evidence like these have suggested the benefits of yoga by altering the neuroanatomical and neurochemical changes in the brain which has therapeutic and strengthening effects on various psychological parameters for an individual.

Psychological Aids With Respect to Yogic Practices

B.K.S. Iyengar, the founder of Iyengar yoga and one of the most prominent yoga gurus in India, asserts that "regular practise of yoga can help you face the turmoil of life with steadiness and stability." The discipline of yoga exerts a lot of focus on the functioning of one's thoughts and emotions. It is believed

Figure 1. Biopsychosocial benefits of yoga leading to mental wellbeing

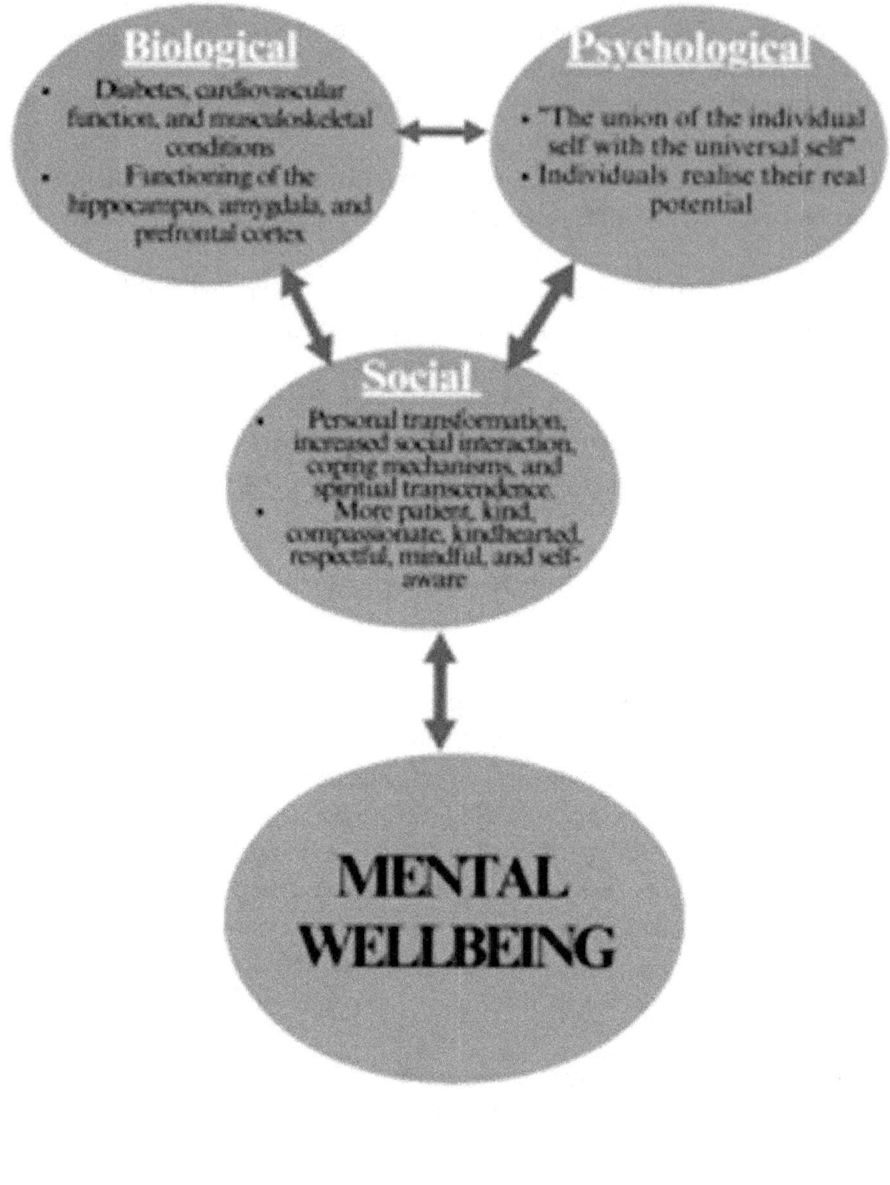

that there are six powers of mind, as illustrated in Table 1, which, when exhibited, make a person self-restrained and help them gain mastery over their passions (Sivananda, 1974).

The greatest Sage Patanjali has described yoga as “the union of the individual self with the universal self,” which complements the idea of self-actualization proposed by Abraham Maslow, an American psychologist. Maslow’s theory has developed a need-based chart that talks about “growth motivation” and enables individuals to realise their real potential as they age and mature. It supports a noble human transition from self-indulgence to altruism and selflessness. (D’Souza & Gurin, 2016).

The positive effects of yogic interventions have been studied globally on demographically different populations. Danielly and Silverthorne’s (2017) Yoga Prison Project in South Carolina implemented a ten-week trauma-focused yoga programme on 33 female inmates. The results were suggestive of a

Figure 2. Six powers of mind explained by yogic discipline

Powers of mind	Associated cognitive process
Vedana Shakti	Power of perception
Smriti Shakti	Power of memory
Bhavana Shakti	Power of imagination
Manisha Shakti	Power of judgment
Ichha Shakti	Power of will or volition
Dharna Shakti	Power to hold

significant decrease in measures of depression and stress and improved self-awareness. Although not statistically significant, there were reduced scores for anxiety as well. However, no results were found for rumination levels. The effects of reduced anxiety extend their boundaries from symptom reduction to overall functioning of an individual. Wood, 2006 conducted a pre-post analysis on 40 students and found that decreased anxiety was predictive of improved school performance and social functioning. Evidence like these gives an indication towards the formation of an interplay between the various factors that affects an individual's functioning.

Social Aids With Respect to Yogic Practises

"*I am a nice person when I do yoga*" was an exclamation made by a participant in the United States of America, where a research study tried to understand the effect of yoga on improving interpersonal relationships with 1,067 yoga practitioners. Ross et al. (2014) identified four major themes in their research: yoga practises contribute to personal transformation, increased social interaction, coping mechanisms, and spiritual transcendence. The participants suggested that apart from the visible physical benefits that yogic practises provide them, they also helped them be more patient, kind, compassionate, kindhearted, respectful, mindful, and self-aware. There was a sense of belongingness to the yogic community, which helped them make new friends.

. Praying yoga gradually inculcates control over body, mind, and speech (Stone, 2009). Michael Stone, author of the book "Yoga for a World of Balance," gives an example of Mahatma Gandhi, who is being followed by millions of people because of his dire passion towards *ahimsa* (non-violence) and *satya* (truthfulness).

Yoga has also been investigated as a method for improving the social functioning of vulnerable populations. 102 pregnant women between 10 and 20 weeks of gestation were randomly assigned to one of two groups: yoga (n = 51) or a control group (n = 51). The yoga group participated in integrated yoga, while the control group participated in conventional antenatal experiences. The outcomes were determined using the WHOQOL-100 (World Health Organisation Quality of Life Scale) and FIRO-B (Fundamental Interpersonal Relations Orientation-Behavior Scale) scores. Yoga practises were found to be an effective method for enhancing the quality of life of pregnant women and enhancing various aspects of their interpersonal relationships, including significant improvements in expressing exclusion, a sense of belonging, and social warmth and closeness (Rakhshani et al., 2010).

Applicability of BPS Model in Yogic Discipline

The biopsychosocial model has been a success as proposed by George Engel in attempting to unify various disciplines of science and it has been widely used in the medical field for gaining a holistic grip over the pathology presented by the patient. From the evidence presented above, it can be well understood how technological advancements gave rise to information in hand about brain structure and functions. Alongside an understanding about psychological disorders, indicate an abnormality in brain functions. However, it is an empirically concluded fact that no psychopathology can be distinguished from social stressors and the effects it has on social functioning. The benefits of yoga have been discussed along the lines of all these continuum making it a suitable subject to understand using the biopsychosocial lens.

Nonetheless there have been critics of the BPS model. One of the major concerns revolving around the model have been its applicability to the field of mental health. Engel's model was proposed as a Biopsychosocial model of medicine and psychiatry. Promoters of mental health and wellbeing have questioned the validity of the BPS model in answering clinical questions pertaining to the field of mental illness. Studies understanding the applicability of BPS model in the medical field have revealed that medical students and professionals rather focus the on biomedical model to explain any illness than using psychological or social lens (Sadler & Hulgus, 1992). From contradictive application based controversies like this around the BPS model it can be said that the doors for understanding yoga from many different theoretical backgrounds are wide open.

YOGA AND PSYCHOPATHOLOGY

Yoga has been used as an adjunctive treatment to enhance well-being and enhance the therapeutic effects of other healing agents. Several yogic practises are based on the stillness of thoughts and mental activities. When a person succeeds in suspending these mental activities, they may attain Yog, and this leads to the establishment of the real self. This is explained in the yoga sutras as the following process: before restraint of mental activities (i.e., before yoga), the individual identifies with the operations of mind, or *vritti,* preventing an individual from identifying their real self. These *vrittis* may be painful (*Klishta*) or non-painful (*AKlisht).* Before the restraint of thoughts, a person is shaped by the quality of these *vrittis, i.e., an* increase in *klishta vritti* may cause worry and suffering. The practise of yoga asanas aids an individual in being sensitive and mindful about the engagement of different muscles and also helps us recognise other *vrittis*. After recognition of these *vrittis*, the task of a yoga practitioner is to calm or suspend these waves of thoughts, which would then aid an individual in establishing the self in its real form.

The above paragraph signifies the importance of the quality of mental thoughts that shape an individual. Maladaptive cognitions, or *klishta vrittis,* have been implicated in the development of several psychopathologies. In psychotherapeutic practises today, recognition of negative and maladaptive cognitions and subsequent restructuring of these cognitions bring relief from the symptomatology of psychopathology. The aim of practising yoga also emphasises calming our mental waves as a way of achieving one's real self, creating a powerful parallel between modern psychotherapeutic practises and the ancient eastern science of yoga in achieving the same goal of identifying with the real self and thus freeing an individual from psychopathologies.

Neuropsychiatric pathologies tend to display a heterogeneous group of symptoms involving biological, social and psychological aspects. Thus, complete reliance on pharmacotherapy is not possible. Therefore, the use of adjunctive treatments such as psychotherapy and yoga is essential, especially for social and psychological well-being. The benefits of practising yoga and the practise of yoga therapy, including but not limited to pranayama, i.e., yogic breathing, relaxation techniques, and meditation forms, have been empirically tested for their therapeutic properties in several psychopathologies.

Among the more common psychiatric disorders are anxiety and mood disorders, with a twelve-month prevalence of the former being 10% and the latter being 7%. Many empirical studies have supported the idea that yoga interventions reduce depressive symptoms. Studies have showcased the effectiveness of *Hatha yoga, asanas, pranayama, mindfulness meditation, and viniyoga in treating* depressive disorders. Today, *Hatha yoga* is widely used in the treatment of depression (Bridges & Sharma, 2017). Apart from this, *sahaj yog,* a form of Kundali Yog or Laya yog, is a meditative technique and is implicated in the improvement of depressive and anxiety disorders. Studies have found that Kundali yoga had significantly lower anxiety symptoms when compared to treatment-as-usual conditions (Gabriel et al., 2018). It is thought that sahaj yoga acts on the limbic system, thus regulating sympathetic activity and endocrine secretion and causing antidepressant effects (Sharma et al., n.d.). Sudarshan Kriya (SK) yoga is also effective in managing dysthymia and depression (Janakiramaiah et al., 1998). SK yoga is a special form of pranayama, and practise of this has elicited seizure-type activity in the brain, i.e., a response similar to ECT, thus bringing about improvement in emotional problems, fatigue, and sleep disturbances experienced in depression (Doria et al., 2015). Pranayama, a controlled breathing exercise, involves the retention and regulation of the inflow and outflow of breath. The practise of pranayama leads the breathing process to become slow and rhythmic. This causes an individual to feel deeply relaxed as slow, deep breaths limit the sympathetic nervous system and HPA activation, leading to less production of adrenaline, noradrenaline, and cortisol and more production of feel-good neurochemicals such as serotonin. Continued practise of pranayama activates brain regions like the cingulate cortex and putamen, which are associated with sustained attention (Betal, 2023). In anxiety and depression-related disorders, GABA levels, an inhibitory neurotransmitter, are deficient. Yoga practitioners experience a surge in GABA levels after one yoga session, which suggests the efficiency of yoga in treating these disorders (Streeter et al., 2007).

Obsessive-compulsive and related disorders (OCD) are another group of disorders characterised by intrusive thoughts (obsessions) and repeated actions, which could be overt or covert, that are performed in response to the obsessions (compulsions). It has a 12-month prevalence of 1.8%. Yogic interventions have been found to reduce anxiety stemming from repeated ego-dystonic thoughts. Patients with OCD were trained in a yoga module and regularly practised 1 hour of yoga. It was seen that the Y-BOCS and HAM-D scores of OCD patients were significantly improved after regular yoga practise (Bhat et al., 2021). A randomised clinical trial attempted to compare the effectiveness of kundali yoga (KY) with relaxation response meditation (RRM), wherein it was found that individuals in the KY group had approximately 40% improvement in Y-BOCS scores when compared to RRM, which showcased 17% improvement (Shannahoff-Khalsa et al., 2019). Rajyoga is another form of yogic meditation that empowers the mind. Rajyoga is believed to work by increasing serotonin levels and decreasing monoamine oxidase, causing a reduction in anxiety. When Rajyoga interventions were given adjunctively to pharmacological treatment, improvement in Y-BOCS was found to be 49% as compared to when pharmacological treatment was given alone (18%) (Mehta et al., 2020).

In psychotic illnesses such as that of schizophrenia, comprising of positive, negative, and cognitive symptoms, practise of yoga has been found to have some relief especially asanas and pranayama(Bangalore & Varambally, 2012). Patients were trained in yoga asanas for one month and it was seen that there was significant improvement in negative symptoms and social dysfunction (Sathyanarayanan et al., 2019). A randomized controlled pilot study found improvement in PANSS score after yoga intervention (Broderick et al., 2018). Schizophrenia is also characterised by deficits in facial emotional recognition. Randomly selected antipsychotic-stabilized patients exhibiting this symptom received yoga therapy, and their Tool for the Recognition of Emotions in Neuropsychiatric Disorder (TRENDS) scores improved significantly, and this improvement was maintained for a period of four months after yoga therapy. (Behere et al., 2011). Therefore, yogic interventions can be recommended in addition to antipsychotics for rapid improvement in patients' symptomatology.

Individuals who have undergone severe trauma, like war veterans, victims of sexual assault, or survivors of natural disasters, may develop post-traumatic stress disorder (PTSD), characterised by sudden repeated flashbacks of traumatic events, and especially in the presence of stimuli related to trauma and subsequent avoidance of these stimuli. They also experience intrusiveness of thoughts, negative moods, cognitions, and altered arousal. In many randomised controlled trials, the efficacy of yoga in improving the symptomatology of PTSD symptoms was found (Gallegos et al., 2017). Non-trauma-focused yoga also yielded significant improvement in patients with PTSD. In a randomised trial, when patients with PTSD were given the intervention of Kripalu yoga, some decline in re-experiencing symptoms was observed (Reinhardt et al., 2018). Hatha yoga, too, has been implicated as an adjunctive treatment for PTSD. The aim is to create mindfulness through breathing exercises and postures. Trauma-sensitive yoga (TSY) practise is a form of hatha yoga designed for trauma and delivered in a gentle and safe environment. TSY aided in personal growth and symptom reduction (West et al., 2017).

The benefits of yoga are not limited to these disorders. Other mental health conditions, such as neurodevelopmental and neurocognitive disorders, eating disorders, sleep and related disorders, and somatic disorders, have also been benefited by different yoga practises. Yoga, being cost-effective and having no side effects, unlike pharmacological treatments, can be used as an adjunctive therapeutic agent in improving symptomatology or otherwise improving mood and reducing stress. Several empirical studies have already established the relationship between yogic practises like asanas and chakras and mental health conditions such as depression.

Whilst there are a number of indications of yoga as an adjunctive treatment in psychiatric disorders, it is also important to explore the contraindications. Yogic interventions may produce adverse effects in certain disorders, however, if used appropriately, this risk is significantly minimized. Walsh and Roche in 1979 through case reports described how intensive meditation in patients with a history of psychosis was a contraindication. From around 3 case reports of patients with history schizophrenia, it was described how intensive meditation along with sleep deprivation and discontinuation of maintenance pharmacotherapy resulted in precipitation of an acute psychotic episode thus contraindicating intensive meditation in patients with history of psychosis (Walsh & Roche, 1979). Such is the case with moderate to severe depression as well, *pratyahara* and advanced meditation should be avoided. Avoidance of high intensity yogic practises in anxiety disorders is recommended. In patients with bipolar affective disorder, it is essential that yogic practise proceeds at an appropriate pace. If too slow it may make the patient agitated. In patients with obsessive compulsive and related disorders, mindfulness based stress reduction program is contraindicated (Dobkin et al., 2012) as is giving precise instructions as it may make the patient more anxious to achieve and perfect the intervention, generalized instructions may give better results (Bhargav et al., 2022). Moreover, in patients with epilepsy it is also recommended to avoid hyperventilation procedure of kapalbhati as it may precipitate the seizure episode. The literature also suggests that it is essential to monitor the interaction of allopathic drugs with the yogic interventions being prescribed (Gangadhar & Varambally, 2011).

Consequently, it is essential to investigate the health benefits of yoga in greater depth and to promote the practise of yoga as an economical, risk-free adjunctive form of treatment or established practise that would assist in the improvement of symptomatology and overall bio-psychosocial health. Emphasis should be put on practise of yoga therapy specifically for neuropsychiatric disorders by licensed professionals as caution needs to be exercised while administering yogic interventions to this special population. Provision of yoga therapy to such a sensitive population therefore requires quality-control. This should include adequate training, accredited courses and ideally certification and licensure. In order to maximize the therapeutic effects of yoga and minimize the adverse ones, 800 hours of certification from an accredited institute is necessary not including the 200 hours of training required to get the title of yoga instructor thus becoming equipped to teach yogic practises and have the knowledge to navigate the sensitive needs of the neuropsychiatric clients. The International Association of Yoga Therapists (IAYT) ensures this quality control by issuing C-IAYT certification through Portfolio Review & Evaluation (PR&E) which has a rigorous eligibility criteria (*C-IAYT Portfolio Review - International Association of Yoga Therapists IAYT*, n.d.).

From this section it is clear that there are numerous psychopathologies wherein use of yoga as adjunctive treatment is implicated. However, it remains essential to understand the types of interventions that can be utilized in enhancing an individual's biopsychosocial health. Keeping the indications and contraindications of yoga in psychopathology in mind, as it may be therapeutic or detrimental to health, delivering tailor made treatments becomes essential which is possible only if comprehensive knowledge of such yogic interventions is available.

YOGIC INTERVENTIONS FOR PSYCHOPATHOLOGY

The Patanjali Yoga Sutras have described the five main *Niyams* of Life (Udupa & Prasad, 1985). Rules, or *'Niyams'*, are regarded as dos and don'ts that result in a standard operating procedure for leading life. But enhancing mind-body harmony also requires a strong ethical foundation. According to study findings, young adults who are properly introduced to the *Niyama* in their practises can develop their psycho-spiritual growth (Xu et al., 2021).

Ivtzan and Papantoniou (2018) have noted that Niyams can be defined by qualities such as self-control, self-discipline, and self awareness. These concepts can be theoretically conceptualized under the discipline of positive psychology, which propagates ideas like flow. Flow, in positive psychology has been understood as individuals becoming fully engaged and immersed in the present moment (Ivtzan & Papantoniou, 2014). When discussing the link between meaning in life and the practice of yoga, the authors highlight the significance of intention, known as Sanklpa, and the process of setting purposeful goals. Together, these elements of discipline and goal- setting play a crucial role in mediating the sense of meaning in one's own life. The following are the *niyams* laid by Yogic philosophers which are to be adhered to in order to achieve the state of flow:

Shaucha

Shaucha represents both internal and external cleanliness and purification. Water should be used every day to purify externally. It also refers to purify the mind through good behaviour and the soul through learning and devotion. For the purification of the mind and soul, one must follow the advice of the saints and sages.

Every individual experiences emotions like guilt throughout their lives. However, the Shaucha practise can be used to clear the mind if one makes mistakes that cause guilt feelings (Shearer, 2010). A person's unconscious mind is constantly filled with negative thoughts, and when these unconscious thoughts try to enter the conscious level through strange channels, they cause issues. Shaucha practise allows one to clear thoughts from the unconscious.

Santosha

The available resources should be used to accomplish one's goals. Contentment is a state of being where one is completely satisfied with the outcomes, does not search for things that are out of reach, recognises the accomplishments made possible by God's grace, and does not aspire for things that are not possible. Happiness is primarily based on satisfaction, while desire and aspirations is the root of unhappiness.

Instead of concentrating on what is absent, Santosha emphasises accepting limitations and cultivating an attitude of gratitude (Shearer, 2010). Santosha emphasises the importance of practising contentment because it helps one focus on the task at hand without being side-tracked by negative self-talk, harsh judgements, or other distractions.

Tapas

Tapas means to put with difficulties. Whatever aches, tribulations, or adversities arise in the path of achieving goals, they should be graciously accepted and should march continuously and without stopping in the direction of the objective.

Tapas, or self-control, sensory training, and effort Tapas has made a commitment to practising yoga and leading a healthy lifestyle in a PTSD yoga study (Schmid et al., 2021). Many people expressed their dedication to their yoga practise by beginning a home practise and using breath work outside of class.

Svadhyaya

Svadhyaya involves paying attention to and reflecting on our attitudes, sentiments, and actions. Additionally, it entails committing to ongoing personal development and turning our attention inward rather than outward. Svadhyaya encourages self-compassion and the exploration of difficult life experiences (Schmid et al., 2021). According to recent research, 10 minutes of contemplation and reflection immediately changed the group for the better, bringing out their enthusiasm, happiness, confidence, a calm smile, and other positive emotions (Verma, 2021).

Ishvara Pranidhana

The name "Ishwar" refers to Sagunbrahma or Paramatma. Pranidhana means "to be submissive with prana" in Sanskrit. The consistent and devoted worship of God as the world's lord is a characteristic of Ishwar Pranidhana (Jadeja, 2020). Yoga can help people with PTSD change their perspective from "this thing happened" to "I am alive" or "I am recovering after this thing (Schmid et al., 2021)." Ishvara Pranidhana might simply be connected to an improved sense of wellbeing and the knowledge that one can be a survivor rather than a victim.

Yoga Therapy

Swami Kuvalayananda is credited for yoga therapy in 1920s. To understand the therapeutic applications of yoga he along with his colleagues used modern medicine methods to study how practise of yoga has physiological effects on our body. However, the use of modern medicine does not implicate alienation of yoga therapy from traditional yoga sharing the goal of 'realization of life.' Thus, yoga therapy does not only focus on the cure of ailment, but also helping individual realize their potential and live their best possible life by integration of various aspects of life (Monro, 1997).

Yoga therapy has been found to be very effective for several common and severe mental illnesses. In general, practising yoga such as kapalbhati kriyas and yoga postures induces calmness, lowering an individual's agitation. It has also been found to increase awareness, attention, and acceptance and provide an individual with a sense of security. Essentially, yoga therapy is delivering yoga tailored to the individual's needs, considering their medical condition and overall lifestyle. Yoga therapy affects the individual in a holistic manner and is not a mere alleviation of symptomatology. A yoga therapy session is inclusive of a balanced set of practises that calm the mind, energise the body, and act upon the ailing area as well. Yoga therapy has been defined by IAYT in the following manner:

Appropriate utilisation of yoga teachings and practises in a therapeutic environment encourages a consistent yoga practise that increases self-awareness and directs the client's or student's energy towards desired goals.

The particular definition puts emphasis on the practise of yoga in a therapeutic context, resulting in the betterment of the individual as a whole. The focus is not on diagnosing and treating the individual and then giving one-size-fits-all solutions; rather, it involves carefully gathering information from the medical professionals and then delivering a range of yoga practises to support the client therapeutically as well as developmentally in physical, emotional, and spiritual areas of their lives. Yoga therapy thus emphasises its goal of working with the whole person, i.e., placing the person in context and encouraging the process of integration within the client.

One of the essential themes of yoga therapy is centering, or finding one's centre. A centered person is balanced in both their physical and mental worlds. Individuals with medical or psychiatric illnesses are ex-centred, and yoga and deep inner acceptance can restore this. Yoga therapy delineates five areas of human life that can become ex-centred: physical, emotional, mental, energetic, and spiritual. Thus, yoga therapy attempts to bring balance to these five facets. Apart from centering, love and acceptance of ourselves is the goal of yoga therapy. After accepting ourselves, we can learn to love and accept others. In yoga therapy, this takes the form of pushing ourselves and being kind to our body and mind. Full potential is reached when we allow our body's separated parts to reconnect. This, in turn, is achieved when we show acceptance to our body and listen to its needs (Foulkes & Barkworth, 2017).

Several empirical studies have provided evidence for the efficacy of yoga therapy (for example, Asanas) and relaxation techniques (for example, Pranayama and progressive muscle relaxation) in alleviating psychophysiological symptomatology. Hence, yoga therapy and relaxation techniques have been used as ancillary management for physical conditions like arthritis, chronic obstructive pulmonary disease, and coronary heart disease. Moreover, it also alleviates psychological symptoms resulting from terminal illnesses like cancer or several neurological diseases. In psychiatric illnesses, certain symptomatology has shown reduction when different types of yoga asanas and breathing techniques are practised.

Relaxation Techniques

Relaxation in yoga, also known as psychic sleep or yoga nidra, is a form of tantric relaxation technique that combines mental imagery and Shavasana. The concept of yoga nidra first appeared in the Upanishads and involves a deep stage of sleep. Shavasana is a corpse-like pose wherein the individual should face upwards and lie flat on the ground. Assuming this position would alleviate normal fatigue and calm one's mind, Yoga nidra aids an individual, as the practitioner of this has their consciousness operating at deep awareness, which is accompanied by immense relaxation. It is not that the practitioner is completely unaware of the surroundings, but in yoga nidra, the person becomes more in touch with their deeper mental activities. In yoga Nidra, arousal of the body is reduced, and the sympathetic nervous system shows a decrease accompanied by dream-like experiences. Many benefits of yoga nidra are seen. Yoga nidra helps with insomnia; in fact, 1 hour of yoga nidra amounts to 4 hours of sleep. It also reduces stress and anxiety, fosters calmness, and releases tension.

One method of relaxation is deep breathing. For this, the practitioner is asked to assume the shavasana posture and calm themselves. The body posture is described as legs being slightly apart, hands slightly away from the body with palms turned upwards, and noses pointing towards the ceiling with their eyes closed. After this position is taken, each part of the body receives attention with the aim of relaxing that part while taking a deep breath. This begins from the eyebrow centre all the way down to the toe tips for both the left and right sides of the body. After each body part has been relaxed, the practitioner takes a five-minute pause and then breathes in and out. They are then told to become aware of their surroundings and to sit up. They first need to roll onto their right side, and with the support of their left hand, they are asked to slowly sit up. Eyes are not open until this moment, and the practitioner is asked to cover their eyes with their palms, then look through gaps in their fingers, and then slowly open their eyes.

Another very popular method is progressive muscle relaxation (PMR). It involves two consecutive steps: contraction and relaxation of muscles carried out systematically for the entire body. The practitioner is first required to tense their muscle groups in the body and then relax those muscles, with emphasis on how they feel after relaxation. Individuals with anxiety spectrum disorders are often tensed throughout the day, unaware of it. Through practising PMR, one can at least become aware of their tensed muscles when anxious and then take appropriate steps to relax their body. Instructions are given starting from the foot all the way to the forehead, which include repeated tensing and relaxing of the muscle groups.

Along the lines of prevention is better than cure, empirical studies suggest that with yoga being indicated in adjunctive and augmentative treatment it can also be used as a preventative measure for several neuropsychiatric disorders. One study looked at integrating yoga specifically targeting eating disorder prevention into ongoing yoga classes promoting self-acceptance messages. Yoga can also be included as a part of intervention specifically designed for eating disorders given to those who had expressed body dissatisfaction (Neumark-Sztainer, 2014). Another disorder in which the role of yoga as prevention is implicated is anxiety and related disorder. State and trait anxiety measured using STAI both showed improvement after a yoga lifestyle intervention was administered significantly reducing the post-intervention scores while no improvement was observed in the no-intervention i.e., control group (Gupta et al., 2006.). Studies have integrated yoga as a school curriculum to evaluate its preventive efficacy. Results suggested improvement in mood and anxiety and yoga receiving groups had significant reduction in negative affectivity (Noggle et al., 2012). Students also reported increased respect for their body and improvement in self image implying prevention for eating disorders. They also reported stress reduction, increased optimism and a tool used for managing negative emotions (Conboy et al., 2013). Thus, yoga should be considered as a preventive treatment for a myriad of psychiatric conditions with yoga therapy being integrated in school curriculum to administering it to those with known genetic predisposition at primary healthcare level.

Feasibility and Limitations of Yogic Interventions

While use of yoga therapy as an adjunctive and supportive line of treatment in psychological disorders has been found to be cost-effective in enhancing the patient's heath it is not completely without its limits especially when evaluating yoga for its feasibility. Firstly, yoga is not without its risks. Many studies have found that yoga can pose a risk for developing hypertension or stroke and involves a risk of personal injury and body aches if not performed correctly. In patients with depression who already present with anhedonia i.e., lack of pleasure in activities, and low motivation adding yoga as self-care may be redundant (Büssing et al., 2012). Like this several mental obstacles to yoga have been identified. Prescribing yoga asanas to those individuals facing these obstacles would be redundant without first working on the obstacles themselves. Maharishi Patanjali delineated obstacles to yoga as mental laziness, procrastination and negligence, presence of false beliefs and delusions, doubts and dullness are described as a blockade to the practice of yoga as they lack the motivation and energy to do so thus pointing towards the necessity of person characteristics in effectiveness of yoga as an adjunctive treatment modality (Bhavanani, 2012).

It is also important to consider the cultural background of the client, especially their religious identity, financial status, and their attitudes and beliefs towards practise of yoga. Studies have investigated that perception of yoga for Indians has been limited to a tool for enhancing physical fitness. It has rarely been viewed as a preventive treatment, or an adjunctive treatment especially for neuropsychiatric treatment. Due to lack of awareness of mental health as such, the Indian population has low consensus on the effectiveness of yoga on mental health and consequently psychiatric disorders. Even though yoga has gained popularity in the recent past among Indians, a knowledge-practice gap is observed with 11.8% of the population practicing yoga (Mishra et al., 2020). Reasons attributed to unwillingness and lack of practice were largely time constraints, lack of knowledge regarding practicing procedure, feeling afraid to practice and lack of company (Sharma et al., 2022). Moreover, yoga interventions should be performed in a spacious and calm environment from experts trained in delivering yoga for it to have its beneficial effects. This is often not followed as yoga is seen as a self-care with the notion that anybody can perform yoga, however, relaxation techniques, asanas, chakras and mudras all require supervision and expertise to be performed in a correct manner and deliver its beneficial effects. Many Indians were also of the opinion that yoga interventions for healthcare should be delivered by trained professionals and were willing to avail these services if it were provided in tertiary care hospitals along with pharmacological treatment (Sharma et al., 2022). As noted, yogic interventions are not without its limitations, hence, it is always a good practice to receive yogic interventions from a trained professional in a setting as discussed earlier.

CONCLUSION

Yoga, one of the ancient practises of human kind constitutes the eight limbs and attempts to promote a lifestyle that is free of maliciousness with emphasis on inculcating qualities that would aid the individual in living a life that is truly actualizing. Practise of yoga is not limited to holding specific asanas, but various components of yoga such as pranayama, pratyahara, samadhi and dhyana all attempt to enhance an individual's biological, psychological and social well-being. Yoga has several benefits, this chapter contextualized yoga therapy, including pranayama, asanas, mudras and chakras to biopsychosocial model of health and has attempted to identify yogic practises that bring enhancement in all three aspects. Yoga, being cost-effective, and having no side effects, unlike the pharmacological treatments, can be used as an adjunctive therapeutic agent in improving symptomatology or otherwise improving mood and reducing stress. Several empirical studies have already established the relationship of yogic practises like yogic asanas and chakras with mental health conditions. However, it is important to note the feasibility and limitations of yoga interventions. It is necessary for yoga therapy to be given by trained professional in order to minimize ill-effects and magnify the benefits gained. Therefore, this chapter attempted to explore the health benefits of yoga in more detail and to promote the practise of yoga, a cost-effective method without any ill-effects as an adjunctive form of treatment which would thereby aid in improvement of symptomatology and general biopsychosocial well-being.

REFERENCES

Adgadanand, S. (2010). *Maharishi Patanjali's - Yog-Darshan: Yoga Sūtras of Patañjali*. Shree Paramhans Swami Adgadanandji Ashram Trust.

Balasubramaniam, M., Telles, S., & Doraiswamy, P. M. (2013a). Yoga on Our Minds: A Systematic Review of Yoga for Neuropsychiatric Disorders. *Frontiers in Psychiatry, 3*. https://www.frontiersin.org/articles/10.3389/fpsyt.2012.00117

Bangalore, N. G. (2012). Yoga therapy for Schizophrenia. *International Journal of Yoga*, *5*(2), 85–91. doi:10.4103/0973-6131.98212 PMID:22869990

Behere, R. V., Arasappa, R., Jagannathan, A., Varambally, S., Venkatasubramanian, G., Thirthalli, J., Subbakrishna, D. K., Nagendra, H. R., & Gangadhar, B. N. (2011). Effect of yoga therapy on facial emotion recognition deficits, symptoms and functioning in patients with schizophrenia. *Acta Psychiatrica Scandinavica, 123*(2), 147–153. doi:10.1111/j.1600-0447.2010.01605.x PMID:20846271

Bhat, S. G. S., Arasappa, R., Jagannathan, A., & Varambally, S. (2021). Yoga therapy for Obsessive Compulsive Disorder (OCD): A case series from India. *Asian Journal of Psychiatry, 62*, 102739. doi:10.1016/j.ajp.2021.102739

Bhargav, H., George, S., & Varambally, S. (2022). Yoga and mental health: What every psychiatrist needs to know. *BJPsych Advances, 29*(1), 1–12. doi:10.1192/bja.2022.22

Bhavanani, A. (2012). OBSTACLES ON THE PATH OF YOGA. *Yoga Life, 43*, 3–9.

Bremner, J. D., Moazzami, K., Wittbrodt, M. T., Nye, J. A., Lima, B. B., Gillespie, C. F., Rapaport, M. H., Pearce, B. D., Shah, A. J., & Vaccarino, V. (2020). Diet, Stress and Mental Health. *Nutrients, 12*(8), 2428. doi:10.3390/nu12082428 PMID:32823562

Brems, C., Colgan, D., Freeman, H., Freitas, J., Justice, L., Shean, M., & Sulenes, K. (2016). Elements of yogic practice: Perceptions of students in healthcare programs. *International Journal of Yoga, 9*(2), 121. doi:10.4103/0973-6131.183710 PMID:27512319

Brenes, G. A., Sohl, S., Wells, R. E., Befus, D., Campos, C. L., & Danhauer, S. C. (2019). The Effects of Yoga on Patients with Mild Cognitive Impairment and Dementia: A Scoping Review. *The American Journal of Geriatric Psychiatry, 27*(2), 188–197. doi:10.1016/j.jagp.2018.10.013 PMID:30413292

Bridges, L. & Sharma, M. (2017). The Efficacy of Yoga as a Form of Treatment for Depression. *Journal of Evidence-Based Complementary & Alternative Medicine*. doi:10.1177/2156587217715927

Broderick, J., Vancampfort, D., Mockler, D., Bennett, K., Waugh, A., McDonough, C., Cramer, H., & Walshe, M. (2018). Yoga for schizophrenia. *Cochrane Database of Systematic Reviews, 2018*(12), CD013213. doi:10.1002/14651858.CD013213

C-IAYT Portfolio Review—International Association of Yoga Therapists IAYT. (n.d.). IAYT. https://www.iayt.org/page/PRE_Eligibility

Capon, H. O., Shea, M., & McIver, S. (2019). Yoga and mental health: A synthesis of qualitative findings. *Complementary Therapies in Clinical Practice, 37*, 122–132. doi:10.1016/j.ctcp.2019.101063 PMID:31587992

Conboy, L. A., Noggle, J. J., Frey, J. L., Kudesia, R. S., & Khalsa, S. B. S. (2013). Qualitative evaluation of a high school yoga program: Feasibility and perceived benefits. *Explore (New York, N.Y.), 9*(3), 171–180. doi:10.1016/j.explore.2013.02.001 PMID:23643372

D'Souza, J., & Gurin, M. (2016). The universal significance of Maslow's concept of self-actualization. *The Humanistic Psychologist, 44*(2), 210–214. doi:10.1037/hum0000027

Danielly, Y., & Silverthorne, C. (2017). Psychological Benefits of Yoga for Female Inmates. *International Journal of Yoga Therapy, 27*(1), 9–14. doi:10.17761/1531-2054-27.1.9 PMID:29131730

Dobkin, P. L., Irving, J. A., & Amar, S. (2012). For Whom May Participation in a Mindfulness-Based Stress Reduction Program be Contraindicated? *Mindfulness*, *3*(1), 44–50. doi:10.100712671-011-0079-9

Doria, S., de Vuono, A., Sanlorenzo, R., Irtelli, F., & Mencacci, C. (2015). Anti-anxiety efficacy of Sudarshan Kriya Yoga in general anxiety disorder: A multicomponent, yoga based, breath intervention program for patients suffering from generalized anxiety disorder with or without comorbidities. *Journal of Affective Disorders*, *184*, 310–317. doi:10.1016/j.jad.2015.06.011 PMID:26142611

Gabriel, M. G., Curtiss, J., Hofmann, S. G., & Khalsa, S. B. S. (2018). Kundalini Yoga for Generalized Anxiety Disorder: An Exploration of Treatment Efficacy and Possible Mechanisms. *International Journal of Yoga Therapy*, *28*(1), 97–105. doi:10.17761/2018-00003 PMID:29698081

Gallegos, A. M., Crean, H. F., Pigeon, W. R., & Heffner, K. L. (2017). Meditation and yoga for post-traumatic stress disorder: A meta-analytic review of randomized controlled trials. *Clinical Psychology Review*, *58*, 115–124. doi:10.1016/j.cpr.2017.10.004 PMID:29100863

Gangadhar, B., & Varambally, S. (2011). Yoga as Therapy in Psychiatric Disorders: Past, Present, and Future. *Biofeedback*, *39*(2), 60–63. doi:10.5298/1081-5937-39.2.03

Gothe, N. P., Hayes, J. S., Temali, C., & Damoiseaux, J. S. (2018). Differences in Brain Structure and Function Among Yoga Practitioners and Controls. *Frontiers in Integrative Neuroscience*, *12*, 26. doi:10.3389/fnint.2018.00026 PMID:29988397

Gothe, N. P., Khan, I., Hayes, J. S., Erlenbach, E., & Damoiseaux, J. S. (2019). Yoga Effects on Brain Health: A Systematic Review of the Current Literature. *Brain Plasticity*, *5*(1), 105–122. doi:10.3233/BPL-190084 PMID:31970064

Gupta, N., Khera, S., Vempati, R. P., Sharma, R., & Bijlani, R. L. (n.d.). Effect Of Yoga Based Lifestyle Intervention On State And Trait Anxiety. *Indian Journal of Physiology and Pharmacology*. PMID:16850902

Ivtzan, I., & Papantoniou, A. (2014). Yoga meets positive psychology: Examining the integration of hedonic (gratitude) and eudaimonic (meaning) wellbeing in relation to the extent of yoga practice. *Journal of Bodywork and Movement Therapies*, *18*(2), 183–189. doi:10.1016/j.jbmt.2013.11.005 PMID:24725784

Jagadeesan, T., R, A., R, K., Jain, T., Allu, A. R., Selvi G, T., Maveeran, M., & Kuppusamy, M. (2022). Effect of Bhramari Pranayama intervention on stress, anxiety, depression and sleep quality among COVID 19 patients in home isolation. *Journal of Ayurveda and Integrative Medicine*, *13*(3), 100596. doi:10.1016/j.jaim.2022.100596 PMID:35693195

Kirk, M. L., Boon, B., & DiTuro, D. (2005). *Hatha Yoga Illustrated*. Human Kinetics.

Maehle, G. (2011). *Ashtanga Yoga: Practice and Philosophy*. New World Library.

Mehta, K., Mehta, S., Chalana, H., Singh, H., & Thaman, R. G. (2020). Effectiveness of Rajyoga meditation as an adjunct to first-line treatment in patients with obsessive compulsive disorder. *Indian Journal of Psychiatry*, *62*(6), 684–689. doi:10.4103/psychiatry.IndianJPsychiatry_401_19 PMID:33896974

Miller, R. (n.d.). *Yoga Therapy: Definition, Perspective and Principles*. International Association of Yoga Therapists (IAYT). https://www.iayt.org/page/YogaTherapyDefinitio

Mishra, A. S., Sk, R., Hs, V., Nagarathna, R., Anand, A., Bhutani, H., Sivapuram, M. S., Singh, A., & Nagendra, H. R. (2020). Knowledge, Attitude, and Practice of Yoga in Rural and Urban India, KAPY 2017: A Nationwide Cluster Sample Survey. *Medicines (Basel, Switzerland)*, *7*(2), 8. doi:10.3390/medicines7020008 PMID:32033426

Monro, R. (1997). Yoga therapy. *Journal of Bodywork and Movement Therapies*, *1*(4), 215–218. doi:10.1016/S1360-8592(97)80047-2

Mooventhan, A., & Nivethitha, L. (2017). Evidence based effects of yoga in neurological disorders. *Journal of Clinical Neuroscience*, *43*, 61–67. doi:10.1016/j.jocn.2017.05.012 PMID:28599839

Neumark-Sztainer, D. (2014). Yoga and eating disorders: Is there a place for yoga in the prevention and treatment of eating disorders and disordered eating behaviours? *Advances in Eating Disorders (Abingdon, England)*, *2*(2), 136–145. doi:10.1080/21662630.2013.862369 PMID:24955291

Noggle, J. J., Steiner, N. J., Minami, T., & Khalsa, S. B. S. (2012). Benefits of yoga for psychosocial well-being in a US high school curriculum: A preliminary randomized controlled trial. *Journal of Developmental and Behavioral Pediatrics*, *33*(3), 193–201. doi:10.1097/DBP.0b013e31824afdc4 PMID:22343481

Patañjali. (1978). *The Yoga Sutras of Patanjali*. Patanjali. http://ci.nii.ac.jp/ncid/BA24616006

Petryszak, N. G. (1981). Tabula rasa–its origins and implications. *Journal of the History of the Behavioral Sciences*, *17*(1), 15–27. doi:10.1002/1520-6696(198101)17:1<15::AID-JHBS2300170104>3.0.CO;2-3 PMID:11608578

Raghuwanshi, A. (2011). A Review: History of Revival of Yoga in the 20th Century and Establishment of Yoga as a Science in the 21st Century. *International Scientific Yoga Journal: Sense, 1*(1).

Rakhshani, A., Maharana, S., Raghuram, N., Nagendra, H. R., & Venkatram, P. (2010). Effects of integrated yoga on quality of life and interpersonal relationship of pregnant women. *Quality of Life Research: An International Journal of Quality of Life Aspects of Treatment, Care and Rehabilitation*, *19*(10), 1447–1455. doi:10.100711136-010-9709-2 PMID:20632115

Reinhardt, K. M., Noggle Taylor, J. J., Johnston, J., Zameer, A., Cheema, S., & Khalsa, S. B. S. (2018). Kripalu Yoga for Military Veterans With PTSD: A Randomized Trial. *Journal of Clinical Psychology*, *74*(1), 93–108. doi:10.1002/jclp.22483 PMID:28524358

Ross, A., Bevans, M., Friedmann, E., Williams, L., & Thomas, S. (2014). "I Am a Nice Person When I Do Yoga!!!" A Qualitative Analysis of How Yoga Affects Relationships. *Journal of Holistic Nursing*, *32*(2), 67–77. doi:10.1177/0898010113508466 PMID:24166108

Sadler, J. Z. (1992). Clinical problem solving and the biopsychosocial model. *The American Journal of Psychiatry*, *149*(10), 1315–1323. doi:10.1176/ajp.149.10.1315 PMID:1530068

Sakthivel, A., Kalyan, P., Bhattacharjee, R., & Ramkumar, A. (2023). Novel Chakra Sadhana Yoga-Based Treatment Approach For Posttraumatic Stress Disorder (Ptsd) And Dissociative Identity Disorder (Did)-A Case Study. *Proceedings of the International Conference on Public Health*. ACM. 10.17501/24246735.2022.7201

Santos, J. L., Bashaw, M. A., Mattcham, W., Cutcliffe, J. R., & Vedana, K. G. G. (2018). The Biopsychosocial Approach: Towards Holistic, Person-Centred Psychiatric/Mental Health Nursing Practice. In *Principles of specialty nursing* (pp. 89–101). Springer International Publishing. https://doi.org/8 doi:10.1007/978-3-319-31772-4_

Sathyanarayanan, G., Vengadavaradan, A., & Bharadwaj, B. (2019). Role of Yoga and Mindfulness in Severe Mental Illnesses: A Narrative Review. *International Journal of Yoga, 12*(1), 3–28. doi:10.4103/ijoy.IJOY_65_17 PMID:30692780

Schmid, A. A., Sternke, E., L, A., DO, Conner, N., Starnino, V. R., & Davis, L. W. (2021). The eight limbs of yoga can be maintained in a veteran friendly yoga program. *International Journal of Yoga, 14*(2), 127. . doi:10.4103/ijoy.IJOY_106_20

Shannahoff-Khalsa, D., Fernandes, R. Y., Pereira, C. A. D. B., March, J. S., Leckman, J. F., Golshan, S., Vieira, M. S. R., Polanczyk, G. V., Miguel, E. C., & Shavitt, R. G. (2019). Kundalini yoga meditation versus the relaxation response meditation for treating adults with obsessive-compulsive disorder: A randomized clinical trial. *Frontiers in Psychiatry, 10*, 793. doi:10.3389/fpsyt.2019.00793 PMID:31780963

Sharma, G., Gujral, J. S., Agarwal, A., Jat, M., Mohanty, S., & Pandey, R. M. (2022). Exploring knowledge, attitude and practice regarding yoga among patients attending cardiology and neurology clinics in a tertiary care hospital in northern India. *The National Medical Journal of India, 34*(4), 201–205. doi:10.25259/NMJI_11_20 PMID:35112541

Sharma, V. K., Das, S., Mondal, S., & Goswami, U., & Gandhi, A. (n.d.). Effect of sahaj yoga on depressive disorders. *Indian Journal of Physiology and Pharmacology*. PMID:16579401

Shetty, K. T., Subbakrishna, D. K., & Meti, B. L., & Raju, T. R. (1998). Therapeutic Efficacy of Sudarshan Kriya Yoga (SKK) in Dysthymic Disorder. *Nimhans Journal*, 21–28.

Shroff, F. M., & Asgarpour, M. (2017). *Yoga and Mental Health: A Review. Journal of Physiotherapy &*. Physical Rehabilitation. doi:10.4172/2573-0312.1000132

Singh, A. D. (2017). Yoga for Mental Health: Opportunities and Challenges. MOJ Yoga &. *Physical Therapy*, *2*(1). Advance online publication. doi:10.15406/mojypt.2017.02.00009

Sivananda, S. (1974). *Mind: Its Mysteries and Control*. Divine Life Society.

Sivananda, S. (1986). *Mind: Its Mysteries and Control*.

Stone, M. (2009). *Yoga for a World Out of Balance: Teachings on Ethics and Social Action*. Shambhala Publications.

Streeter, C. C., Jensen, J., Perlmutter, R. M., Cabral, H., Shu, G., Terhune, D. B., & Ciraulo, D. A. (2007). Yoga Asana Sessions Increase Brain GABA Levels: A Pilot Study. *Journal of Alternative and Complementary Medicine (New York, N.Y.), 13*(4), 419–426. doi:10.1089/acm.2007.6338 PMID:17532734

Streeter, C. C., Jensen, J. E., Perlmutter, R. M., Cabral, H. J., Tian, H., Terhune, D. B., Ciraulo, D. A., & Renshaw, P. F. (2007). Yoga Asana sessions increase brain GABA levels: A pilot study. *Journal of Alternative and Complementary Medicine (New York, N.Y.), 13*(4), 419–426. doi:10.1089/acm.2007.6338 PMID:17532734

Suresh, N. C., & Srilakshmidevi, N. B., & Suresh, V. (. (2020). Yogic Diet, Trigunas and Mental Health: Implications for Research. *Indian Journal of Health Studies, 02*(02), 64–73. doi:10.56490/IJHS.2020.2204

Udupa, K. N., & Prasad, R. (1985). Stress and its management by yoga. In *Motilal Banarsidass eBooks*. https://ci.nii.ac.jp/ncid/BA47667811

Vancampfort, D., Vansteelandt, K., Scheewe, T., Probst, M., Knapen, J., De Herdt, A., & De Hert, M. (2012). Yoga in schizophrenia: A systematic review of randomized controlled trials. *Acta Psychiatrica Scandinavica, 126*(1), 12–20. doi:10.1111/j.1600-0447.2012.01865.x PMID:22486714

Verma, G. (2021). The Effect of Swadhyay on the Mental Health Using Statistical Approach. *IOSR Journal of Humanities and Social Science, 26*(3). doi: 2603051921 doi:10.9790/0837-

Walsh, R., & Roche, L. (1979). Precipitation of acute psychotic episodes by intensive meditation in individuals with a history of schizophrenia. *The American Journal of Psychiatry, 136*(8), 1085–1086. doi:10.1176/ajp.136.8.1085 PMID:380368

West, J., Liang, B., & Spinazzola, J. (2017). Trauma Sensitive Yoga as a complementary treatment for posttraumatic stress disorder: A Qualitative Descriptive analysis. *International Journal of Stress Management, 24*(2), 173–195. doi:10.1037tr0000040 PMID:28458503

Wood, J. J. (2006). Effect of anxiety reduction on children's school performance and social adjustment. *Developmental Psychology, 42*(2), 345–349. doi:10.1037/0012-1649.42.2.345 PMID:16569172

Woodyard, C. D. (2011). Exploring the therapeutic effects of yoga and its ability to increase quality of life. *International Journal of Yoga, 4*(2), 49. doi:10.4103/0973-6131.85485 PMID:22022122

Xu, W., Itagi, R. K., & Thaiyar, M. S. (2021). Impact of yama and niyama on psychospiritual factors in young adults: A randomized controlled trial. *International Journal of Yoga - Philosophy Psychology and Parapsychology, 9*(1), 32. doi:10.4103/ijoyppp.ijoyppp_17_20

Chapter 9
Mahabharata Immersion: The Praxis of Antaranga Sadhana – A Pathway to Personal Transformation

Ananthanarayanan Raghu
Ritambhara Ashram, India

Noa Schwartz Feuerstein
Ritambhara Ashram, India

ABSTRACT

This chapter traces the theory and practice of the Mahabharata Immersion (MI) process. It draws from autoethnographic documentation of the participants of more than 20 MI programs. It also explores the parallels with Jungian approaches to inner transformation as experienced by Noa Schwartz Feuerstein (a Jungian Psychotherapist) as a participant observer in one of the programs. The process of deep introspection aided by mirroring oneself through the Mahabharata stories is the central process of the MI. By working with Indian dance and theatre, as well as drawing, introspective practices, and discussions, the participants discover how to practice a meditative witnessing of their inner processes. The MI participants write a reflective journal on their experience of each day. The themes that emerged in the self-reflective essays and the data analysis form the concluding part of the chapter.

INTRODUCTION

It is a dark and dingy room. Not been opened for quite some time. Windows have remained closed too.

Open the door & windows with some effort.

There is a mirror on the wall. Quite old - its coating has faded. And, there is a thick layer of dust and & grime.

With some difficulty, I open the door and the window.

DOI: 10.4018/978-1-6684-9778-4.ch009

Fresh air comes in slowly as if with some caution.

I look in the mirror.

I can't recognise myself.

Gently clean the mirror - remove all the dust and grime. Hold the mirror steady. I see myself now - yes it is me.

I smile.

"Must allow fresh air and clean the mirror regularly"

I say to myself.

Thank you, Raghu and all you wonderful people.

In gratitude

This chapter is divided into 3 parts. Parts 1 and 2 are authored by Raghu Ananthanarayanan and part 3 by Noa Schwartz. Atul Sapre provided the conceptual framework for the chapter and analyzed the data:

- Part 1: Outlines the philosophical underpinnings of the work: the theory of self that is found in Yoga and Sankhya as well as some of the frameworks derived from dance and theatre.
- Part 2: Goes into the details of the programme design. It describes the way the Mahabharata Immersion is conducted. It includes some details on the way each day was planned. Critical parts of the discussions that ensued as the Immersion progressed are also shared.
- Part 3: Comprises a self-reflective piece from a Jungian perspective. We also present an analysis of the self-reflective narratives written by each of the participants of the MI conducted for the Barefoot Academy of Governance.

AN OVERVIEW AND BACKGROUND

The idea of an "immersion" is inspired by the notion of a dip in the Ganges that rids one of their *pApa*. The word *pApa* means going against the flow or the grain. The disappointment, hurt and struggle that characterize one's *vyAvahArika* or transactional life in the marketplace, leaves residues and provokes defence mechanisms. It also conditions one to a combative and maybe even an acquisitive stance. The outcome of this is a life that is in *duHkha*, one that is not replenishing.

The "immersion" assumes that each of us has within a stream of Intelligence and compassion and by clearing up the blocks to the flow of this life-giving spring we can wash away our *pApa*. We will therefore discover a way of living that is more in tune with our true selves, more vibrant and filled with rasa.

The aspiration with which we are offering the immersion is:

- To provide a space for the participants to access the inner dynamics of the psyche.
- To provide them with a map through which to navigate the inner space/ archetypal energies.
- To enable them to discover the "*shAntam*" location (the still space beyond the archetypal energies) from which to access healing energies.
- To equip them with practices that they can take forward into their life spaces.

HOW DOES THE "IMMERSION" WORK?

A Few Key Ideas From the Yoga Sutras

The Yoga Sutra speaks about four stages through which we can delve into the more subtle (*sUkshma*) aspects of our psyche. We start a serious enquiry with intellectual probing. This is characterised by interpretation, judgment, liking and disliking and so on. This stage is called *vitarka*, argumentative. As we engage further, an attitude of examination and seeking takes over and we enter a self-reflective inquiry. We observe the phenomenon with curiosity and care. This stage is called *vichAra*, dialogic. This yields insights and one experiences delight. We touch the stage of *Ananda*. The insight causes deep shifts in our being and our processes of thinking, feeling and acting change spontaneously. This stage is called *asmita*, identity.

The Immersion Process

In the 6-day learning laboratory, we create the context where a person can go through these stages of introspection. Each part of the "immersion" has the space for the participant to experience all four stages. We start with examining our prevailing *rasa*. Are we in touch with them? Are we blocking them? Are we indulging in them? and so on. Through this encounter, we also discover the space of *shAntam*, quietude, that is aware, balanced and calm. Learning how to observe our inner processes from *shAntam* is the primary objective of the immersion. We then encounter our archetypal energies and the mental landscapes that we have created within us. We use a lot of practices from traditional theatre and dance to enable us to examine these inner processes. This gives us an insight into our *antaranga,* our inner faculties and how we create our inner drama, our habitual patterns of feeling, thinking, and doing. The next movement occurs when we use the Mahabharata to reflect ourselves off, like mirrors to ourselves. We start by engaging with one of the heroes that we feel attracted to. For instance, let's say BhIshma. Our enquiry starts with an attempt to understand him intellectually. A small group of us who are all drawn to this character join together and take up one context in which the inner drama of BhIshma plays out. We slowly enter the phase of dialogue. When we enact the inner drama of BhIshma as we see it, and do so with intensity, we see how we are playing out the BhIshma in us, in our lives. The mirror has done its job, we have entered a space where we observe our processes and insights pop up. There is intense sharing and joining in by the other members of the group and many facets of the drama and the BhIshma in us get revealed. If we engage in this dialogue from an inner space of curiosity and compassion accompanied by sufficient intensity, the insights that emerge wash away our conditioned ways of being and burn away the seeds of *avidya* (erroneous perception and action). New perspectives, possibilities and potentials emerge. We can act from a new self. A new being emerges.

WHAT ARE THE FOUNDATIONS OF THIS WORK?

A Brief Story of the Seeding and the Growth of the Offering

There is a bit of a story behind the evolution of the "immersion". I started studying Yoga with Shri T K V Desikachar ("T. K. V. Desikachar," 2017) and his father Yogacharya Krishnamacharya from 1978. In the year 1980, I met Prof Pulin Garg (Patel, n.d.) and started my engagement with Process work (I-Groups as Dr Garg called them). In '81 Prof. Garg spent 6 weeks in Chennai specifically to study Yoga with Desikachar and to engage with him in discussions on the convergence between the Yoga Sutra and Psychology. We started a project called "Inner Work Through Yoga". About 60 Sutras were selected from the various chapters as the key idea that was both pragmatic and profound without being esoteric. I kept the dialogues alive through my engagements with both Shri Desikachar and Prof. Garg. After 4 years, we produced a first-cut version of a manuscript. This was vetted and approved by Shri Desikachar. This became the basis of my work with labs ever since. In 2010 I conducted a 6-day seminar called "Inner Work Through Yoga" where I shared the work I was doing with a larger group of Process workers (R&C Dialogue- Sumedhas).

The Other Influences in the Work as it Has Evolved

Three important influences have shaped the lab design. Firstly discussions and dialogues I have had with Na Muthuswamy ("Na. Muthuswamy," 2015) (founder of the experimental theatre group Koothu P Pattarai) primarily and Anmol Velani (Mekong Cultural Hub, n.d.) on the Indian Theatre traditions. The Koothu traditions enact various episodes from the Mahabharata, and weave in deep philosophy based on the text into their very vibrant (usually all night) performances. Secondly, my dialogues with Jyotsana Narayanan a dance teacher from Kalakshetra and a long-time student of Desikachar. The parallels between the profound insights from the Yoga Sutra and the training that went into the preparation of the performers were striking. With Anmol's help, I designed the "Learning Theatre". This experiment, where I brought a convergence between the Yoga Sutra and laboratory learning processes, has now become the "immersions". So, it is a journey of about 4 decades.

The Journey in a Little More Detail

My experimentation with the process work modality merging theatre and Yoga began with the "Learning Theatre" laboratory learning programme. In these labs, I reversed the process that characterised the laboratory learning methodology of Prof. Garg. He based his work on a concept from Sankhya that he enunciated as follows: "Articulating the unarticulated, seeing the invisible, owning the disowned and acting the withheld". This was based on the Sankhyan aphorism *"vyakta avyakta gnya vignyAnam" (Sāṃkhya Kārikā Verse 2 - Centre for Yoga Studies, 2023)* having an insight into the nature and process of the tangible, the intangible and the seer as the way to end *duHkha*. In my understanding, since the process involved speaking as the primary mode of initiating self-reflexivity, it afforded the participant the possibility of escape and fantasy. At this time I was helping Na Muthuswamy and his theatre group called "Koothu-p-pattari" in their physical and psychological preparation for their performances. It became very clear to me that the body does not lie!

Often my work involved the observation of the actor in their practice and working with them through process methods to enable them to dissolve their inner blocks and bring authenticity and power into their performance.

Let me illustrate: while working for a play, one of the actors (who was very skilled) found it very difficult to be authentic in playing the role of a person showing compassion to a woman in distress. When we delved deeper, it became apparent that there was a space within that he was guarding. He had felt used and discarded by a woman he fell in love with. When we "worked" with this further, he pictured himself bleeding and with raw skin. He could neither extend touch nor could he tolerate touch when he was in this inner space. I also discovered many practices found in traditional Indian theatre and dance that combine breathing techniques and meditative practices that enable the dissolving of inner structures of feeling and thought thus making the actor flow into the characters they take. For example, the actor we discussed earlier would get into laboured and intermittent breathing when he entered his difficult space. Enabling him to "stay with" the trauma while observing the body and the breath would quieten him. This inner observation allowed him to reenter the space and recover the parts of him that he felt alienated from.

Theatre and dance focus on the portrayal of Archetypal Heroes. The portrayal brings out the profound humanness of the hero, a person grappling with the pulls and pushes of inner contradictions. Their counterpoint mirrors the struggle but ends up acting out of compulsion and not out of heroic choice. The actor/ dancer who plays the role has to struggle with their inner demons if they are to touch the energetic point that enlivens the *"pAtra"*, the vessel, with their authentic struggle. This re-experiencing of the archetypal drama of life makes the portrayal evocative and makes it possible for the audience to resonate with the inner experience. In dance, this is the moment when the *rasa* portrayed unites the dancer and the *rasika* in a shared space. In the dance tradition of south India, the stages through which a *nAyika* (the heroine) develops as she matures into a person capable of being one with her *nAyaka* (the divine hero) is very similar to the process of maturity of a person growing from an ordinary distracted mind to one with a mind capable of *samAdhi*. Maturing is the process of dissolving the various elements that make one's mind gross and outward-oriented i.e., dissolving the veil that covers her divine Self.

Exploring the Parallels With the Yoga Sutras of Patanjali

My study of Yoga Sutra formed the basis of my study with Shri Desikachar and his father Yogacharya Krishnamacharya. The parallels between the work of Prof Garg the Yoga Sutras are profound. In Yoga there is a distinction between outer work (*bahiranga sAdhana*- practices like *yama, niyama, Asana* and *prANAyAma*), Inner work (*antaranga sAdhana*- practices like *pratyAhAra, dhAraNA* and *samAdhi*) and work with even more subtle inner processes (*nirbIja samAdhi*). The final 62 sutras (out of 195) selected by Shri Desikachar and Dr Garg fall into the space of *antaranga yoga*.

With the help of Anmol Velani and Rudraprasad Sengupta (*Rudraprasad Sengupta*, 2012), I designed the "Learning Theatre" in 1996. I brought in the elements of Yoga, Indian dance and theatre as well as process work to develop this methodology. After about two decades of shaping the Learning Theatre Lab, I launched the Mahabharata Immersion. The "theory of self" that I use to design this process is based entirely on Yoga, dance and theatre. The Mahabharata Immersion endeavors to play out the particular drama we are drawn to from the Mahabharata and view it from an inner location of *shAntam* to gain insights into ourselves. *shAntam* is the location from which we can watch inner confusions and compulsions being transformed.

THE KEY IDEAS FROM THE YOGA TRADITION THAT THE IMMERSION IS BASED ON

The key Sutra I am basing the inner work on is *"dhyAna heyAH tad vrttayaH"* (Chapter 2- Sutra 11). Through the practice of *dhyAna* the seeds of suffering are de-potentized The Yoga Sutra speaks about two ways of bringing about a change in one's behaviour: firstly *karmajam karma* which is an effort that is undertaken with a consequence in mind. One sets a goal in one's mind and to achieve that one shapes and manipulates oneself. Secondly, *dhyAnajam karma* where the changes in one's psyche and behaviour are the outcome of meditative insight. The Yoga Sutra says that this change is lasting while the one brought about by stiving for consequences is impermanent. Also, when changes come out of meditative insight, a greater Intelligence is in operation and potentials that lie latent get awakened. When one sets goals, one is focusing on consequences drawn from one's present level of understanding of oneself and one's world. It is limited by *avidya* (erroneous knowing). The immersion is therefore an attempt to create a space where one can get in touch with one's meditative self.

Exploring the Convergence Between Dance and Yoga shAdhana

Dance offers a very beautiful framework of the *nava rasa*. One of the key insights we work with is that the ability to touch *shAntam* (one of the nine *rasas*) is synonymous with the ability to be in a state of vulnerability; to be in touch with one's potential; to be in deep attentiveness and quietude all at the same time. We fear touching our vulnerable selves, we therefore create structures of thought, feeling and action to protect ourselves as well as to grasp and cling to what we think is safe and comforting. Yoga Sutra says that these structures of the self, the feelings of desire and aversion to the world that are based on feelings of threat and opportunity are built on the ground of *avidya*. *Avidya* comprises mistaken ideas about permanence and impermanence, good and bad, the healthy and unhealthy, and enlivening and deadening. Our ability to feel the range of *rasa* is therefore completely conditional to these inner structures built upon mistaken ideas about ourselves and our world. When one is enabled to feel safe, and senses that one is in the company of people intent on being compassionate, it becomes possible to let go of the vicelike grip we have on our *avidya* and its creations. Slowly, one moves away from a suspicious and judgmental interface with one's world and begins to savour one's experience of the world and others as they arise spontaneously and therefore experience *rasa*. One begins to be self-reflective, and gradually one touches *shAntam*. The Yoga Sutra describes this process as moving away from an *udAra* level (where ones defensive/ aggressive structures are fully energised) and entering the *tanu* level of experiencing oneself (a state where the inner structures are just starting to form) or even the *prasupta* state (latent and sleeping). When a person experiences Their inner motivations/ emotions/ *rasa* in the *tanu* or *prasupta* stage, the person is in *dhyAna* and has insights into the whole structure and nature of one's psyche. (This process is described in detail in the 2nd Chapter Sutra 2.3 to 2.14 and the 4th chapter Sutra 4.8 to 4.11 of Patanjali's Yoga Sutras).

Integrating the Ideas With Theatre

While working with the actors of Koothu-p-Pattarai, I found that each of the actors was very fluid with one set of expressions but frozen and forced with another set. It was only by sensitising them to their subtle processes through *rasa* exercises that were they able to see how some of the partial selves were held. For example one of the actors had created strong defence/ offence patterns around his "Victim", and could not empathise with the pain of others. Any expression of compassion became "fake". It was only when he discovered an ability to touch his helplessness without an instinctive recoil could he begin to find an authentic expression of empathy with another's suffering.

The Design of the Immersion

The immersion starts with the participants being sensitized to the *navarasa.* They then learn the practice of acting from a core of *shAntam*. Therefore, they are capable of being with others in what dance refers to as the *sakhi bhAva-* relating to the other with curiosity and compassion. The participants are then introduced to the "Archetypal Inner Figures" (AIF) that populate one's inner landscape. Both theatre and dance explicate the drama that takes place between these archetypes. In theatre, they are externalised and treated as separate entities. In reality, they are our inner personalities shaped by our circumstances. All of us have experienced hurt, and that part of us that holds on to hurt is the essence of the victim's archetypal figure. All of us have an inner judge, an inner fighter and so on. Our external behaviour is just a manifestation of the inner drama. As we observe ourselves from a meditative state, the way we have built an Archetypal Inner Figure around each of our *rasa* becomes clear: *bhayAnaka* (fear) feeds the victim, *roudram* (anger) feeds the fighter, *adbhutam* (wonderment) feeds the escapist and so on. When we observe this drama in its *tanu* (sprouting) state, our inner reality becomes very clear to us, our inner mirror is getting cleansed, and our minds become insightful. Yoga Sutra states that the intensity of *dhyAna* (meditative insight) will release the frozen inner patterns.

The Mahabharata as the Mirror

The group is now ready to explore how these inner energies and archetypes manifest. We ask the participants (who have prepared for the immersion by reading the Mahabharata) to choose the character that attracts them/ troubles them the most. Usually, a group of four or five gather around this central figure. The obvious choices are Draupadi/ Arjuna and Karna. But we have had people exploring Shakuni or BhIshma or Ekalavya too. By now it is clear to the participants that behaviour does not arise in a vacuum, nor is a human being a robotic entity with fixed attributes and responses. Behaviour emerges in a context and in response to the way one perceives oneself, others, and the context. Also, in the Indian *itihAsa purANa*, no character is wholly good or bad. For example, Duryodhana is a great warrior and an equal of BhIma in courage and mace craft, but he is caught with envy of his cousins and therefore deploys his immense potential in destructive ways. The group chooses a situation replete with *dharma sankata* (double binds and severe emotional and ethical dilemmas) to explore. In these contexts, the inner drama and the pull of both the *dharmic* and *adharmic* forces become apparent. We ensure that every member of the group explores/ enacts all the characters, and we ask them to see how the *dharmic* options can be enhanced by changing the script in the last enactment of the play. This not only ensures that each one sees that every character is potentially within each of us, but it also completely breaks the process of projection and "othering". Often the participants come up with exciting twists to resolve the tension. To illustrate, a group that explored BhIshma decided to end the Mahabharata war by making Krishna become many (as he did with the Gopika) and befriend BhIshma while simultaneously being with Arjuna! BhIshma is then able to let go of the terrible vows he has taken and see how much *adharma* is created by his so-called *dharmic* act of adhering to his idea of right conduct. BhIshma's eyes are opened as he receives his

Gita, and he calls out Duryodhana and DhritarAshtra! BhIshma finds legitimacy to act, he awakens his psychological ownership of the land and its people. He leaves behind his impotence that is held on too firmly under the excuse of having to uphold the throne which is being occupied by a person committed to being blind to *dharma* despite having advisors like Vidura in his court!

These resolutions are great breakthroughs for the whole group and not just for the people exploring the characters through the enactment. The play recedes into the background. Participants face up to their ways of disowning responsibility, of having made commitments or come to conclusions about themselves or others and mortgaging their lives to old and irrelevant promises. The BhIshmas, Dronas and Karnas inside each of us playing out our inner battles become the focus of the enquiry.

A whole Life Saga is Replayed Through the Process!

Yes, that's the way it feels. If there are 20 participants in the immersion, it is really like delving into the deepest recesses of twenty lives! And in this deep dive, the springs of compassion and meditation are regenerated. Healing takes place; The victim selves become inner healers; The fighters discover what it means to be dharmic warriors; Judges become wise and the escapist within becomes a seeker of truth. This is the discovery and change brought out by observing oneself in *dhyAna*. When this inner transformation is touched, there is a great release of energy. Huge potentials that were used as protective barriers or as acquisitive probes get freed, *rasa* that is locked up gets released. One discovers new ways to be, and a new identity that was full of hidden potential takes the place of old defensive structures of feeling, thought and action.

PART TWO: THE FACILITATION OF THE IMMERSION

There are three levels at which one can work with oneself using the Mahabharata: conversation, exploration, and immersion.

- Conversation: examine frameworks of the mind and formulate thought processes
- Exploration: examine the basis of action, identity and choice making
- Immersion: go to the deep layers of the self and watch how we construct our identities and action choices.

Unlike the laboratory or workshop format, the immersion does not rely on extensive dialogues. The expectation from the participants is that each individual works with his or herself through the enactments and theatre/ dance/ drawing exercises and discovers how to locate oneself in a contemplative space while engaging with others.

A literal understanding of the Mahabharata is not the basis for the immersion. We constantly engage in the process of meaning-making and choice-making that is unique to each of us. All the Mahabharata characters are looked at from their Archetypal locations and their implications for each of us. Unfortunately, with the advent of television serials, these characters have been concretized in each of our minds. We tend to see them as stereotypes because of this and prevent ourselves from understanding their quintessential attributes or looking at them as archetypal energies. If we can separate the popular meanings and stay with the essential flavor of these characters, then it's possible to get in touch with our primal energies. The more we engage with this process the more we bring alive the collective immersion space. We avoid the didactic storyline and dive into the inner meanings we give the characters in relation to our life contexts. Embodied exploration is the key. It is only through this that transformation can take place, otherwise, we will fall back into old behaviours and perspectives.

INVOKING THE BHARATA KOOTHU TRADITION

Traditional Indian theatre and its exploration of the Mahabharata in the village context is our guideline. Bharata Koothu has been performed in Tamil Nadu for more than a thousand years. The Western theatre and its proscenium stage have a specific impact on the spectator, it has an outside-in orientation. The stage is set at a higher level and demarcates the audience space and the actor space. Traditional Indian theatre on the other hand is more inclusive and the spectator and actor are constantly in a relationship of equity in the here-and-now space that they share. The screen is used to make a temporal division between the time past and the time present. The actors seek to invite the archetypes into themselves and see themselves as a "*pAthiram*" or "*bhUmika*" i.e., a vessel that is filled with other energy. The process of donning the make-up is ritualistic and is a time when the "transcendent" is invited to enter the actor. The stage is the space for bridging time past and time present. The actor too comes from behind the screen as if in a process of birth and joins the audience in a contemporary time-space. The "*sUtradhAr*" (the Jester/ narrator) links the archetypal energies with the here and now and threads the narrative into the lives of the audience.

We learn how to simulate this process through the explorations we engage with. We are the actors and the audience. We learn to observe ourselves and our inner drama from a place of *shAntam*.

SOME FOUNDATIONAL IDEAS

The exploration is founded on exploring the *navarasa* and Archetypal Inner Figures as discussed in part 1 of the paper. In MI we are attempting to look at the self-construct and the processes by which we continuously recreate and reinforce this construct. By becoming attentive to this process from its subtle origins to its tangible manifestation, we transform the process.

The self is being shaped through constant engagement with the world. The self creates the construct/ idea of the 'Me' through responses to challenges. Can one become aware of the ground from which this 'me' is being created? The various forms that one creates for oneself come from the assumption that "if I am like .... then I will be viable?" This is a habit we develop for self-preservation. The constructed sense of self is kept intact and inviolate. In MI we strive to create a context for deep insight into this process.

We watch our bodily processes, our emotional processes and our psychological processes with compassion, attentiveness and curiosity. We discover the location of *dhyAna* and a state of *shAntam*. The intensity and insight that this profound observation creates burn the seeds of *avidya* and ends *duHka* .

- Axiom 1: The *navarasa (liminal emotional cathexis)* are the subtlest form in which we can experience ourselves. This requires a release of energies locked up in the body due to the concretisation of one's conditioning.

- <u>Axiom 2:</u> These *navarasa* gather force and substance as they start to manifest. We experience them as Archetypal Inner Figures(AIF) at this stage of their formation. The various AIF are - the actor, guardian, judge, beckoner, victim, friend, dreamer, nurturer, and meditator. The "actor" is the persona that encounters the world and is experienced by others. This AIF exemplifies *vIryam* (courage) since it is that part of the self that is resolute and shows up to act in the world day after day regardless of whether yesterday held up to one's expectations or not. However, the actor can be energized by the other AIFs:

When we contemplate our inner chatter (stories), it becomes clear to us that a drama is being enacted within. The most prominent dramatis personae are the Victim, the Guardian, and the Judge (and his able assistants namely, the Prosecutor and the Defendant). To escape the cacophony of this chatter, we listen to the seductive fantasies of the Beckoner. This inner drama/chatter is our story.

The 'script' that these Archetypal Figures play out is very repetitive. If we distill the lines (litany) that each of these figures/ voices, they sound something like this:

- The Victim (*bhayAnakam*- fear): poor me!.....I am always misunderstood! .....watch out, I will be hurt again.....!
- The Guardian (*roudram*- anger): I am ready and vigilant.......; the world is full of potential danger.....
- The Judge (*bhibatsam*- aversion): I should not ......! I must.....! I deserve to be punished......!
    - Prosecutor: I am guilty because.....;
    - Defendant: I am not guilty because.....;
- The Beckoner (*adbhutam*- wonderment): The world is full of pleasurable possibilities, let me just run away, just have fun.....!

When the Meditator and the Friend are awakened then the Dreamer has a space to emerge and manifest through the actor.

- The Friend (*shrngAram*- Love): I am affectionate, accept the actor as is and confront with honesty....
- The Dreamer (*hAsyam*- Joy): Here are the gifts and talents you are endowed with. Can you hear my gentle voice? My subtle visions...
- The Nurturer (*karuNa*- compassion): I will heal all your wounds, and help you grow....
- The Meditator (*shAntam*- quietude): I am tranquil, silent, Conscious, compassionate and aware waiting with infinite patience for you to embrace me....

When the self is not anchored in the Meditator and Friend locations, the Victim, the Guardian, the Judge and the Beckoner dominate the Actor. The Actor takes on forms that are either defence mechanisms or instruments of acquisitiveness.

- <u>Axiom 3:</u> The process of witnessing with compassion and curiosity comprises three aspects: action, reflection and observation. As we learn how to anchor ourselves in the Meditator and Friend, our observation becomes a meditative enquiry into the processes of the Actor. The intensity of this observation yields insight as well as healing.
- <u>Axiom 4</u>: The most easily observable form of our action is our role-taking in relationship to others in a context. This choice is mediated by a subconscious process of meaning-making which is trig-

gered by the *navarasa* and AIF at a deeper level. Thus the “role” we choose to play is conditioned by processes that are normally invisible to us. The acculturing epics like the Mahabharata create symbolic Role-identities that can be used as mirrors to the self.

- Axiom 5: The process of enactment sensitizes us to our bodies, our emotions and our inner processes allows us to observe ourselves from the Meditator and Friend location. We can reflect our inner processes to ourselves and gain insights into the nature of our psyche.

DETAILS OF THE FACILITATION PROCESS

Day One Theme: Exploring the *Navarasa and Annamaya Mandala*

The objective: enable the participant to become conscious of the deep patterns of congealed feelings that characterize our psychic structures. The participants are enabled to melt the frozen inner self.

- Various movements to break the ice
- Facilitated walking exploring associations with various landscapes
- Exploring the living processes in these landscapes
- Introducing the *navarasa* through guided imagery
- Introducing the *navarasa* through theatre exercises
- Exploring the masculine and feminine expression of the *navarasa*
- The *annamaya mandala:* “Self-portrait” based on the *navarasa* exploration: Drawing one’s body and locating the *navarasa* in the parts where it was felt strongly either in flow or blockage; *navarasa* not experienced or ‘faked’ drawn outside the body
- Sharing the day’s experience in triads: speaker (describing the action), mirror (enabling reflection) and a silent observer (enabling meditativeness)
- Large group sharing

Day Two Theme: Exploring the Archetypal Inner Figures and *prANamaya mandala*

The objective: enable the participant to see their inner drama from a space of compassion. This enables them to understand the inner tensions and envisage new possibilities.

- Exploring the masculine and the feminine through different types of walking
- Facilitated exploration of the Archetypal Inner Figures using the “Greek theatre” mode: The participants are requested to treat the room as their space, locate themselves in a place that “feels like” the AIF briefly described; AIF is voiced in the first person singular while the participants listen blindfolded; the narration links the AIF with the dominant *navarasa* that evokes/ provokes the AIF; participants are encouraged to intensify the experience, find their litany and assume postures that get evoked; a card is given to the participants and they represent their experience symbolically; Each AIF is explored for about 10mins
- The *prANamaya mandala:* Once the exploration of the individual AIF is completed, the participants arrange the cards in a way that reflects the inner drama: AIF that dominate the inner dialogue are

given more space, the suppressed voices are hidden, relative positions that they occupy in ones inner landscape gets reflected in the arrangement

- The participants then draw a "river of life": the key turning points in their life and how these challenges/ interactions with significant others evoked/ provoked the AIF and shaped the inner drama
- Sharing in triads

Day Three Theme: Exploring the Inner Landscape and *Manomaya Mandala*

<u>The objective:</u> enable the participant to understand how they create their world as they encounter others. What inner patterns sustain interpersonal interfaces and how to expand one's behavioral repertoire?

- Exploring the inner drama through simple theatre exercises
- The *manomaya mandala:* (explained in appendix-1)
- Koothu performance: the participants are exposed to a performance of an important episode of the Mahabharata by a traditional Theatre Group
- The participants then choose a character and groups get formed around a central theme proposed by one of them; 5 groups are formed
- Preparation time

Days Four, Five Theme: Inner Exploration of *the pAndava Mandala* Through the Mahabharata

<u>The objective:</u> enable the participant to uncover their archetypal patterns and own up to their heroic potential.

- Each group is given a whole session of 2 hrs
- The group enacts the chosen play
- The inner drama and its outer expression through the *pAndava* enactments is explored
- The audience responds to the enactment by "voicing the unarticulated, making the invisible visible, owning up to the disowned" by playing out the "alter-egos" of the character that awakened them to their own hidden selves
- Pulling together all the enactments and relating the insights to the frameworks discussed

Day Six, The *hAnopAya mandala*: Consolidation and the Covenant

<u>The objective:</u> enable the participant to consolidate the learning, define their dream and make a covenant unto oneself.

- The *manomaya mandala* is revisited through a process of psychic recalibration that enables *prAyashchitta* - reclaiming one's innocence
- The participants make a *sankalpa* - a covenant to oneself to invest in "the best that one can be" and awaken to their heroic potentials
- The participants experience a symbolic rebirth

PART THREE: EPILOGUE AND CONCLUSION

Reflections of a participant observer from a Jungian Perspective (Author- Noa Schwartz Feuerstein)

The archetypal level in the psyche is the collective unconscious, the deepest inner substratum that one is born with, composed of all human experience since its beginning and the whole of human potential. The building blocks of the collective unconscious are the archetypes, which are the main clusters around which the human experience is assembled. The Self is the central archetype, and the other major archetypes are the Big Mother, the Father, Anima, Animus, Persona, Shadow, Puer and Senex, the Wounded Healer and more.

According to the map of the psyche that Raghu is drawing, at the archetypal level are residing 9 archetypal patterns, depicted as 9 differentiated inner personalities, or archetypal figures. Those 9 figures are describing 9 psychic potential tendencies and functions. Each individual, according to their life circumstances, will experience and color each of those inner personalities differently and will identify with some of those personalities, will be assisted by some and be injured by some.

According to Jung, in the process of Individuation, which is life's goal, one should aspire to come to know all the parts of his psyche and fulfill them to live as complete life as possible in a way that renders his life and the world around him meaningful and fulfilling.

But when we look deeply into our life and our functioning, we realize that we are not in touch with all those parts and that our potential is far from being fulfilled because of that. A crucial role is played by the environment in which one grew up, and one's early life experiences in causing this insufficiency.

For understanding the environmental effect on one's process of individuation, Raghu created an additional set of typologies, the '*manomaya mandala*' which describes 5 possible outer structures of one's life. The interaction that takes place between the environmental structure and the individual personality, influences, and even determines the way one's personality will be consolidated out of the archetypal collective level.

The space of the *manomaya mandala* is where the critical encounter happens. The movement from the archetypal level to the personal level takes place. The archetypes are consolidated and become individual complexes. The complexes, according to Jung, are created and crystalized along life encounter between the archetypes of the inner world and the objects of the outer world. Thus, for example, out of the inner holistic 'big mother' archetype, the individual will experience just a limited part, which corresponds with his own personal mother and the qualities of their interaction. This may become a mother complex, which is their personal conscious and unconscious experience and image of their mother, which its roots are in the archetypal big mother. limited by the encounter with the outer world experience. In yoga, this meeting will be named the meeting of *Ashraya* (subtle inner structures) and *Alambana* (subtle outer ground) (*Sutras Ch 4 PH Notes*, n.d.).

Koodam: The Village tradition of playing out the Mahabharata in which the whole village becomes both spectators and actors is referred to as a *Koodam*- the trusted collective. The presence of the group as a trusted container enhances the power of the *manomaya mandala.* The projections, complexes, internalizations and introjects that one has been unconscious off get reflected off others. One begins to accept and embrace the disowned parts of oneself. The unconscious is made conscious through the encounter with others in a space of compassion.

Amplification - A therapeutic tool which Jung developed, which uses myth as an amplifier and guide in the personal inner state, conflicts, and challenges which one meets along one's "heroic journey". The collective myth can embrace the confused and lonely individual in their personal life situation, help them to understand their hidden inner motives, wishes. fears, wounds, and hindrances in fulfilling himself. The myth may help them find the solution and their way. The Mahabharata is a fertile field for amplification, as it is being said the Mahabharata encompasses all human experience. This inner work through mythological amplification is what MI offers the participant.

The transcendent Function, - is an unconscious psychic function which comes to help as one finds himself in an unsolvable conflict. Jung states that staying and waiting, holding the opposites, instead of choosing a one-sided solution will evoke the transcendent function; then a new entity, a third; a solution will arise. this will happen in a creative act, out of the unconscious. The MI offers the participant to live and experience inner conflict, through a *dharma sankata* being enacted in the myth or hero one chose to explore. The creative act (drama) of the deep symbolic level of the myth, will enable the participant to observe in *shantam* his inner world illuminated by the myth. Thus, in- *shantam* observation helps to hold the inner opposites and create through the transcendent function one's answer.

ANALYSIS OF THE REFLECTIVE NARRATIVES OF AN MI COHORT

The MI was conducted for 15 participants of a Diploma course called "Dignity and Development" offered by the Barefoot Academy of Governance and the Tata Institute of Social Sciences.

About an hour was set aside every day through the 5.5 days for participants to reflect on the day. They were asked to

1. reflect on their inner responses
2. look at what evoked them
3. look at disconnects
4. examine what enabled a reconnect
5. any insights

The reflections along with their review after 3 months were collated and studied. We took up the reflections of A (male) and V (female) for detailed analysis. The patterns that we saw in the reflections of A & V were then correlated with the self-reflections of the others.

THE PATTERNS

The reflections followed a pattern. The initial exercises and explorations largely helped the participant gain an acceptance of who they were and what was happening to them at the level of body, emotion, and deeper sensing of the AIF. Those participants who did not plumb this depth also found insights difficult to come by. They ended up with "lessons learnt" more than experiencing transformative changes. However, 12 out of the 15 participants reported significant insights and transformation. Many of them were able to take these back to their "work-a-day world" and implement significant changes. For example,

"A" reported a recalibration of his relationship with his wife. Their recalibration provided the space and energy needed to redefine his work. "V" reported a fundamental review of her work world and a renewed interface with her family. On the whole, participants reported the discovery of meaning in life and therefore renewed energy in their work. Many reviewed their definitions of the central purpose of their life.

Every participant's review contained at least a few statements in each of these stages. There was some progression in the narrative as we went from day 1 to day 5, along the dimension of self-acceptance to inner shifts. Often, a deeper acceptance of self especially of the disowned sides occurred on the 3rd or 4th day. This seems to indicate a cyclic process of self-discovery: self-acceptance leads to self-exploration, this in turn allows for an acceptance of the disowned parts of the self. As the disowned parts are embraced the inner patterns seem to become clear to the person. The next stage includes an exploration of new possibilities and goes back to new levels of self-acceptance. Many participants got into the grips of their inner blocks, double binds, and *dharma sankata*. The struggle with the *dharma sankata* was made more visible through the enactment of the self-selected dramatic incidents from the Mahabharata. Watching others perform their drama seems to be as helpful as one's enactment in finding inner healing. The discovery of inner healing and the realising of hidden potentials seem to go hand in hand.

The review narratives suggested the following stages of inner movement:

1. Accepting self as is: Most of the early reflections of the participants centred around the discovery of themselves in ways that were surprising to them. This awareness and acceptance in a "safe" context is the ground on which the space of the immersion is built.
    a. Through the Body
    b. Through Emotions
    c. Through Archetypal Inner Figures
2. Exploring and expanding the idea of self: Once there is an acceptance of oneself, the participant feels free to explore further inward, looking at new parts of the self.
3. Awareness and acceptance of shadows: - "the parts I have hidden/ avoided": The ability to look at hidden parts of the self seems to be a critical threshold that needs to be crossed for real insights to emerge.
4. Understanding internal patterns/ Interlinking events and responses: Once the participant discovers the ability to accept one's shadows without reacting to them, they seem to understand the inner and the outer worlds as reflections of each other.
5. Playing with possibilities/ Alternate ways of dealing with situations: The participants seem to dabble with "ways out" of what they experience as negative patterns as the understanding of inner patterns grows.
6. *Dharma Sankata* (double bind/ paradox)- feeling stuck / the central knot: The second critical threshold is the discovery of double binds. Some of the participants described it as a loop, some as being stuck in a deep pattern and some as a knot. In the Yoga Sutra crossing this internal vortex is considered a key for releasing *prANa* that is trapped in negative structures.
7. Discovering the basic inner drama, and the ground of being: The acknowledgement of the *dharma sankata* within seems to allow the participants to take a holistic view of themselves in their context.
8. Realizing higher potential/ healing – New Voices: At different points in the exploration, but more often in later stages, participants release long-held hurts and discover healing energies. This is accompanied by some catharsis.

9. Powerful Internal Shifts - New possible ways of being – Resolves and Commitments: Intuitive leaps into new ways of being in the world emerge at various points in the self-reviews, but very often come in the form of a commitment to the "new self" that they have experienced in the Immersion.

REFERENCES

Wikipedia. (2017). *T. K. V. Desikachar*. Wikipedia. https://en.wikipedia.org/wiki/T._K._V._Desikachar

Mekong Cultural Hub. (n.d.). *Anmol Vellani*. Mekong Cultural Hub. https://www.mekongculturalhub.org/people/anmol/

Wikipedia. (2015). *Na. Muthuswamy*. Wikipedia. https://en.wikipedia.org/wiki/Na._Muthuswamy

Patel, B. (n.d.). Pulin K Garg. *Archives*. https://archives.iima.ac.in/faculty/Pulin-K-Garg.html

Rudraprasad Sengupta. (2012). Wikipedia. https://en.wikipedia.org/wiki/Rudraprasad_Sengupta

Centre for Yoga Studies. (2023, May 14). *Sāṃkhya Kārikā verse 2*. Centre for Yoga Studies. https://yogastudies.org/samkhya/samkhya-verse-2/

Sutras Ch 4 PH Notes. (n.d.). Sanskrit Documents. https://sanskritdocuments.org/sites/athayoga/sutra_ch4phn.html

APPENDIX ONE

About the Quadrants of the Manomaya Mandala

The living process is very dynamic. However, to enable one to introspect about the nature of one's behaviour and one's experience we use the framework called the *manomaya mandala*. The mandala framework highlights four life spaces by juxtaposing the self and the other. One can be fully self-expressive or become progressively self-contained till one is completely non-expressive. The other in whose presence one expresses oneself can either be fully receptive or become progressively non-responsive till they become actively rejecting. We can therefore conceptualize our lives in four different ways, namely, the four quadrants of the *manomaya mandala*.

First, the quadrant of Nurturance: when one is fully expressive and the other/context is fully receptive and appreciative, one experiences great freedom to be and act. There is flow and love, mutuality and play, give and take. This is the ideal nurturing space, a garden where one experiences belonging and one can grow roots and feel safe. The lover is the role archetype that plays out in this space. *shringAram* and *hAsyam* are the *rasa*-s that dominate the space.

Second, the quadrant of Challenge: when one is fully alive and expressive, but the other/ context is unwilling to receive the expression. One experiences challenges and feels provoked to force acceptance. One experiences resistance and flow is blocked, there is a struggle to dominate and to avoid being imposed upon. This is the space testing one's capabilities and proving one's power, an arena as it were. One strives for progress and victories and seeks to acquire wealth and power. The hero overcoming great odds is the role archetype that plays out. *roudram* and *vIryam* are the *rasa*-s that dominate this space.

Third, the quadrant of Search: when one feels empty of resources and motivation to express oneself and the other/ context is also hostile or indifferent. One experiences loneliness and meaninglessness. There is a retreat from engagement both from the world of loving connectedness as well as from antagonizing confrontation. There is space to rest and recoup. Perhaps one can search for new resources within oneself, and meanings not defined either by affirmation or by disaffirmation of the other. The seeker encountering the uncharted is the role archetype that plays out. *adbhutam* and *bhibhatsam* are the *rasa*-s that dominate this space.

Fourth, the quadrant of Experimentation: when one feels empty and resourceless, but the other/ context is inviting and willing to foster growth. One experiences hope and the stirrings of will. Inner resistances can be overcome, and one can learn how to relate and connect in ways that are appropriate and meaningful. There is space to act, make mistakes, experiment and gain self-confidence. The new and unformed capabilities can be shaped, and one develops competencies. The disciple eager to learn is the role archetype that plays out. *karuNa* and *bhayAnakam* are the rasas that dominate this space.

Fifth, the meditative centre from which one can witness the whole drama with stillness and tranquility- *shAntam*.

APPENDIX TWO

Some Sample Statements

1. Accepting self as is:

a. Through the Body:

i. One of my first observations is that all the emotions are in my body. I used to feel I am indifferent to disgust but today, during the activity I felt a deep feeling of disgust in my abdomen and throat.

ii. Different emotions dominate different parts of my body. For Eg:

1. Anger – Palms and the soles of my feet
2. Sorrow – Deep inside my chest
3. Disgust – Stomach
4. Love – Shoulders and Chest
5. Courage – Backbone, Face, Shoulder
6. Fear – Deep inside my chest
7. Happy – Face, shoulder, hand

iii. The part of my body I identified with is a representation of the sharp feeling of disgust that comes and during which, I refuse to look beyond. The heart palpitates when it feels fearful; the legs might also shake, and sweat might pour.

b. Through Emotions

i. I find myself in a space of equanimity with everything that's inside me and outside me through a defense mechanism, which is shutting myself down from the external stimuli that I am not comfortable with.

ii. It seems like the actor is holding the emotions inside him and does not want others to see the emotions.

c. Through Archetypal Inner Figures

i. Another insight which I received from my Meditator is that because the fear is so deeply rooted, my actor is protected by my Guardian and is very close to Victim. This position of my Guardian and Victim makes it difficult for my actor to engage with my Dreamer and Meditator.

ii. The Guardian manifests in the form of a volcano that puffs out anger on people who are in my close vicinity and makes me think I am superior to others around me.

iii. The Judge waits for the weak moment of the opponent and helps me in the plot to attack.

2. Exploring and expanding the idea of self:

a. I understood how the different *rasa*, different shadows, Actor and the Meditator are placed in our life. This will guide me to explore my inner dynamics further.

b. I could feel the sensation in my body so I understood that statement like consciousness is in my brain – are partial truth. Emotions are in every part of my body.

c. I have been falling sick often in the last year and I am starting to doubt whether it is attributed to the choices I have made in my life.

3. Awareness and acceptance of shadows - the parts one has hidden/ avoided:

a. I observed that my Victim was fully awake and super active. It was so active that it made it impossible for the Guardian to calm down as if it always was ready for a fight.

b. I never thought I judge people. I used to think everyone has their part of the story so let's not be biased. But I was wrong. I had a deep-rooted and strong judge whose idea of wrong and right is very strong. Another dangerous perception of the Judge is – everything is bad, everyone is bad. This perception makes the Judge very rigid to reason, evolve or listen.

c. At the subconscious level, I used to hope someone or some passion would make me get out of the shell I had constructed around me. It seemed that I had gotten so comfortable in the shell that nothing succeeds to get me out of the refuge.

4. <u>Understanding internal patterns/ Interlinking events and responses:</u>

a. I found it easier to give love than receive it. My compassion did not come from my deep being and it seemed quite superficial I could not think of a real-life situation where I felt deeply compassionate about anything.

b. I am a vicious commander who leads his force in a battle, he loves to break the pattern, go against the status quo, takes care of his community and also loves to solve the problems of others. This warrior has strong principles. They are so strong principals that they can't be compromised.

c. I consciously try to hide my true self from people - I hold myself back from expressing emotions to avoid feeling vulnerable later. Unless I ask for help, others have no clue about what I am going through. This makes me feel secluded from others and the events around me.

d. I get extremely uncomfortable when someone loves me madly or expresses intense love, even if it is my mother. I had opposed my dad's wrath in a very subtle way, but I have always gauged the intensity of his anger before I countered it.

5. <u>Playing with possibilities/ Alternate ways of dealing with life challenges:</u>

a. The idea of the Meditator emerging from its cocoon and undergoing a different kind of *tapas* is indispensable to further the pursuit towards a joyous life - to be vulnerable and go through the *rasa* while effectively coming back without a *bogha.*

b. *Shantam* and Compassion, both stem from the whole of my being. If my whole being is in a state of *Shantam*, it automatically leads to a wholesome sense of compassion of which, the part that love holds is a big one and an extremely crucial one.

c. The problem, I believe, does not lie in the ascetic quadrant. It lies in the lack of movement between the quadrants. Perhaps I am trying to jump to acceptance directly from rejection without maneuverings around the shit in the middle and this is causing a certain dislocation and a false sense of detachment which needs to be understood

6. <u>*Dharma Sankata* (double bind/ paradox/ feeling stuck / the central knot):</u>

a. My dominant force is highly charged in this context. This is the reason why my Actor was always super active, always in a war-like situation and never it reflected on what it is actually doing. This is the reason why I don't have a dream or why it is always a blur.

b. My Actor fails to listen and thus never learns completely. Thus it fails again and again and this loop continues. After some time it retreats and shuts himself down but gets bored quickly in solitude and quickly returns to the fighting space with much more frustration and rage and deep disgust. Sometimes it seeks love and approaches it, but there also he fights to change norms in the family. The actor is so stiff that he doesn't let the love sink in. This constant tussle or struggle has never let the Actor be at peace.

7. <u>Discovering the basic inner drama, and the ground of being:</u>

a. I heard something which I have never anticipated. I heard about my family, and I also heard about my regret of not settling down in my life. I don't have a fixed job, no fixed income and I don't even talk to my family properly. I behave so mechanically with them. I realized I never spoke with my mother or wife with compassion and love. I always wanted to correct them, correct their thinking, correct their belief system and their behavior. I never accepted love from them. I believed that love is for weak people, someone who doesn't have the strength to deal with things

b. After the four plays, I realized that I have become more comfortable in the group and felt accepted the way I am. During the sharing about my new Dreamer, my group members pointed out that the thorns of my Victim are black and hurtful to the outside world. Yet I still have a beautiful core which is reflective and filled with love. It was also pointed out that the black in my painting came out in all the archetypes – thorns of the Victim, the core of the volcano of my Guardian, Dreamer, the wall of the Guardian and the head of the Beckoner all had the same black. I realise it was an unpleasant heartbreak from a close friend/relative three years ago, that influenced my current choices in life. I gave up meditation because I felt that my spirit guides did not stop me from trusting him. I started eating meat again and drinking because I felt the discipline that I followed gave me more pain.

8. <u>Realizing higher potential/ healing – New Voices:</u>

a. The Victim in me has seen a shift, yes. It is aware of the bruises, but now it is also aware that he is not the only one who is in pain. He has realized that no one is away from pain. Pain is a part of the world and everybody has a share of it. The Victim in me is not only bold and beautiful, it does not reject love or compassion nor does it vibrate any dark worldview. It is sensing a power. It feels like the Victim in me is transforming into a steady, strong, bold and calm and composed Hero.

b. I felt like I was in a middle of a *kirtan* and I was dancing. I was enjoying every single note in my head. I did feel empty but this emptiness was the presence of a lot of space in me. I wanted to keep quiet and enjoy the feeling as long as possible.

c. I looked into the eyes of the audience and felt safe (this is very strange) to expose my vulnerability. A part of me wanted to be de-robed to expose my true self in front of people. It was like feeling totally safe in a place where others felt unsafe.

9. <u>Powerful Internal Shifts - New possible ways of being – Resolves and Commitments:</u>

a. In the quest to seek the eternal self, I need to begin with a deep exploration of my physical self.

b. My new Dreamer is fluid yet grounded, with large feet on the ground, absorbing all the essence of the ground and transforming it. This Dreamer is full of joy and happiness, but it is not loud. It activates the friend in me and keeps the friend awake. I dream and I am ready to transform my Actor to a much larger perspective. Yes, I want to contribute, but not like a leaf. More like a tree which is grounded, and the roots go deep inside.

c. I began to cry; silent heavy tears taking their time to drip down. The state of people in my surroundings and at large moved me. The fact that in chasing what we chase throughout our life we are running away from true joy, while constantly unable to understand this dichotomy. These tears subsided soon and in came the realization that any change I want to see in the world has to first take root in me; for the tree to grow tall and bloom, it first has to go deeper. The seed needs to shed its layers to embrace the earth around it and strive.

d. I have a hero inside me waiting to bring out the best of myself – I know what I am against, but I don't know what I should strive for.

Chapter 10
Management Practices on Execution Effectiveness of Strategies Based on Thirukkural

Priyadarshini Srinivasan Moharkonda
https://orcid.org/0000-0001-8442-3198
Christ University, India

Rithani
Christ University (Deemed), India

S. Shakshitha
Christ University (Deemed), India

ABSTRACT

Thirukkural by Thiruvalluvar contains couplets that speak about the morale necessary for an individual based on the roles played in various circumstances of life. These are applied to various fields including management even today. In this chapter, the authors conduct a narrative analysis on two major aspects of management skills to be inculcated in managers for successful progression of the organization. Execution is one such important aspect of management which plays a significant role in constructing effective doable strategies and executing the strategies without delay after proper analysis, thus sustaining the motivation level of the team and progress.

INTRODUCTION

Thirukkural, an iconic Tamil literary work, is notable for its concise description of values and ways of life that stands on the sands of time (Durai, 2023). The author, Thiruvalluvar, has written this text with 133 chapters, and each chapter has ten verses and, each consisting of 7 words, totaling 1330 verses. The entire 133 chapters are categorized into three major aspects governing human life – Aram - Virtue (Fundamental Principles of Life), Porul - Wealth (Management) and Inbam - Love (Love in a Family). These

DOI: 10.4018/978-1-6684-9778-4.ch010

couplets (Kurals) talk about the morale needed in an individual based on the roles played in varied life contexts and certain social and political topics. Although Thirukkural was originally written in Tamil, it has now been translated into multiple Indian and European languages. Utilising this translation, numerous scholars started exploring the text to apply it to various life settings including organizational contexts.

The number 7 was considered magical and of great significance to the Greeks. This has been followed and accepted by a multitude of management practices and books (Krishnamurthi, 2018). Thirukkural has a total of 1330 kurals. When we add these numbers together, we get a 7, and similarly, each Kural consists of 7 words. These 7 words are still relevant and have been used as a moral and life guide for over seven ages (Krishnamurthi, 2018).

Krishnamurthi (2018) used two hundred and forty-six Kurals to explain thirty-four management practices. Some of the management practices covered by him are public speaking, communication, employee recruitment, and selection, the art of delegation, ethical practices, and decision-making. He discloses in his book saying these Kurals were chosen based on his exposure and education and that there are more Kurals that contain great management lessons (Krishnamurthi, 2018).

PROBLEM STATEMENT

In this chapter we aim to focus on analyzing two major aspects of management skills to be inculcated in managers for the successful progression of the organization.1. Chapter 67 on Vinaithitpam – Execution Focus 2. Chapter 68 on Vinai Seiyalvagai – Mode of Execution. Execution is one such important aspect of management which plays a significant role in constructing effective doable strategies and in maintaining the motivation level of the team.

Snippet

Before starting to discuss the thirukkural concepts, I would like to illustrate a short story about 100 lazy travelers and 1 fruit seller. Once a group of 100 people decide to go on a long trip, they planned and strategize the entire trip and finally one day they began their journey, but halfway through the journey, they lost felt tired, lost interest in the journey, nobody wanted to move further and they just decided to stay there.as they were resting a fruit seller came by that way and people started to buy fruits from him and it tasted delicious, the taste was so unique and none of them had ever tasted any fruit like that before. They asked him if they could get more of it, to which the fruit seller said if you could come with me to my place which is little further, I will get you even more delicious fruits. Hearing this some of the lazy travelers decided to forgo their desire for fruits and stay back in the same place, as they didn't want to walk further. But many others decided to go with the fruit seller and started their journey with him. After going some distance, a few of them didn't want to walk further so they decided to return back to their friends. So, the rest continued the journey with the assurance of the fruit seller. As they moved down further, they came across an oasis, some of them felt happy seeing that place and didn't want to proceed further, so stayed back there. Now the fruit seller and the remaining few people alone continued their journey. Within a few minutes, they all reached the place mentioned by the fruit seller. The place was like heaven, with delicious fruits, fragrant flowers, peaceful serenity filled with positive energy and happiness. This story is to remind us how most of us plan, strategize and try to execute but only very few become successful in achieving what they planned, some of us lose motivation in the beginning itself, some feel happy and convinced with minimal fulfillment, only very few strive till the end and succeed and earn the fruit of rewards. Organizations which don't execute the plans and have it only on paper at the right time with the right blend of resources will never survive. Some organizations do survive with compromises in execution style and format. But only organizations that plan, strategize and execute it completely win the business market.

Today we are in a 4.0 industrial revolution, there is lot of changes in the workplace environment, workforce, customer need and requirement, technology advancements etc., if an organization doesn't strategize and execute to implement the strategies at the right time with proper analysis of the scenario, it would end up as a failure. Keeping these in context let us investigate chapters 67 and 68 of Thirukkural and how it relates to the current scenarios in organizations.

Chapter 67: VINAITHITPAM—Quality of Action

Execution Focus

This chapter focuses on certain virtues that are important to be considered when we are executing strategies for development. The couplets brief about the importance of determination one possesses in executing the plan and action, if there is no determination one can't achieve anything even if there is a well-designed plan. One should also not lose motivation to execute when he/she faces hurdles and plan in such a way that there are no challenges, but in case any unforeseen challenges come in the way of execution, one should not lose his/her motivation and strive for the implementation at any cost. This chapter further cautions that one shouldn't keep discussing plans and strategies until it is finally executed, if not there could be hindrances to the execution of plans causing difficulty to execute the plan. Further the chapter states that in management it is very important to "walk the talk", it is easy to say but, in many cases, it is hard to practice what one preaches. If a person's talk and actions correlate highly then he/she will be highly successful and appreciated by all, even by the top management. Another important lesson the chapter teaches us is, if any person is determined to put his productive thoughts into action, he is sure to win. At the same time, one should be cautious about the role everybody plays in accomplishing a task and not to ignore or neglect people based on their levels/ significance of role, even if it is minor or minimal, because even the smallest contribution is very significant for greater success and it shouldn't be ignored. Once a well-planned task is taken up it should be implemented without losing motivation or interest at any cost, even if the task execution is faced by tough and unpleasant demands/challenges. If anybody fails in executing the planned task, even if they are people in power positions, society will no longer respect them. Thus, this chapter focuses on how this chapter throws light on the most significant aspects of "Execution focus". Further in this chapter we will discuss the various couplets relating to the current management scenario.

661) Vinaiththitpam Enpadhu Oruvan Manaththitpam

Matraiya Ellaam Pira..

Meaning- The firmness of one's action depends on the firmness of mind.

Goal Setting Theory offers important insights into how "firmness of action" depends on "firmness of mind." Setting clear, demanding, and doable goals for oneself and one's team is more likely for a manager who is resolute and motivated. The basis for focused and deliberate activity is this clarity and commitment. According to Edwin Locke and Gary Latham's goal-setting theory, achieving particular, difficult goals might boost performance. It emphasizes the significance of dedication, difficulty, and clarity in setting goals. Furthermore, Locke and Latham emphasize that success depends on a strong dedication to a goal (Locke & Latham, 2006). Baron et al. (2016) reveal that entrepreneurs typically have high levels of self-efficacy. This indicates that they have confidence in their capacity to complete demanding tasks. While this self-assurance is important, it can also cause business owners to establish objectives that are extremely challenging, often to the point of being unreasonable or unreachable.

Here is where self-control, a key component of self-regulation, comes into play. Entrepreneurs that possess self-control are better able to manage their ambition and realism. It motivates them to set challenging goals that are within their realm of possibility. This suggests that an entrepreneur's behaviors depend on how strong and disciplined their attitude is. Baron et al. (2016) corroborates this idea by showing that business owners who use self-control while setting goals are more likely to choose ambitious yet attainable goals. This comprehensive approach to goal-setting may have a good effect on business performance.

662) Oororaal Utrapin Olkaamai Ivvirantin

Aarenpar Aaindhavar Kol.

Meaning- Doing flawlessly and even more steadily when there is a flaw are paths shown by the learned. The learned (in management context, the leader) needs to have the competency of guiding the subordinates to succeed. According to Adams & amp; Webster, 2021, task-oriented leaders, their gender and their emotional management play a role in the subordinates' performance. The authors combined leadership and gender theories with trust research to develop a model that connects interpersonal emotion management (IEM, relational leadership) and task-oriented (T-O) leadership to follower adaptive performance. The authors also investigate the indirect influence of IEM and T-O on adaptive performance via trust and the potential moderating function of gender in these connections. The results confirmed the IEM model since it was directly and indirectly associated (by trust) to adaptive work performance (even after controlling for transformational leadership), and these correlations were more beneficial for female leaders. T-O leadership was associated with adaptive work performance as expected, but not to trust or, through trust, to adaptive performance. Findings also imply that. women direct leaders may gain more trust and adaptive performance from followers by engaging in higher levels of IEM, while not incurring backlash for engaging in more agentic T-O behaviors during a crisis.

663) Kataikkotkach Cheydhakka Thaanmai Itaikkotkin

Etraa Vizhuman Tharum.

Meaning- Virility (strength – basically masculinity) lies in completing a task, giving up. midway causes misery.

Victor Vroom's Expectancy Theory (Lawler, 2005) postulates that a person's willingness to put forth effort towards a specific job or goal is determined by their perception of three crucial elements:

Expectancy: The conviction that hard work will produce successful results.

Instrumentality: The idea that good performance will lead to the desired results or rewards.

Value: The value or significance a person attaches to the anticipated benefits.

A person's confidence in their capacity to execute a task effectively might be compared to "Virility" or strength in the context of the quoted Kural. An individual demonstrates a sense of confidence and self-efficacy when they are determined to finish a task, both of which are essential elements of anticipation (Lawler, 2005). They are certain that their efforts will produce successful results.

On the other hand, giving up in the middle shows a lack of willpower and perseverance. The word "misery" refers to the negative psychological and emotional effects of giving up on a task, which is where it comes into play. This is consistent with the idea of instrumentality, in which a person recognises that foregoing a task will result in unfavourable outcomes, in this example, a feeling of sadness or dissatisfaction (Lawler, 2005).

The Kural essentially emphasizes the significance of dedication and drive in achieving achievement. It emphasizes the value of creating a work atmosphere that motivates people to persevere in their efforts and finish tasks, realising that this sense of accomplishment and achievement is essential for their motivation and overall job satisfaction.

664) Solludhal Yaarkkum Eliya Ariyavaam

Solliya Vannam Seyal.

Meaning- It is easy to say but hard to do exactly as said.

As a leader, it is important to walk the talk. An exploratory study on authentic leadership during the Covid-19 pandemic in India showed that one of the best strategies of leading their organizations was by proactively working to inspire and motivate the employee. This is best defined as leading by example (Chully et al., 2022).

The study emphasizes that demonstrating distinct behaviours, which call for more than simply verbal expression, is a requirement for real leadership. It entails execution and actual action. While discussing or expressing real leadership may be simple, actually practising it, particularly in a disruptive environment, is a considerably more difficult task. Genuine leaders must go beyond empty platitudes; they must show their devotion by their actions.

For instance, Chully et al. (2022) recognised the necessity for leaders to reexamine themselves as one of the key elements of authentic leadership. This requires reflection, self-awareness, and the readiness to make changes to oneself. Although it is simple to talk about self-reflection, the difficult part is really making the time and effort to do so.

Chully et al. (2022) also emphasize how crucial it is for genuine leaders to restate the organizational goal. This entails acting in accordance with the organization's mission and values and verbally stating them as well. Speaking about an organization's purpose is one thing, but continuously aligning one's behaviour with that purpose is quite another, especially in a disruptive climate.

The kural emphasizes that genuine leadership requires the commitment and effort to turn words into meaningful actions, especially in the face of disruptive circumstances. It does not simply involve verbalising objectives or ideas.

665) Veereydhi Maantaar Vinaiththitpam Vendhankan

Ooreydhi Ullap Patum.

Meaning- Those who have gained praise, bring good name to their rulers and thus are highly respected.

This Kural emphasizes the value of thanking people for their contributions and recognising them. It stresses that those who are praised not only build a positive reputation for themselves but also favourably represent their superiors or leaders. This concept is directly related to the compensation agenda, notably in the areas of recognition and incentive in workplace environments.

The motivation of employees is what propels their devotion and dedication to their jobs. People become more motivated and engaged when they believe their efforts are recognised and appreciated. Consequently, their work becomes more excellent and precise. A culture of continuous improvement can be developed by using recognition as a potent tool for reinforcing desired behaviours and performance goals.

This idea is supported by the study of Hooi and Chan (2022), which emphasizes the value of rewards and recognition when used in conjunction with transformative leadership. Through the creation of a vision, the setting of high standards, and the provision of support, transformational leaders inspire and drive their colleagues. This leadership style encourages an environment favourable to creativity when coupled with a strong incentives and recognition programme.

This strategy is even more important in today's digitally-driven world, when quick adaptability and innovation are essential for organizational success. It fosters an inventive culture where workers are not only encouraged to complete their work accurately but also to think creatively and contribute to the expansion of the company.

Essentially, this Kural and the related research stress the fact that rewarding employees not only benefits them personally but also improves the standing and productivity of their leaders. In today's dynamic corporate climate, it fosters innovation and organizational success when combined with transformational leadership and a strong rewards system.

666) Enniya Enniyaangu Eydhu Enniyaar

Thinniyar Aakap Perin.

Meaning- An individual can achieve whatever he/she seeks to as long as he/she is steady and enduring (of firm resolute).

This aligns with the principles of contingency theory. According to the contingency theory, there is no one management strategy that works for everyone. The success of a management approach or strategy instead rely on a number of contextual variables. It recognizes that various circumstances call for various answers, and good management is one that can modify their strategy in light of the unique conditions (Moniz, 2010). The Kural's emphasis on the need to be steady and enduring illustrates how crucial consistency and persistence are to accomplishing one's objectives. A manager using the contingency theory, for instance, would consider the special conditions and traits of their team or organization before selecting the best management approach (Moniz, 2010). They are aware that certain circumstances can call for a more directive approach, while others would necessitate a more participative or laissez-faire attitude.

667) Uruvukantu Ellaamai Ventum Urulperundherkku

Achchaani Annaar Utaiththu.

Meaning- A small linchpin holds the big chariot. Thus, we should not judge someone by their appearance. The Halo effect in Psychology talks about the cognitive bias due to which we tend to influence judgements positively or negatively about a person/company. This cognitive bias tends to exist during the recruitment processes (Bicer, 2022).

A study was conducted to investigate the relationship between critical thinking and the halo effect among managers in corporate Human Resources (HR) departments. The findings also show that salary level modifies this link, with lower-income HR managers having a larger association between negative perfectionism and the halo effect than higher-income HR managers. These findings add greatly to our understanding of the interaction between critical thinking and the halo effect in business contexts. The identification of negative perfectionism as a mediating component illuminates the underlying mechanisms between critical thinking and the halo effect, while the moderating effect of compensation level emphasizes the need of taking contextual factors into account. This study's application practically includes the importance of fostering critical thinking abilities among HR managers in order to reduce the halo effect in job recruitment and performance evaluation. Furthermore, organizations should prioritize fairness and consistency in pay levels to reduce the impact of negative perfectionism and its impact on the halo effect (Lv et al., 2023)

668) Kalangaadhu Kanta Vinaikkan Thulangaadhu

Thookkang Katindhu Seyal.

Meaning- Do the task with clarity of thought, without procrastination and unwaveringly. Transactional leaders in managerial levels give importance to structure in doing work and set clear goals for the teams to achieve. When the plan is executed with such clarity, it smoothens the process for everyone involved (Dhar et al., 2022).

(669) Thunpam Uravarinum Seyka Thunivaatri

Inpam Payakkum Vinai.

Meaning- Even if it causes distress during the process, if the result shall give happiness, do it with determination. An interdisciplinary science called 'Modern Management Psychology' is successfully used in work environments today.In order to help individuals become effective and capable of working in the management system, management psychology's main objective is to understand the psychological conditions and features of management activities. It places emphasis on system management principles: determination of the condition of management subsystem changes; the creation of a strategy for the activities of the subordinates with the intention of changing the status of the management objects for a particular objective; Organization of the decision's execution. To encourage workers to carry out more important tasks, management systems need motivation (Koleci & Koleci, 2022). According to self-determination theory, motivation is an essential factor in cultivating self-determination (Gagné & Deci, 2005). Relating this to the Thirukkural above, self-determination is fueled by motivation and when the end goal provides happiness, an individual innately is motivated to work with determination to achieve it.

670) Enaiththitpam Ey Thiyak Kannum Vinaiththitpam

Ventaarai Ventaadhu Ulaku.

Meaning- Despite worldly abilities one has acquired, the world shall not desire an individual who does not wish to execute resolutely. Conscientiousness can be defined as individual differences in an individual's ability to conform to socially established norms for control of emotions, to be focused on goals, planful, able to delay satisfaction, and to adhere to norms and rules (Jackson et al., 2010). By encouraging orderly, responsible, diligent, ambitious, devout, and rule-abiding behaviour, conscientiousness affects task performance. This characteristic is linked to a variety of positive outcomes, such as longevity, longevity at work, and lawfulness. Goal setting theory states that conscientious people are more likely to create detailed, difficult goals and to stick with them in the face of challenges. Additionally, they are more inclined to plan ahead and prepare, which might support them in overcoming obstacles and achieving their objectives. In general, conscientiousness plays a significant role in encouraging efficient task completion and goal achievement (Bates et al., 2023).

Vinai Seiyalvagai: Mode of Execution—Chapter 68

Let us look into what this chapter 68 of Thirukurral has in store regarding the management practices on mode of execution. The 10 couplets in this chapter provide guidelines on the importance of execution of strategies, with proper analyses, at the right time, right place with the support of right people to yield the expected outcome.

The first COUPLet "Soozhchchi Mutivu Thuniveydhal Aththunivu"

"Thaazhchchiyul Thangudhal Theedhu" (671) states the importance of analyzing the pros and cons of strategies in depth before being executed and once it is done there shouldn't be any delay in the execution, if delayed it might end up in grievous fault. According to Miranda, Eduardo. (2002) Statistically Planned Incremental Deliveries offer an approach that addresses problems like requirements often gets slashed halfway through the project, thus resulting in missed deadlines, customer frustration, and wasted effort, in time bound projects by combining ideas from critical chain planning, incremental development, and rate monitoring into a practical method for planning and executing time-bound projects, which aligns with the couplet's emphasis on the importance of executing on time once proper analysis has been done, to avoid grievous faults.

The next couplet

"Thoonguka Thoongich Cheyarpaala Thoongarka

Thoongaadhu Seyyum Vinai": (672)

denotes that there should be no delay in executing strategies that need immediate attention. Following this the next couplet

"Ollumvaa Yellaam Vinainandre Ollaakkaal

Sellumvaai Nokkich Cheyal" (673),

in this chapter, further explains on how it is important to find ways to execute actions even when the path looks impossible rather than waiting ideally. The next couplet in kural in this same chapter:

"Vinaipakai Endrirantin Echcham Ninaiyungaal

Theeyechcham Polath Therum"(674),

further explains it is very important to complete a task undertaken, unfinished task is like smoldering fire and it will ruin all the efforts.

All the above 3 couplets emphasize the importance of implementing strategies immediately without delay and leaving no space for incomplete work. An intervention study conducted by Eerde, 2003 provided employees training in time management. After the intervention employees noted a significant reduction in stress and avoidance behaviour as well as an improvement in time management skills. The findings imply that time management interventions and training are beneficial in reducing anxiety and procrastination at work.

"Porulkaruvi Kaalam Vinaiyitanotu Aindhum

Iruldheera Ennich Cheyal". (675)

Denotes that both tangible and intangible resources should be thoroughly examined before taking action.

"Mutivum Itaiyoorum Mutriyaangu Eydhum

Patupayanum Paarththuch Cheyal".(676)

Denotes that the end goal should be clear and communicated well before the beginning of a project.

According to a study by Schaap (2012), higher levels of organizational performance is due to clearly developed implementing plans, indicating specific tasks for individuals, with clear-cut deadlines, and identifying the people responsible for task completion. Smith et al. (1990) found that organizational performance and planning quality were both positively correlated with the establishment of specified organizational goals. When planning quality was high, higher performance was related with more total planning time; however, when planning quality was low, lower performance was associated with more total planning time. According to Zenger & Folkman (2016), many employees who are enthusiastic about execution tend to dive right into activities and take action before organizing themselves, making a plan, or connecting what they're doing to the organization's strategy. Execution is improved by having the discipline to coordinate people, gather resources, and then develop a strategy that everyone can agree on. According to Chamorro-Premuzic & Lovric (2022). Establishing organizational clarity and placing the appropriate personnel in the appropriate roles are two techniques for effective execution. Pre-mortem exercises, which let executives discover the strategy's weak points and, consequently, its main execution risks, are one way to obtain this clarity. In order to implement a strategy effectively, strategic clarity is necessary. The first step is to explicitly define the fundamental organizational capabilities that the new approach would demand – one needs to develop capabilities that others can't readily imitate.

Overall, these studies highlight the necessity of a holistic approach that includes organised planning, focused execution, and smart people allocation for successful strategy implementation. Achieving strategic success also requires the formation of organizational clarity and the awareness of potential execution risks. Organizations can position themselves for improved performance and a long-lasting competitive edge in the fast-paced business world of today by following to these principles.

"Seyvinai Seyvaan Seyanmurai Avvinai

Ullarivaan Ullam Kolal".(677)

Denotes that it is always best to consult the experts in the field to understand all of the duties nuances and responsibilities.

"Vinaiyaan Vinaiyaakkik Kotal Nanaikavul

Yaanaiyaal Yaanaiyaath Thatru".(678)

These above kural couplets states that, one should procure required resources (money), and have clarity in means, time, place and execution. To be more profitable one should know the benefits to be gained at the end of the project and what kind of obstacles will be hindering the performance before executing the strategies to maximize the performance. Despite the fact that organizations recognise the importance of strategy and its efficient implementation, most organizations' implementation frequently falls short of the objectives that the firm has set for itself. Shah, 2005 found that organizations should concentrate on developing sound strategies, allocating enough resources to them, ensuring management commitment and leadership, managing employee understanding and commitment, linking financial rewards with performance, and establishing efficient information systems in order to remove barriers and encourage successful strategy implementation. Businesses that can handle these issues will avoid numerous implementation issues and promote success (Shah, 2005). The couplets also, states that one should first get the inputs and suggestions from the person who have through experience in the task. An effective strategist should try to get multiple tasks done at the single stroke, like using an elephant to control and catch another elephant.

"Nattaarkku Nalla Seyalin Viraindhadhe

Ottaarai Ottik Kolal".(679)

Denotes that befriending enemies is more important than helping out friends. This aligns with the principles of Stakeholders theory of management given by Dr. R.E.Freeman in 1984.

According to the stakeholder theory, a business or organization should take into account the requirements and interests of all parties involved, not just shareholders or close allies. Employees, shareholders, suppliers, consumers, the community, and even rival companies (Szwajkowski, 2000).

"Befriending enemies" in the Kural refers to appreciating the value of interacting with stakeholders who might not always share the organization's objectives or may have competing interests. It indicates that developing connections with rivals, detractors, or enemies can be strategically advantageous in order to establish common ground or work together on shared goals. Stakeholder Theory posits that managing relationships with a wide range of stakeholders is crucial for long-term organizational success (Szwajkowski, 2000). Ignoring or alienating certain stakeholders, even if they may be considered "enemies" in a competitive sense, can lead to negative consequences for the organization. Therefore, it is necessary to maintain and manage a good relationship with different stakeholders to ensure long-term success of the organization.

"Uraisiriyaar Ulnatungal Anjik Kuraiperin

Kolvar Periyaarp Panindhu". (680)

Goes on to explain that the smaller state will yield to a strong authority when their concerns are addressed.

These above kural couplets state that, it is always better to keep our enemies closer and if it is profitable having alliance with enemies / competitors can prove to be a good strategy to execute. Current research studies and organizational theories also show support to the couplets stated in the chapter 68 on mode of execution, clearly linking the relevance of the thirukurral couplets to organizational behavior. According to Zenger & Folkman (2016), teams functioned effectively when the following conditions were met. Clear job assignments, a logical methodology, strong but reasonable deadlines, and lots of feedback are all present. Many employees who are enthusiastic about execution tend to dive right into activities and take action before organizing themselves, making a plan, or connecting what they're doing to the organization's strategy. Execution is improved by having the discipline to coordinate people, gather resources, and then develop a strategy that everyone can agree on Zenger & Folkman (2016) They also noticed that on these teams, team members are motivated by expectations from peers on the team as well as their supervisor. As a result, developing this kind of team culture is crucial to successful implementation. Management by Objective by Peter Drucker, MBO promotes employees' active participation in the goal-setting process. Together with their staff, managers create goals that are both challenging and doable. This participatory strategy encourages employee ownership of the objectives as well as involvement and dedication and helps in successful implementation of strategies. Employees who are highly committed to their work with required KSAO's will contribute to the execution of strategies with low cost, high quality innovations and superior service. MBO places a strong emphasis on the requirement for ongoing goal-related monitoring and measurement. Leadership too plays an important role in crafting and implementing strategy. Employee commitment majorly depends on leadership style, planning quality, appropriate perception and learning. To evaluate performance, precise performance metrics and key performance indicators (KPIs) are established. Employees receive regular feedback on their development, enabling course correction and performance enhancement.

One of the ancient poems Agananuru and Purananuru written by Neduman Anji in the sangam era, there were a total of 2381 poems, in that 206th poem talks about management and leadership, reflects the importance of time management in executing tasks on time without delay. The poem talks about the process of planning and organising to achieve specific tasks on time. It further states that failing to manage time and scheduling tasks effectively might lead to harming organizational effectiveness. The poem further implores that even if the manager or leader posses all the qualities of leadership but fails to execute tasks on time and with swift action, then the leader will fail to guide the followers in execution of task. This is in line with the Thirukural chapters 67 and 68 we discussed above. The ancient scriptures thus presents to us the significance of execution focus and modes of execution on leadership and organizational effectiveness.

CONCLUSION

Thirukurral's chapter 67, "VINAITHITPAM - Quality of Action," offers insightful explanations on the significance of management's execution focus. The couplets highlight how important it is to be determined, motivated, and steadfast in order to carry out strategies successfully. It emphasizes the necessity for leaders to set an example by matching their words and deeds, which is crucial for earning followers' respect and trust.

The importance of honouring people' efforts at all levels of an organization is also emphasised in this chapter. It emphasizes the value of each team member's work and emphasizes that even the smallest role plays a crucial role in achieving bigger success.

Additionally, the Kural couplets in this chapter make comparisons to elements of Transactional Leadership as well as management theories like Expectancy Theory and Contingency Theory. These theories support the notion that achieving organizational goals requires tenacity, consistency, and clear communication. The chapter ends with a potent reminder that, whatever the difficulties encountered, steadfast execution is crucial. It emphasizes the significance of perseverance and completing things as intended to gain credibility and respect.

In conclusion, Chapter 67 acts as a road map for good management techniques. In order to accomplish organizational goals, it emphasizes the importance of tenacity, consistency, and alignment between words and deeds. Following these guidelines can help leaders create a culture of accountability, drive, and quality within their teams, which will ultimately result in success and expansion for the organization.

Chapter 68 of Thirukurral, focusing on the mode of execution, provides profound insights into effective management practices. It emphasizes the significance of precise and prompt strategic implementation. The couplets in this chapter emphasize the need for careful planning before action, for acting quickly when a strategy calls for it, and for not leaving work unfinished. They also emphasize the value of resource evaluation, clear goal communication, and consulting experts to make educated decisions. Studies on management conducted recently support these ideas. The effectiveness of an organization is positively correlated with well-developed implementation plans, specified tasks, and certain dates, according to studies by Schaap (2012) and Smith et al. (1990). Zenger & Folkman (2016) stress the need of methodical planning, implementation, and coordination. Additionally, for efficient implementation, Chamorro-Premuzic & Lovric (2022) promote organizational clarity and strategic risk assessment.

The idea of "befriending enemies" is consistent with stakeholder theory, which emphasizes the value of taking into account the interests of all parties. The strategic importance of alliances, even with rivals, is also emphasised in this chapter.

In conclusion, Chapter 68 encapsulates timeless wisdom on strategy execution. It outlines the process for achieving good organizational performance through careful planning, methodical implementation, and stakeholder involvement. Businesses may overcome obstacles, promote innovation, and achieve long-term success in the dynamic and cutthroat business environment of today by paying attention to these insights.

REFERENCES

Adams, G. A., & Webster, J. R. (2021, November 18). Relating supervisor interpersonal emotion management- and task-oriented leadership to adaptive performance: A moderated-mediation model incorporating trust and gender. *Equality, Diversity and Inclusion: An International Journal*. https://www.emerald.com/insight/content/doi/10.1108/EDI-07-2021-0174/full/html

Baron, R. A., Mueller, B. A., & Wolfe, M. T. (2016). Self-efficacy and entrepreneurs' adoption of unattainable goals: The restraining effects of self-control. *Journal of Business Venturing*, *31*(1), 55–71. doi:10.1016/j.jbusvent.2015.08.002

Bates, T. C., Enkhbat, T., Gray, E., Lee, J., & Zakharin, M. (2023, July 14). How to get things done: Tight linkage of conscientiousness with twelve mechanisms of goal setting theory. *Personality and Individual Differences*. Science Direct. https://www.sciencedirect.com/science/article/pii/S0191886923002544

Bicer, C. (2022, January 1). *Avoiding halo effect in employee selection: Implementing effective techniques in hiring*. Fiscaoeconomia. https://www.ceeol.com/search/article-detail?id=1046177

Chamorro-Premuzic, T., & Lovric, D. (2022, June 20). How to move from strategy to execution. *Harvard Business Review*. https://hbr.org/2022/06/how-to-move-from-strategy-to-execution

Education World. (2013, September 7). Chapter 68: Mode of execution. *Thirukkural in English*. https://thirukkural133.wordpress.com/2013/09/07/chapter-68-mode-of-execution/

Chully, A. A., Jose, J., & M, L. (2022, August 4). *Authentic leadership in a pandemic world: An exploratory study in the Indian context*. Journal of Management Development. https://www.emerald.com/insight/content/doi/10.1108/JMD-10-2021-0281/full/html?casa_token=6U6Idw9AS5AAAAAA%3ALfnipb5fIGa2lJ-UYJa-PxqFVC4dcIc6du1qyuVPF_iBiwfek3C-u-lo8j1yOurLeLSKhF_852PKW7NIWRaTkRDrNo-pVwcQBn2OmvkxP3g-CgkSfyI

Dhar, B. K., & Stasi, A. Döpping, J. O., Gazi, M. A. I., Shaturaev, J., & Sarkar, S. M. (2022, July 14). *Mediating role of strategic flexibility between leadership styles on strategic execution: A study on bangladeshi private enterprises - global journal of flexible systems management*. Springer. https://link.springer.com/article/10.1007/s40171-022-00310-3

Durai, S. (2023). Truth-based leadership: Lessons from thirukural. In A. K. Maheshwari (Ed.), Consciousness-Based Leadership and Management, Volume 1: Vedic and Other Philosophical Approaches to Oneness and Flourishing (pp. 319–338). Springer International Publishing. doi:10.1007/978-3-031-06234-6_14

Eerde, W. V. (2003). Procrastination at work and time management training. *The Journal of Psychology*, *137*(5), 421–434. doi:10.1080/00223980309600625 PMID:14629073

Gagné, M., & Deci, E. L. (2005). *Self-determination theory and work motivation*. Wiley Online Library. https://onlinelibrary.wiley.com/doi/abs/10.1002/job.322

Hooi, L. W., & Chan, A. J. (2022, September 20). Innovative culture and rewards-recognition matter in linking Transformational leadership to workplace digitalisation? *Leadership & Organization Development Journal*. https://www.emerald.com/insight/content/doi/10.1108/LODJ-07-2021-0349/full/html?casa_token=E5olx2zLS6QAAAAA%3Av9IS4q9Efyr8WvZO4_CAUC0Pkz0J9rXD3QmpfIkg-TrDIJFVNdrwhn3HUwvHbc1dP1tcRpMAIfuTm4bGECkJgJ9LFbYy7CwmpgR7-Op7q3cjduz0XA40

Jackson, J. J., Wood, D., Bogg, T., Walton, K. E., Harms, P. D., & Roberts, B. W. (2010, August 1). What do conscientious people do? development and validation of the behavioral indicators of conscientiousness (BIC). *Journal of research in personality*. https://www.ncbi.nlm.nih.gov/pmc/articles/PMC3028204/

Koleci, V., & Koleci, R. (2022). *(PDF) objectives of Modern Management Psychology*. Research Gate. https://www.researchgate.net/publication/364642679_Objectives_of_modern_management_psychology

Lawler, V. V. & Lyman Porter, E. (2005). Expectancy theories. In Organizational Behavior 1. Routledge.

Locke, E. A., & Latham, G. P. (2006). New directions in goal-setting theory. *Current Directions in Psychological Science*, *15*(5), 265–268. doi:10.1111/j.1467-8721.2006.00449.x

Lv, J., Sun, Z., Li, H., & Hou, Y. (2023, June 26). *The role of negative perfectionism and the relationship between critical thinking and the halo effect: Insights from Corporate Managers in human resources*. MDPI. https://www.mdpi.com/2076-328X/13/7/533

Miranda, E. (2002). Planning and executing time-bound projects. *Computer*, *35*(3), 73–79. doi:10.1109/2.989933

Moniz, R. J. (2010). 1 - History of managerial thought: A brief overview. In R. J. Moniz (Ed.), *Practical and Effective Management of Libraries* (pp. 1–18). Chandos Publishing. doi:10.1016/B978-1-84334-578-7.50001-3

Rao, P. S. (2010). *Organizational behaviour*. Himalaya Publishing House.

Schaap, J. (2012). Toward strategy implementation success: An empirical study of the role of senior-level leaders in the nevada gaming industry. *UNLV Gaming Research & Review Journal*, *10*(2). https://digitalscholarship.unlv.edu/grrj/vol10/iss2/2

Shah, A. M. (2005). The foundations of successful strategy implementation: Overcoming obstacles. *Global Business Review*, *6*(2), 293–302. doi:10.1177/097215090500600208

Sivachandrakumar., A. (2019, January). Classic Poem (Puram - 206) – A Management view. *International Journal of Emerging Technologies and Innovative Research*, .*6*(1), 42-46. https://www.jetir.org/papers/JETIRT006007.pdf

Smith, K. G., Locke, E. A., & Barry, D. (1990). Goal setting, planning, and organizational performance: An experimental simulation. *Organizational Behavior and Human Decision Processes*, *46*(1), 118–134. doi:10.1016/0749-5978(90)90025-5

Szwajkowski, E. (2000). Simplifying the principles of stakeholder management: The three most important principles. *Business & Society*, *39*(4), 379–396. doi:10.1177/000765030003900403

Zenger, J., & Folkman, J. (2016, May 23). 4 ways to be more effective at execution. *Harvard Business Review*. https://hbr.org/2016/05/4-ways-to-be-more-effective-at-execution

Chapter 11
Mindfulness-Based Interventions:
Applications in Western and Indian Psychology

Ranjit Singha
https://orcid.org/0000-0002-3541-8752
Christ University (Deemed), India

Surjit Singha
https://orcid.org/0000-0002-5730-8677
Kristu Jayanti College (Autonomous), India

ABSTRACT

This chapter examines mindfulness-based interventions (MBIs) in Western and Indian psychology. It begins with a summary of MBIs, their historical origins, and their theoretical frameworks. The empirical evidence then examines the efficacy of MBIs, emphasizing their impact on both Western and Indian psychology. It probes deeper into the specific applications of MBIs in each cultural context, focusing on adapting mindfulness practices to accommodate cultural differences. Case studies demonstrate the efficacy of MBIs in reducing anxiety, depression, and work-related stress. The significance of cultural sensitivity and inclusiveness, in addition to the implications of MBIs for psychological practice and future research directions, is discussed. It highlights the significance of MBI and provides recommendations for future advancements. It provides an overview of the applications of MBIs, emphasizing their potential to improve well-being, reduce psychological distress, and promote a more inclusive approach to psychological practice.

1. INTRODUCTION

Mindfulness-based interventions (MBIs) are a continuum of therapeutic approaches incorporating mindfulness practices to promote well-being and resolve various psychological difficulties. Mindfulness

DOI: 10.4018/978-1-6684-9778-4.ch011

derives from ancient contemplative traditions and involves focusing on the present moment, cultivating nonjudgmental awareness, and adopting an accepting attitude. Typically, MBIs consist of mindfulness meditation, body awareness exercises, and incorporating mindfulness into daily activities. These interventions aim to improve self-awareness, reduce tension, regulate emotions, enhance cognitive functioning, and promote overall psychological health. In recent years, MBIs have become increasingly prominent in Western and Indian psychology due to their prospective benefits and adaptability across diverse populations. The cross-pollination of ideas and practices from various cultures has become a hallmark of progress in an increasingly interconnected world. Integrating MBIs into Western and Indian psychology is a cross-cultural exchange that has received considerable attention recently. This chapter examines the profound influence of mindfulness practices on therapeutic and strategic models in these distinct but interconnected disciplines.

The discipline of mindfulness, originating from ancient Buddhism, has expanded beyond its original context and gained worldwide recognition. Mindfulness entails cultivating an elevated state of consciousness about one's cognitive processes, affective states, and bodily experiences in the immediate present while upholding a non-evaluative stance. Initially confined to Buddhist monastic settings, this technique has assimilated into Western psychology, particularly mental health and overall well-being (Lee et al., 2021). Mindfulness-Based Stress Reduction (MBSR) and Mindfulness-Based Cognitive Therapy (MBCT) have surfaced as practical approaches for alleviating conditions such as anxiety, depression, and chronic pain due to the Western adoption of mindfulness. Mindfulness has become a prominent tool in Western psychotherapy due to its ability to improve emotional regulation and overall psychological well-being (Kraines et al., 2022; Querstret et al., 2020). Zindel Segal, Mark Williams, and John Teasdale developed MBCT in 1989 when these three individuals met at the World Congress of Cognitive Therapy. They pondered why even ostensibly effective remedies for depression, such as cognitive therapy and pharmacotherapy, did not prevent future relapses. It led to the development of MBCT; mindfulness-based Cognitive treatment (MBCT) integrates cognitive-behavioural treatment strategies alongside mindfulness meditation practices and other relevant psychological methodologies. Mindfulness-Based Cognitive Therapy (MBCT) is influenced by traditional East Asian formative and functional medicine with philosophical and spiritual principles (Salmon & Loo, 2023). In the 1970s, Professor Jon Kabat-Zinn devised MBSR at the University of Massachusetts Medical School. MBSR combines mindfulness meditation, body awareness, yoga, and investigating patterns of behaviour, thought, emotion, and action1. It is essential to note that although MBSR originates in the teachings of Zen Buddhism, Hatha Yoga, Vipassana, and Advaita Vedanta, the program itself is secular. The ancient Buddhist mindfulness practice has transcended its origins to become a global phenomenon. Mindfulness entails cultivating an elevated state of consciousness characterized by an intensified perception of one's cognitive processes, affective states, and somatic experiences within the immediate temporal context while upholding a disposition of impartial acceptance devoid of evaluative tendencies. Once exclusive to Buddhist monasteries, this practice has permeated Western psychology, particularly mental health and well-being (Lee et al., 2021). MBSR and MBCT have surfaced as practical approaches for alleviating conditions such as anxiety, depression, and chronic pain due to the Western adoption of mindfulness. Mindfulness has become a prominent tool in Western psychotherapy due to its ability to improve emotional regulation and overall psychological well-being (Kraines et al., 2022; Querstret et al., 2020).

MBIs, derived from ancient Buddhist practices, have evolved into powerful modern therapeutic tools, exemplified by MBSR, which substantially improves mental health (Cillessen et al., 2020). Ancient India and the profound teachings of Siddhartha Gautama, the Buddha, serve as the origins of MBIs. In the complex tapestry of Buddhist philosophy, mindfulness, referred to as "sati" in Pali, constitutes a fundamental concept. The practice entails developing a heightened consciousness regarding the current moment and impartially examining one's thoughts, emotions, and physical sensations. The inception of this practice was conceptualized as a method to attain enlightenment and undergo significant internal metamorphosis. Jon Kabat-Zinn, a renowned scientist and meditator, popularized MBSR in the late 20th century, thereby secularizing mindfulness for clinical use. The eight-week MBSR program incorporates mindfulness meditation, cognitive-behavioural techniques, and various meditation practices, such as the body scan and yoga. It promotes the incorporation of mindfulness into daily life and incorporates reflective exercises for self-discovery and self-compassion (Janssen et al., 2018).

Woods et al. (2021) state that the MBSR program reduces tension and enhances overall well-being. It effectively treats chronic pain, reduces the need for pain medication, and shows promise in treating anxiety and depression (Gold et al., 2009). MBSR equips individuals with emotional modulation skills, enhancing their resilience in facing life's obstacles (Keng et al., 2021). A wealth of empirical research supports the efficacy of MBSR across various populations and conditions. It alleviates anxiety, depression, and pain symptoms while reducing perceived tension and enhancing psychological well-being. MBSR has also demonstrated efficacy in preventing relapse in recurrent depression and enhancing pain management in chronic pain states. Based on extensive research, MBSR, rooted in Eastern mindfulness traditions, excels at stress reduction, pain management, and emotional regulation (Lengacher et al., 2021).

The primary objective of this chapter is to examine the global integration of Indian psychology, concentrating on incorporating mindfulness-based practices into both Western and Indian psychological landscapes. The objectives include examining how mindfulness, deeply rooted in Indian and Buddhist traditions, has found its place within Western psychological frameworks, its therapeutic applications in addressing mental health issues, and its function as a strategic tool for personal and societal development. Case studies and research findings from the real world will illustrate its practical cross-cultural impact. In addition, this chapter will shed light on the cultural and psychological nuances that influence the adaptation of mindfulness practices and highlight its transformative potential as a unifying force that transcends geographical and cultural boundaries, ultimately contributing to individual well-being and societal harmony. This exhaustive investigation will examine mindfulness's historical origins, therapeutic efficacy, and broader global significance to create a holistic understanding of its diverse therapeutic and strategic applications.

To thoroughly examine the incorporation of MBIs into Western and Indian psychology, it is necessary to explore the pertinent theories and historical context underpinning this synthesis. The mindfulness theory is at the centre of this investigation, which contends that cultivating nonjudgmental awareness of one's present-moment thoughts, emotions, and bodily sensations can lead to increased self-awareness, emotional regulation, and a heightened sense of well-being. This foundational theory originates in Buddhist and contemplative traditions and is the basis for mindfulness practices. Understanding the philosophical foundations of mindfulness is also essential. Buddhist and Indian traditions, including Zen Buddhism and Vipassana, emphasize mindfulness as a path to enlightenment and self-realization. Not only do these ancient traditions provide historical context, but also profound philosophical insights that influence the essence of mindfulness practices. Incorporating mindfulness into Western psychology is intricately interwoven with several psychological models, including cognitive-behavioural therapy (CBT) and positive psychology. These models gave rise to well-known mindfulness-based approaches such as MBSR and MBCT, which are firmly rooted in using mindfulness to improve psychological well-being. Jon Kabat-Zinn's importance in the 1970s and 1980s cannot be exaggerated. His pioneering work, particularly the development of MBSR, played a transformative role in introducing mindfulness to the Western therapeutic landscape, with the mission of secularizing mindfulness and making it accessible to a broader audience. Indian psychology, rooted in ancient texts such as the Vedas and the Upanishads, provides an alternative lens to comprehend mindfulness integration. This perspective explores concepts such as yoga, meditation, and the essence of consciousness to provide unique insights into the Indian mindfulness practice. Adapting mindfulness to various cultural contexts, whether Western or Indian, requires careful consideration of cultural norms, values, and beliefs. Acknowledging these cultural nuances is pivotal for the effective integration of mindfulness practices. Recent developments in the field of neuroscience have provided scientific validation for the benefits associated with the use of mindfulness techniques. Studies conducted in several fields, such as neuroplasticity, the default mode network, and the effects of mindfulness on brain structure and function, have significantly enhanced the scientific comprehension of the profound neurological implications associated with mindfulness.

Globalization has been instrumental in facilitating the exchange of cultural ideas and practices. The globalization of mindfulness underscores the interconnectedness of our world and the adaptability of ancient practices to contemporary contexts. In addition, an extensive body of research supports mindfulness's therapeutic and clinical applications. It includes studies demonstrating its effectiveness in treating anxiety, depression, and chronic pain and fostering overall well-being and resiliency. In light of this complex context, the ethical dimensions of mindfulness, including issues related to cultural appropriation, authenticity, and ethical conduct in mindfulness instruction, are of critical importance. These theories and contexts provide a comprehensive framework for comprehending how MBIs have found a place in Western and Indian psychology and evolved. They illuminate the distinct contributions and challenges associated with this integration in each context, thereby augmenting our knowledge of the global spread of mindfulness practices.

Western Psychology

Mindfulness-Based Interventions (MBIs) have garnered attention as empirically supported therapeutic approaches for many mental health disorders within Western psychology. Numerous therapeutic approaches, such as Cognitive Behavioral Therapy (CBT), Dialectical Behavior Therapy (DBT), and Acceptance and Commitment Therapy (ACT), have incorporated mindfulness as a fundamental component within their treatment modalities. Research has produced positive results in reducing anxiety, sadness, and chronic pain symptoms and improving general psychological well-being (Zhang et al., 2021). Steven C. Hayes, a professor at the University of Nevada, created ACT, a form of psychotherapy. ACT began its development around 1982. Developers created it to integrate essential elements of cognitive therapy and behaviour analysis, particularly behaviour analytic data on the frequently adverse effects of verbal rules and how to mitigate them. In addition to Kelly Wilson and Kirk Strosahl, other psychologists like Kirk Strosahl and Kelly Wilson also contributed to its development (Webster, 2011). In the late 1980s, Dr. Marsha Linehan created DBT. Self-harm, suicidal behaviour, Post-Traumatic Stress Disorder (PTSD), Substance Use Disorder, Eating Disorders (specifically Binge Eating Disorder and Bulimia), Depression, and Anxiety are among the mental health conditions for which DBT has proven effective. This therapeutic approach combines traditional cognitive-behavioural strategies for emotion regulation and reality assessment with elements of distress tolerance, acceptance, and mindful awareness primarily derived from meditative practices. DBT is the first empirically supported treatment for Borderline Personality Disorder (BPD) based on the biosocial theory of mental illness (Tan et al., 2022).

Incorporating Indian mindfulness practices into Western psychology represents a significant development in the field. In ancient Indian traditions such as Buddhism and Hinduism, mindfulness was practised to cultivate self-awareness, insight, and spiritual growth. In recent years, Western psychologists have acknowledged the value and potential for promoting the psychological health of these practices. Western psychology has incorporated mindfulness of Indian origin through MBIs. These interventions adapt Indian mindfulness principles and techniques to the West's cultural context and therapeutic approaches.

Developed in the late 1970s by Jon Kabat-Zinn, MBSR is one of the most well-known MBIs in Western psychology. It combines mindfulness meditation, yoga, and body awareness to cultivate acceptance and understanding of the present moment, devoid of judgment. MBSR has been utilized effectively in various clinical settings, including treating stress, anxiety, depression, and chronic pain (Baldo et al., 2021). MBCT is an additional mindfulness-based intervention that includes Indian mindfulness. MBCT integrates mindfulness practises with cognitive therapy techniques and is notably effective at preventing relapse in those with recurrent depression. It helps individuals develop new relationships with their thoughts and emotions, thereby decreasing the likelihood of relapsing into negative thought patterns (Kraines et al., 2022). Accentuate the importance of MBRP for postpartum smoking cessation in women. Despite limited research, the positive results of studies on substance addiction support the use of mindfulness-based approaches, particularly in India, where their efficacy is evident (Vadivale & Sathiaseelan, 2022). Emphasize the significance of confronting cultural barriers and gender disparities in pursuing gender equality. Based on Buddhist principles, mindfulness empowers women to surmount obstacles and promote equality (Soumya & Sathiaseelan, 2021). In addiction recovery, the combination of MBSR and CBT is highly effective. Mindfulness is essential for managing cravings and tension, whereas cognitive-behavioral therapy addresses negative beliefs. Their research highlights the efficacy of this combined approach in reducing relapse rates and promoting long-term health (Vadivale & Sathiaseelan, 2019). The principles and concepts of mindfulness in India have influenced and enriched other Western therapeutic approaches. DBT, frequently used to treat borderline personality disorder, involves mindfulness as one of its central components. DBT teaches individuals to observe and accept their experiences without judgment, facilitating emotional regulation and distress tolerance. ACT is another mindfulness-based therapeutic approach. The Embrace and ACT emphasize the acceptance of one's thoughts and emotions and encourage individuals to act following their values. Mindfulness practices help individuals become more present and aware of their experiences, allowing them to make decisions consistent with their values.

Incorporating mindfulness practices with Indian roots into Western psychology has played a crucial role in expanding the therapeutic tools available to mental health professionals. MBIs have provided new avenues for promoting psychological well-being and addressing mental health problems by integrating the knowledge of Indian traditions with Western psychological theories and methods. The incorporation of mindfulness practices into Western psychology necessitates cultural sensitivity and adaptation. Mindfulness practices have been translated into secular and accessible forms to ensure their applicability and relevance for individuals from various cultural contexts. Respecting their cultural origins enabled the integration of Indian mindfulness practices into Western psychological frameworks. Western psychology has incorporated mindfulness practices of Indian origin by introducing MBIs and acknowledging their influence on various therapeutic approaches. This integration has enhanced our comprehension of mindfulness's role in promoting psychological well-being and broadened the array of treatment alternatives accessible to individuals. Mindfulness practices have become an indispensable part of the therapeutic landscape, providing individuals with powerful tools for self-awareness, healing, and personal development.

Indian Psychology

Mindfulness-based practices have profound historical roots in Indian psychology. For centuries, ancient Indian traditions such as Yoga and Buddhism have utilized mindfulness to cultivate inner peace, self-transformation, and spiritual growth. In the Indian context, mindfulness frequently associates itself with concepts such as self-realization, self-observation, and the study of consciousness. Integrating mindfulness into therapeutic models is consistent with the mind-body integration and holistic approach of Indian psychology. MBIs are significant in Western and Indian psychology because they have the potential to bridge the gap between ancient knowledge and modern therapeutic practices. These interventions provide individuals with easily accessible tools for cultivating self-awareness, enhancing emotional regulation, and fostering personal growth. In addition, MBIs provide a forum for intercultural dialogue and integrate various one-dimensional psychological perspectives. Incorporating mindfulness practices into the conceptual frameworks of Indian psychology has a long history. In addition to other ancient Indian philosophies and spiritual traditions, Buddhism, Yoga, and Vedanta are the origins of mindfulness. In Indian psychology, mindfulness is fundamental to self-realization, self-transformation, and achieving elevated states of consciousness. In Indian psychology, mindfulness is typically called "sati" or "smriti," which includes focus, awareness, and recollection. Mindfulness entails being fully present in the present moment and observing one's thoughts, emotions, and bodily sensations with nonjudgmental awareness and without establishing attachments to them.

In its original form, mindfulness practice centrally focused on purification, regarded as cultivating self-awareness, fostering insight, and promoting a deeper understanding of oneself and the essence of reality. However, as time passed, mindfulness practice adaptations made it more accessible for laypeople. Most contemporary forms of mindfulness have removed compassion, an integral practice element. The original mindfulness practice primarily targeted monks residing in Buddhist monasteries, creating challenges for its adoption by laypeople and family members. Monastic life for monks included voluntary renunciation of worldly attachments, adherence to ethical guidelines known as Vinaya, meditation, dedicated study and reflection, reliance on alms for material needs, and communal living in monastic communities or monasteries. To accommodate laypeople's diverse situations and circumstances, they introduced modifications to make mindfulness practice accessible and practical.

Compassion practice in mindfulness involves begging for alms and subsisting solely on alms, ideally leading to the development of a compassionate society and the monk's realization of compassion. Forgiveness is a central component of ancient mindfulness practice and a central component of modern self-compassion practice. In other words, a practice called "Compassion" is now distinct from mindfulness. Over time, mindfulness practice has become secularized; it originated in monastic life and is now widespread. It has undergone alterations from its original state. There are advantages and disadvantages to each system and modification. The change has separated the ancient practices of purification and compassion from the modern approach. Today, however, there is virtue. Singha & Kanna (2022) state that nuns do not receive equal privilege in certain Buddhist monastic practices to advance their spiritual learning and obtain elevated monastic positions. Tara is a powerful female deity in Tibetan Buddhism. She is known as Tara in Sanskrit and Dol-ma in Tibetan, where "Dol" means liberation and "ma" means female or mother, giving her the meaning "female liberator." Nuns and other female lay practitioners continue to encounter obstacles as they develop within a monastic lifestyle or a spiritual foundation intended for lay practitioners. In other words, anyone can now practice mindfulness as a positive sign.

Considering the word "smriti," which signifies remembrance, ideally connotes a positive memory and a joyous event. Buddha spoke of cultivating "right" mindfulness, implying that it is possible to cultivate "wrong" mindfulness. Integrating mindfulness practises into Indian psychology has broader implications for social and spiritual development than individual well-being. Mindfulness is a significant concept, viewed as a means of transcending the ego and establishing a connection with a larger universal consciousness. Individuals can experience a sense of interconnectedness and unity with all beings through mindfulness, thereby cultivating compassion, empathy, and harmony in relationships and society. Indian psychology highlights the importance of mindfulness in obtaining mental balance and overcoming suffering. Practices such as Vipassana meditation, which originated in India and has gained worldwide popularity, emphasize the cultivation of mindfulness and perception of the nature of reality. These practices intend to purify the mind, liberate it from attachments and delusions, and cultivate stability, compassion, and wisdom. Recently, there has been an increased interest in incorporating Indian mindfulness practices into Western psychological frameworks. Scholars and researchers have investigated mindfulness's therapeutic applications for various psychological disorders and found promising results. Mindfulness-based interventions, anchored in Indian mindfulness practices, have been utilized in Western contexts for stress reduction, anxiety, depression, addiction, and other mental health issues. Incorporating Indian mindfulness practices into Western psychology offers a holistic and comprehensive approach to mental health and well-being. It recognizes the function of mindfulness in fostering self-awareness, emotional control, and psychological resilience. Incorporating Indian mindfulness practices into Western psychology also promotes cultural exchange and dialogue. It improves the field of psychology by incorporating diverse wisdom traditions. Indian psychology recognizes the importance of mindfulness practices for personal growth, self-realization, and spiritual development. Incorporating Indian mindfulness practices into Western psychology expands the therapeutic options available to individuals and provides valuable tools for self-awareness, emotional health, and personal transformation. By incorporating Indian mindfulness practices, psychologists can promote mental health and foster a deeper understanding of human consciousness and well-being.

2. ORIGINS AND DEVELOPMENT OF MINDFULNESS PRACTICES AND INTERVENTIONS

Understanding the origins of mindfulness practices requires tracing their historical roots. Ancient contemplative traditions, primarily from India and East Asia, are the source of mindfulness. Mindfulness dates back to India's Vedic period (1500-500 BCE) when meditation and self-inquiry were the foundations of spiritual development and self-realization (Sharma et al., 2021). The Upanishads, written between 800 and 200 BCE and utilizing contemplative practices, investigate the essence of consciousness and the ego (Freud, 2015; Piparaiya, 2003). Meditation and self-inquiry played crucial roles in pursuing self-realization and understanding of the nature of consciousness during the Vedic period, characterized by a long history of spiritual exploration and inquiry. According to Sathiyaseelan et al. (2022), the most important discovery of the Upanishads is that mindfulness practice has its antecedents in Hindu traditions. Mindfulness involves practising silence meditation to cultivate acceptance and calm the mind. It increases directed awareness, facilitating a multidimensional understanding of problems and fostering insights. The benefits of mindful leadership include creating a safe environment for creativity, recognizing team efforts, demonstrating humility, being receptive to feedback, and adapting to change. Mindfulness enables leaders to effectively engage, interpret situations, and pose pertinent questions. Hindu mindfulness practice contributes to effective leadership by cultivating clarity, creativity, and adaptability in a calm and receptive mind. Although "mindfulness" may not have been used explicitly, numerous texts and teachings from that time contain concepts and practices associated with mindfulness. The Vedas, the earliest sacred texts in Hinduism, contain hymns and verses emphasizing the significance of focused attention, awareness, and introspection. These practices aimed to cultivate a deeper understanding of the self and ultimate reality. The Upanishads, which emerged later in the Vedic period (around 800–200 BCE), explored more deeply into consciousness and self-realization. Sages and seekers of the truth frequently present these texts' philosophical and spiritual teachings through dialogues. Through contemplative practices and self-inquiry, the Upanishads investigate the nature of the mind, the ego, and the essence of consciousness, although the term "mindfulness" is not explicitly mentioned. Xu (2020) noted that the Upanishads, for instance, contain discussions about the essence of the ego (Atman) and its relationship to the universal consciousness (Brahman). These dialogues emphasize the significance of self-awareness, introspection, and cultivating a focused and clear mind to comprehend the true nature of existence. They imply that meditation, concentration, and self-reflection are methods for cultivating heightened awareness and insight.

While the term "mindfulness" may not have been used during the Vedic period or in the Upanishads, we can trace its essence back to the contemplative practices and teachings of that time. The emphasis on present-moment awareness, self-inquiry, and cultivating a clear and focused mind is consistent with the modern understanding of mindfulness' fundamental principles. Notably, the concept and practice of mindfulness continued to evolve and develop after the Vedic and Upanishad periods. In later centuries, traditions such as Buddhism, Yoga, and Jainism refined and elaborated upon the teachings and practices associated with mindfulness in Indian psychology. By advancing the understanding and application of mindfulness, these traditions contributed to the intricate tapestry of ancient and modern Indian thought. Buddha, also known as Siddhartha Gautama, popularized mindfulness through his teachings around 500 BCE (Keown, 2022). Mindfulness meditation, especially Vipassana (insight) meditation, became essential to the Buddhist path to enlightenment (Farb, 2014). Buddhist traditions such as Theravada, Zen, and Tibetan Buddhism have refined mindfulness practices over the centuries. The Eightfold Path is a fundamental concept in Buddhist philosophy and practice, and one of its integral components is mindfulness, according to Aich (2013). The path, as taught by Siddhartha Gautama, also known as the Buddha, provides a systematic framework for overcoming suffering and escaping the cycle of rebirth and death (samsara). As part of the Eightfold Path, mindfulness meditation, notably Vipassana (insight) meditation, plays an essential role in cultivating mindfulness, according to Huxter (2015). According to Marques (2022), the Eightfold Path is a profound framework of eight interconnected factors or practices that serve as governing principles for attaining enlightenment or awakening. These factors illuminate the path to a more profound understanding of reality by highlighting all phenomena' inherent impermanence and interdependence. They begin by cultivating noble and compassionate intentions, free of greed, hatred, and delusion. The journey continues with mindful and skilful communication, characterized by truthful, kind, and beneficial speech.

The Eightfold Path extends to a person's actions, requiring moral behaviour consistent with the principles of compassion and mindfulness. Earning a living through honourable means following the ethical foundations of the path is another essential aspect. The path also requires constant effort to abandon unwholesome qualities while cultivating healthy ones while maintaining a state of consciousness and equilibrium. Integral to this path is the internal and external cultivation of moment-to-moment awareness and a nonjudgmental focus on one's current experiences. The journey culminates in developing focused and concentrated mental states, predominantly through meditation practices such as mindfulness, which ultimately lead to enhanced wisdom and insight. The Eightfold Path is, in essence, a profound roadmap to self-discovery and enlightenment, incorporating ethical conduct, mental discipline, and deep contemplation as essential components of the transformative journey (Anlayo, 2022). As a component of the Eightfold Path, mindfulness meditation, specifically Vipassana meditation, is a well-known method for cultivating mindfulness. Vipassana meditation involves meticulously observing the body, sensations, thoughts, and emotions to gain insight into phenomena' transience, contentment, and selflessness. By cultivating mindfulness through meditation, an individual gains clarity, stability, and a profound understanding of the nature of reality. Notably, although the eightfold path and mindfulness have deep roots in Buddhist philosophy, their principles and practices have transcended religious boundaries and been integrated into nonreligious contexts.

Daoism in China emphasized coexistence with the natural order of existence (Hwang & Chang, 2009). Daoist meditation and qigong involve cultivating mindfulness to align with the present moment and increase awareness of the self's interconnections with the universe. Taoism, an ancient Chinese spiritual and philosophical tradition, centres around Dao, which can be interpreted as the universe's governing fundamental principle or primordial force and is central to Daoist teachings. Miller (2003) explains that Daoism prioritizes living in harmony with the natural flow of existence, embracing simplicity, and cultivating a profound connection with nature and the world. Mindfulness is essential in Daoist practices for cultivating heightened awareness and aligning with the present moment. In Daoist meditation and qigong, mindfulness promotes inner tranquillity, balance, and harmony (Cohen, 2015). Diverse Daoist meditation techniques seek to calm the mind, sharpen perception, and foster a profound state of presence.

Practitioners strive to attain a state of tranquillity and absence by focusing their attention, allowing thoughts and distractions to dissipate and cultivating heightened awareness. This state of mindfulness enables individuals to acquire a greater appreciation for the interdependence between themselves, the natural world, and the larger cosmic forces at play. Qigong is a holistic system of body-mind exercises that incorporates movement, control of respiration, and focused attention. It seeks to cultivate and balance the body's vital energy, known as Qi, while cultivating awareness and inner harmony. Focusing on being fully present and attuned to the body's subliminal sensations and energy flow, practitioners engage in gradual, deliberate movements and breathing techniques. Through consistent practice, individuals cultivate a profound awareness of their physical, mental, and energetic states, which enhances their overall health and sense of interconnectedness with their surroundings. Daoist meditation and qigong emphasize mindfulness as a means of dissolving attachments, resting the mind, and cultivating a profound sense of oneness with nature. By harmonizing with the natural rhythms and aligning with the present moment, individuals can develop a profound understanding of themselves and their place in the more excellent web of existence. In addition, Daoism considers the individual an integral part of the interconnected fabric of life, emphasizing the interdependence and interaction of all beings and phenomena. Mindfulness allows Daoist practitioners to recognize and embrace this interconnectedness, dispelling the illusion of separateness and cultivating a sense of unity with the universe. Its heightened awareness and comprehension of connection can result in a profound shift in how people perceive themselves and their position in the world.

It is worth noting that Daoist mindfulness practices have not remained exclusive to China but have also influenced and found incorporation into other East Asian cultures like Japan, Korea, and Vietnam. While there may be variations in techniques and approaches, the fundamental principles of nurturing mindfulness, embracing the present moment, and fostering interconnectedness with the natural world remain at the core of Daoist-inspired practices across East Asia. In Indian psychology, particularly in schools of thought like Advaita Vedanta and Kashmir Shaivism, there is a strong emphasis on non-dualism and the interconnectedness of all entities and phenomena. These philosophies recognize the essential unity of existence and advocate transcending dualistic perceptions to realize the oneness of all things. Similarly, Daoism emphasizes the interconnectedness of all aspects of the universe and the necessity of living in harmony with the natural order of things.

In addition, both Indian psychology and Daoism emphasize cultivating present-moment mindfulness and awareness. Indian traditions utilize meditation, self-inquiry (e.g., "Who am I?"), and contemplation to cultivate self-awareness, insight, and direct experiential comprehension of one's true nature. Similarly, Daoist practices like meditation and qigong aim to cultivate awareness of the present moment, inner tranquillity, and mindfulness. Despite these philosophical and practical similarities, it is essential to recognize that Daoism and Indian psychology have distinct cultural and historical roots. Daoism is deeply rooted in Chinese traditions, while Indian psychology comprises numerous philosophical, spiritual, and psychological practices developed over thousands of years on the Indian subcontinent. Daoism is a tradition within the philosophy and spirituality of East Asia, distinct from the specific schools of thought and practices that constitute Indian psychology.

Modern MBIs owe a great deal to influential figures and their pioneering contributions. In the late 1970s, scientist and seasoned meditator Jon Kabat-Zinn created the MBSR program. This secular program integrated mindfulness meditation, yoga, and body awareness to help individuals manage tension, discomfort, and chronic illness. (Carmody et al., 2009) MBSR established the essential groundwork for incorporating mindfulness into Western psychology, marking a significant milestone. In the 1990s, researchers advanced the discipline by introducing MBCT, building upon Kabat-Zinn's pioneering work. The primary goal of this approach is to prevent relapse in conditions such as depression and other mental health disorders by emphasizing the integration of mindfulness practices and cognitive-behavioural techniques (Apolinário-Hagen et al., 2020). In addition to MBSR and MBCT, the landscape of MBIs has expanded. Innovations such as MBRP, Mindful Self-Compassion (MSC), and ACT integrate mindfulness with specific therapeutic approaches to address various needs and contexts (Sun et al., 2021). MBRP is an intervention that incorporates mindfulness practices and cognitive and behavioural-based relapse prevention techniques. Marlatt and Gordon conceived it in 1985. Andrea Konig, Christopher J. Gioia, Vivian M. Rodrguez, John A. Starr, William Meese, Danielle Worthington-Stoneman, Karen Kersting, Eva Natanya, and J. Kim Penberthy reviewed the development of MBRP specifically for alcohol use disorders and its implementation details. To promote a compassionate approach based on acceptance and openness as opposed to remorse, blame, and humiliation regarding one's behaviour, they combined techniques and strategies from RP with mindfulness-based methods, resulting in the manualized intervention known as MBRP. This investigation originated in the early 2000s at the Addictive Behaviors Research Center of the University of Washington (Penberthy et al., 2013). Kristin Neff originated the concept of Mindful Self-Compassion, developed in 2010. It consists of three essential components: self-kindness, humanity, and mindfulness. The creator of the Self-Compassion Scale, Kristin Neff, has utilized it extensively in self-compassion research. This scale measures individuals' self-kindness versus self-judgment, common humanity versus isolation, and mindfulness versus over-identification. However, it is essential to note that mindfulness originates in ancient Eastern and Buddhist philosophy dating back approximately two millennia. Mindful Self-Compassion (MSC) is a multifaceted technique with numerous applications. Enhancing emotional resilience by nurturing a receptive and curious attitude toward challenging emotions is crucial. MSC promotes healthy lifestyle choices by enhancing happiness and decreasing anxiety and depression. MSC can augment therapists' skills in the domain of self-care and protect against compassion fatigue. It has found a position in educational settings, where it serves as an invaluable tool for learning and growth. Furthermore, MSC can motivate behaviour change, offering a new perspective on personal development. It also offers techniques to reduce caregiver fatigue, offering valuable assistance to individuals in caregiving positions. Finally, the Mindful Self-Compassion program aims to enhance therapists' skills, broadening its range of applications (Jiménez-Gómez et al., 2022).

MBI practices have profound roots in Buddhist philosophy; they incorporate cognitive-behavioural principles to promote cognitive flexibility, emotional regulation, and adaptive coping. Mindfulness practices entail the development of self-regulation and attentional control abilities. Models such as the Three-Process and Attention Regulation Model imply that mindfulness improves metacognitive awareness, attention stability, and the capacity to disengage from automatic thought patterns. Neuroscientific research has uncovered the neural mechanisms underlying mindfulness, including the Default Mode Network, prefrontal cortex, and insula. Understanding the effects of mindfulness on the brain requires grasping neuroplasticity, which is the brain's capacity to change. By integrating these theoretical frameworks, MBIs offer a conceptual comprehension of how mindfulness practices influence individuals' psychological well-being, cognition, emotion regulation, and behaviour. Mindfulness practices and interventions have evolved and merged with contemporary psychological models. This integration has facilitated the adoption of MBIs in Western and Indian psychology, thereby making them valuable instruments for improving diverse populations' mental health and well-being.

3. EMPIRICAL EVIDENCE FOR THE EFFECTIVENESS OF MINDFULNESS-BASED INTERVENTIONS

In Western psychology, empirical research has produced compelling evidence supporting the efficacy of MBIs. Significant findings indicate that these interventions effectively alleviate anxiety, depression, and tension symptoms, among other psychological disorders. Participation in programs such as MBSR and MBCT has been associated with substantial improvements in psychological well-being and quality of life overall (Kraines et al., 2022). Moreover, mindfulness-based interventions, particularly MBCT, effectively prevent depression relapse in recurrently depressed individuals. Combining mindfulness practices with cognitive-behavioural strategies increases self-awareness, cognitive flexibility, and emotion regulation while decreasing the risk of relapse (Williams & Kuiken, 2012). Research has shown that mindfulness improves cognitive functioning, including attention, working memory, and executive functions. Mindfulness training regularly enhances cognitive flexibility, problem-solving, and decision-making skills (Whitfield et al., 2021). Researchers have demonstrated that mindfulness improves cognitive functioning, including attention, working memory, and executive functions. Regular mindfulness training enhances cognitive flexibility, problem-solving, and decision-making skills (Whitfield et al., 2021).

In addition, MBIs have demonstrated positive effects on physical health outcomes, such as reduced pain intensity and improved immune function (Howarth et al., 2019). The multifaceted advantages of MBIs for improving mental and physical health are evident in these findings. Although research on MBIs in

Indian psychology remains limited, traditional mindfulness practices, particularly Vipassana meditation, have yielded promising results. These practices, deeply rooted in Indian psychology, have been linked to profound self-transformation, heightened self-awareness, and spiritual development. Practitioners frequently describe experiencing increased emotional stability, a deeper understanding of reality, and a heightened sense of interconnectedness (Frank & Marken, 2021). In Indian psychology, mindfulness practices emphasize cultivating emotional balance while reducing attachment and aversion. Initial research suggests that these practices may increase emotional well-being, decrease emotional reactivity, and promote greater acceptance (Chandna et al., 2022). In addition, integrating mindfulness practices from Indian psychology with Ayurveda, the traditional Indian medical system, has shown promise for improving physical health. Mindfulness-based Ayurvedic interventions, such as mindful eating and mindful movement, have been linked to enhanced digestion, stress reduction, and overall well-being (Tatta et al., 2022). Despite the limited research, these findings demonstrate the potential for Indian-rooted mindfulness practices to positively contribute to mental and physical health. MBIs have demonstrated efficacy in various cultural contexts, but it is essential to recognize the influence of cultural nuances on their implementation. These nuances include mindfulness practices rooted in particular cultural frameworks and beliefs, necessitating culturally relevant adaptations. In addition, the cultural context, which includes social support, therapeutic relationships, and attitudes toward mental health, substantially impacts the intervention outcomes. Customizing interventions to cultural preferences and communication styles is essential for engagement and efficacy. Research across cultures necessitates careful consideration of measurement instruments and culturally-adapted outcome measures. Recognizing cultural complexities is crucial for maximizing the accessibility and efficacy of MBIs in diverse cultural environments.

4. MINDFULNESS-BASED INTERVENTIONS (MBIS) IN WESTERN AND INDIAN PSYCHOLOGY

Mindfulness practices have acquired widespread acceptance and incorporation into numerous therapeutic approaches in Western psychology. Here is a summary of Western psychology's mindfulness practices. Jon Kabat-Zinn created MBSR, an eight-week program integrating mindfulness meditation, body awareness exercises, and mild yoga. It seeks to cultivate a nonjudgmental awareness of the present moment, reduce stress, and enhance well-being overall. MBSR has been extensively utilized to treat numerous mental and somatic health conditions, According to Ong & Smith (2017). The MBCT combines mindfulness practices and CBT techniques. It emphasizes developing awareness of negative thought patterns and cognitive flexibility to prevent relapse into depression and other mental health disorders. Sipe and Eisendrath (2012) found that MBCT effectively reduces the risk of relapse and enhances emotional well-being. ACT integrates mindfulness practices to aid in developing psychological flexibility and accepting challenging emotions and thoughts. It focuses on aligning actions with personal values and committing to significant life changes. ACT has addressed several psychological conditions, such as anxiety, depression, and chronic pain (Dindo et al., 2017). MBIs in Education practices have been incorporated into educational settings to promote the well-being of students and improve their learning outcomes. In educational contexts, programs such as Mindfulness-Based Cognitive Education (MBCE) and MBIs for Teachers (MBIT) seek to improve attention, emotion regulation, and overall psychological functioning (MacPherson et al., 2022).

Mindfulness practices have a lengthy history in Indian psychology and are firmly rooted in ancient traditions. The following is an overview of mindfulness practices within Indian psychology. Vipassana, which translates to "insight," is a form of meditation that cultivates non-reactive awareness of bodily sensations, thoughts, and emotions. It is frequently practised in the context of silent retreats and seeks to cultivate an understanding of the transient and selfless nature of experience. According to Dreeben et al. (2013), Vipassana is a prominent practice in Buddhist and Indian contemplative traditions. Yoga incorporates mindfulness into its larger framework, including physical postures (asanas), respiration control (pranayama), and meditation. Yoga emphasizes the union of body, mind, and spirit, with mindfulness enhancing self-awareness, concentration, and spiritual development. Various varieties of yoga, including Hatha, Raja, and Kundalini, incorporate mindfulness (Kwok et al., 2017). Within the context of Ayurveda, mindfulness integrates into various aspects of daily life, encompassing mindful eating, movement, and self-care practices. Ayurvedic mindfulness aims to nurture awareness of the body, senses, and environment, promoting equilibrium and well-being (Pyles, 2018). Adapting mindfulness practices to various cultural contexts is essential for ensuring their effectiveness. Here are some cultural adaptation considerations.

The efficacy of mindfulness practices in diverse cultural contexts, it is essential to use culturally relevant language, terminology, and adaptations. It includes translating mindfulness concepts and instructions in a way that correlates with the cultural beliefs and values of the intended audience, thereby enhancing comprehension and engagement. Incorporating cultural metaphors, examples, stories, symbols, and idioms into mindfulness instruction increases students' connection to the practice. In addition, it is essential to adapt mindfulness to incorporate cultural values, such as collective well-being or spiritual elements. Adaptation is refined further by addressing specific cultural challenges and stressors while considering social, economic, and environmental contexts. By harmonizing mindfulness with traditional practices, these interventions become more accessible and effective at promoting psychological development and well-being among diverse populations.

5. IMPLICATIONS AND FUTURE DIRECTIONS

The extensive incorporation of MBIs into Western and Indian psychology has substantial implications for psychological practice and research. Research has demonstrated the effectiveness of these interventions in reducing psychological symptoms, preventing relapse, and promoting well-being. They can complement various therapeutic approaches and enable mental health professionals to assist clients in developing crucial skills such as self-awareness, emotional regulation, and adaptive coping mechanisms. In addition, MBIs advocate a holistic approach to well-being that includes physical, psychological, and spiritual dimensions. This alignment with the understanding of interconnected human experiences promotes a more inclusive view of mental health and well-being. These interventions also hold promise for preventive programs and wellness initiatives, potentially contributing to early intervention, stress reduction, and improving psychological well-being among individuals without specific mental health diagnoses. Moreover, by adapting mindfulness practices to diverse cultural contexts, MBIs can bridge cultural divides, promoting inclusivity and cultural responsiveness in mental health care. This cultural awareness paves the way for more accessible and equitable mental health care.

Additional research is required to understand the intricate mechanisms underlying mindfulness-based interventions' therapeutic effects. Exploring the neurobiological, cognitive, and psychological processes involved in mindfulness practice promises a deeper understanding of how these interventions affect the well-being of individuals. Research should prioritize the cultural adaptation of MBIs and their efficacy across diverse cultural environments. Investigating the impact of these adaptations and dissecting the cultural factors that influence outcomes can be helpful in the development of culturally sensitive mindfulness interventions. The significance of longitudinal studies cannot be exaggerated, as they can shed light on the lasting effects of MBIs that extend beyond the immediate treatment outcomes. It is crucial to examine the long-term effects of mindfulness practice on mental health, general well-being, and quality of life.

Diverse populations, such as infants, adolescents, older adults, individuals from marginalized communities, and those with comorbid conditions, merit targeted research. Examining the benefits and potential obstacles within these groups can inform the development of interventions that suit their specific requirements. In addition, comparative research should investigate the similarities and differences in the efficacy of MBIs across diverse cultural and psychological frameworks. By doing so, we can elucidate the universal aspects of mindfulness practice while respecting and appreciating the cultural variations that influence its implementation and outcomes. MBIs have established themselves as valuable instruments in Western and Indian psychology, supported by substantial empirical research. They have promising implications for psychological practice, including promoting well-being, reducing symptoms, and preventing relapse. Future research should focus on comprehending mechanisms, cultural adaptations, long-term effects, specific populations, and cross-cultural comparisons within a holistic and culturally sensitive approach to mental health care. These endeavours are poised to advance the discipline and improve the efficacy and accessibility of mindfulness-based interventions, which will ultimately benefit individuals worldwide.

6. CASE STUDIES OF MINDFULNESS-BASED INTERVENTIONS (MBIS) IN WESTERN AND INDIAN PSYCHOLOGY

Case Study One: MBSR for Well-Being in Western Psychology

BK, a 21-year-old female, seeks assistance to improve her well-being and life satisfaction. BK has been feeling overwhelmed by the demands of modern life, experiencing stress and a lack of equilibrium despite not being diagnosed with a specific mental health disorder. BK enrols in an eight-week well-being-enhancing MBSR program. This program includes meditation, body awareness exercises, and mild yoga. Its primary objective is to assist individuals such as BK in cultivating a nonjudgmental awareness of the present moment, managing tension, and cultivating a sense of contentment and fulfilment.

BK develops greater self-awareness and a deeper connection to the richness of each moment as a result of his consistent engagement in mindfulness practices. She discovers the power of accepting and appreciating the present moment. As a consequence, BK experiences decreased stress, enhanced emotional well-being, and an overall improvement in life quality. She reports feeling more in control of her emotions, better equipped to deal with life's obstacles, and more satisfied with her daily experiences. This case study illustrates the versatility of MBSR in Western psychology, not only for treating conditions but also for promoting general well-being and life satisfaction. It demonstrates how mindfulness practices can enable people like BK to lead more fulfilling and balanced lives.

Case Study Two: MBCT for Addiction Recovery in Indian Psychology

AC, a 21-year-old male, has been battling a chronic dependence on nicotine for several years. The effects of his addiction on his physical health, intimate relationships, and overall quality of life have been severe. Despite numerous attempts to quit, he has repeatedly relapsed and struggled with cravings. AC enrols in an eight-week MBCT program designed for addiction rehabilitation in the Indian psychological context. This program combines mindfulness with cognitive-behavioral techniques. The primary objective is to assist individuals like AC in developing an understanding of their addiction's triggers, cravings, and habitual thought patterns, thereby promoting long-term recovery.

AC begins to recognize the fundamental causes of his addiction and the automatic thought patterns that fuel his cravings due to the MBCT program. Mindfulness practices provide him with the tools necessary to observe his cravings without judgment and to respond to them with greater self-compassion and emotional regulation. AC experiences a decrease in the frequency and intensity of his desires over time. In addition, he learns adaptive coping strategies to supplant unhealthy behaviours, substantially improving his overall health. This case study demonstrates the efficacy of MBCT for addiction recovery within the context of Indian psychology. By combining mindfulness and cognitive-behavioural techniques, individuals such as AC can obtain valuable insights, improve self-regulation, and embark on a path to long-term addiction recovery.

Case Study Three: Mindfulness-Based Interventions (MBIs) for Cultivating Mindfulness in Both Western and Indian Psychology

Two undergraduates, LR and MN, embark on a voyage to improve their mindfulness and well-being amidst the demands of their studies. As they navigate the challenges of their coursework, they recognize the need to cultivate qualities such as presence, focus, and emotional resilience. LR and MN engage in mindfulness meditation, mindful breathing exercises, and daily mindfulness practices after opting for a mindfulness-based program designed to increase mindfulness. This program seeks to instil the transformative power of mindfulness, fostering a deeper connection to the present moment and one's inner self, irrespective of culture.

Consistently engaging in mindfulness practices profoundly transforms the lives of LR and MN. Their increased self-awareness allows them to approach daily experiences more clearly and purposefully. Emotional regulation becomes an easier-to-learn skill, resulting in decreased tension and enhanced emotional health. In addition, mindfulness permeates their academic pursuits, enhancing their concentration, creativity, and sense of purpose. LR and MN report a significant increase in mindfulness, resulting in enhanced well-being, reduced tension, and a profound connection with themselves and the world. Their academic pursuits benefit from increased concentration and creative thinking, resulting in higher grades and a greater appreciation for the learning process. This case demonstrates the universal applicability of MBIs for increasing mindfulness in both Western and Indian psychology. By cultivating self-awareness, emotional regulation, and an unwavering connection to the present moment, these interventions offer a valuable path to enriching one's life and transcending cultural boundaries.

7. DISCUSSION

The debate surrounding MBIs in Western and Indian psychology is significant in global psychology. Throughout this chapter, we have scrutinized several crucial details, shedding light on the applications and significance of these interventions. A crucial factor is the acceptance and incorporation of MBIs into Western psychology. MBSR and MBCT effectively reduce psychological symptoms, prevent relapse, and promote overall well-being. This recognition has resulted in incorporating mindfulness practices and interventions into conventional psychological practices and interventions. Mindfulness practices have deep roots in Indian psychology, including Vipassana meditation and incorporating mindfulness into yoga and Ayurvedic practices. These practices aim to cultivate self-awareness, perception, and balance. By recognizing these historical and cultural foundations, MBIs can contextualize and enrich India's psychological framework. MBIs have several advantages and disadvantages. On the positive side, MBIs are highly effective in improving various biopsychosocial conditions, including depression, anxiety, stress, insomnia, addiction, psychosis, pain, hypertension, weight management, cancer-related symptoms, and prosocial behaviours. They are generally safe and cost-effective in treating some health conditions. Online MBIs have shown significant improvements in anxiety symptoms in adult populations. However, there is limited or preliminary data on the effects of MBIs on conditions such as PTSD, ADHD, ASD, eating disorders, loneliness, and the physical symptoms of cardiovascular disease, diabetes, and respiratory conditions. Researchers have reported higher attrition rates in online MBIs. Numerous systematic reviews and meta-analyses on mindfulness demonstrate the poor quality of the included studies. MBIs have shown marginally positive effects on cognitive and socioemotional processes, but these effects have not translated to behavioural or academic outcomes. It is essential to emphasize the need for additional research into the efficacy of MBIs for various issues. Required are high-quality studies with sufficient sample sizes and extended follow-up periods.

MBIs must prioritize cultural sensitivity and adaptability above all else. Adapting these interventions to various cultural contexts, considering language, metaphors, and values, increases their applicability and accessibility to diverse populations. It fosters cultural sensitivity in psychological practice, addressing individual requirements across cultures. Significantly, the preventive nature of MBIs shifts the emphasis from treating mental illness to promoting general well-being, resiliency, and relapse prevention. They promote international cooperation and cross-cultural understanding, thereby enriching the field of psychology. MBIs undeniably impact global psychology, promoting cultural awareness, prevention, and collaboration. However, additional research is required to comprehend their mechanisms, ensure cultural adaptation, and improve accessibility, ultimately fostering a more inclusive and culturally sensitive approach to psychological practice around the globe.

8. CONCLUSION

This chapter has investigated the complex landscape of MBIs in both Western and Indian psychology. In Western psychology, MBSR and MBCT have gained recognition for effectively reducing psychological symptoms and preventing relapse. In addition, we have examined the historical significance of deeply rooted mindfulness practices in Indian psychology for cultivating self-awareness and equilibrium.

The adaptability of MBIs to diverse cultural contexts, with an emphasis on linguistic, symbolic, and contextual considerations, has been a central theme. Empirical evidence supports their efficacy, encompassing holistic well-being, cultural sensitivity, resilience-building, and preventive mental health care. Recommendations include enhanced mechanistic comprehension, longitudinal and comparative research, cultural adaptation, professional training, and increased accessibility. This chapter concludes by highlighting the profound significance of MBIs in Western and Indian psychology, providing a comprehensive overview of their origins, evolution, and empirical support. It is undeniable that they have the potential to improve well-being, alleviate psychological distress, and promote inclusivity in global psychological practice.

REFERENCES

Aich, T. K. (2013). Buddha philosophy and Western psychology. *Indian Journal of Psychiatry, 55*(6), 165. doi:10.4103/0019-5545.105517 PMID:23858249

Anālayo, B. (2022). Eightfold Path in Early Buddhism. Springer eBooks. doi:10.1007/978-3-030-90465-4_38-1

Apolinário-Hagen, J., Drüge, M., & Fritsche, L. (2020). Cognitive behavioural therapy, mindfulness-based cognitive therapy and acceptance commitment therapy for anxiety disorders: integrating traditional with digital treatment approaches. *Anxiety Disorders: Rethinking and Understanding Recent Discoveries*, (pp. 291-329). Springer. https://link.springer.com/chapter/10.1007/978-981-32-9705-0_17

Baldo, J. V., Schendel, K., Lewis, S. J., Herron, T. J., Dempsey, D. G., Muir, J. J., Curran, B., Paulraj, S., Chok, J. M., & Cole, M. (2021). Mindfulness-Based Stress Reduction Intervention in Chronic Stroke: A Randomized, Controlled Pilot Study. *Mindfulness, 12*(12), 2908–2919. doi:10.100712671-021-01751-0

Carmody, J., Baer, R. A., & Lykins, LB, E., & Olendzki, N. (. (2009). An empirical study of the mechanisms of mindfulness in a mindfulness-based stress reduction program. *Journal of Clinical Psychology, 65*(6), 613–626. doi:10.1002/jclp.20579 PMID:19267330

Chandna, S., Sharma, P. K., & Vasudevan, M. (2022). The Mindful Self: Exploring Mindfulness in Relation with Self-esteem and Self-efficacy in Indian Population. *Psychological Studies, 67*(2), 261–272. doi:10.100712646-021-00636-5 PMID:35125522

Cillessen, L., Compen, F., & Speckens, A. E. M. (2020). Mindfulness-Based interventions. In Springer eBooks (pp. 1396–1399). Springer. doi:10.1007/978-3-030-39903-0_101983

Cohen, E. (2015). The hold and release practice: A new way into meditation and mindfulness. *Transpersonal Psychology Review, 17*(1), 9–19. https://eprints.leedsbeckett.ac.uk/id/eprint/3470/. doi:10.53841/bpstran.2015.17.1.9

Dindo, L., Van Liew, J. R., & Arch, J. J. (2017). Acceptance and commitment therapy: A transdiagnostic behavioural intervention for mental health and medical conditions. *Neurotherapeutics; the Journal of the American Society for Experimental NeuroTherapeutics, 14*(3), 546–553. https://link.springer.com/article/10.1007/s13311-017-0521-3. doi:10.100713311-017-0521-3 PMID:28271287

Dreeben, S. J., Mamberg, M. H., & Salmon, P. (2013). The MBSR body scan in clinical practice. *Mindfulness*, *4*(4), 394–401. https://link.springer.com/article/10.1007/s12671-013-0212-z. doi:10.100712671-013-0212-z

Farb, N. A. (2014). From retreat centre to clinic to boardroom? Perils and promises of the modern mindfulness movement. *Religions*, *5*(4), 1062–1086. doi:10.3390/rel5041062

Frank, P., & Marken, M. (2021). Developments in Qualitative Mindfulness Practice Research: A Pilot Scoping Review. *Mindfulness*, *13*(1), 17–36. doi:10.100712671-021-01748-9

Freud, S. (2015). Beyond the pleasure principle. *Psychoanalysis and History*, *17*(2), 151–204. https://www.euppublishing.com/doi/full/10.3366/pah.2015.0169. doi:10.3366/pah.2015.0169

George, A. J., John, R., & Rajkumar, E. (2021d). Mindfulness-based positive psychology interventions: A systematic review. *BMC Psychology*, *9*(1), 116. doi:10.118640359-021-00618-2 PMID:34362457

Gold, E., Smith, A. M. S., Hopper, I., Herne, D., Tansey, G., & Hulland, C. (2009). Mindfulness-Based Stress Reduction (MBSR) for primary school teachers. *Journal of Child and Family Studies*, *19*(2), 184–189. doi:10.100710826-009-9344-0

Howarth, A., Smith, J. G., Perkins-Porras, L., & Ussher, M. (2019). Effects of Brief Mindfulness-Based Interventions on Health-Related Outcomes: A Systematic Review. *Mindfulness*, *10*(10), 1957–1968. doi:10.100712671-019-01163-1

Huxter, M. (2015). *Mindfulness and the Buddha's noble eightfold path*. Buddhist Foundations of Mindfulness. https://link.springer.com/chapter/10.1007/978-3-319-18591-0_3

Hwang, K. K., & Chang, J. (2009). Self-cultivation: Culturally sensitive psychotherapies in Confucian societies. *The Counseling Psychologist*, *37*(7), 1010–1032. doi:10.1177/0011000009339976

Janssen, M., Heerkens, Y., Kuijer, W., Van Der Heijden, B., & Engels, J. (2018). Effects of Mindfulness-Based Stress Reduction on employees' mental health: A systematic review. *PLoS One*, *13*(1), e0191332. doi:10.1371/journal.pone.0191332 PMID:29364935

Jiménez-Gómez, L., Bernabé, J. R. Y., Crego, A., Ventola, A. R. M., & Gómez-Martínez, M. Á. (2022). Effectiveness of the Mindfulness-Based Stress Reduction (MBSR) vs. the Mindful Self-Compassion (MSC) Programs in Clinical and Health Psychologist Trainees. *Mindfulness*, *13*(3), 584–599. doi:10.100712671-021-01814-2

Keng, S., Tong, E. M. W., Yan, E. T. L., Ebstein, R. P., & Lai, P. (2021). Effects of mindfulness-based stress reduction on affect dynamics: A randomized controlled trial. *Mindfulness*, *12*(6), 1490–1501. doi:10.100712671-021-01617-5

Keown, D. (2022). Origins of Buddhist ethics. Encyclopedia of Religious Ethics, (pp. 602–610). Wiley. doi:10.1002/9781118499528.ch71

Kraines, M. A., Peterson, S. K., Tremont, G., Beard, C., Brewer, J. A., & Uebelacker, L. A. (2022). Mindfulness-based stress reduction and cognitive therapy for depression: A systematic review of cognitive outcomes. *Mindfulness*, *13*(5), 1126–1135. doi:10.100712671-022-01841-7 PMID:36059888

Kwok, J. Y. Y., Kwan, J. C. Y., Auyeung, M., Mok, V. C. T., & Chan, H. Y. L. (2017). The effects of yoga versus stretching and resistance training exercises on psychological distress for people with mild-to-moderate Parkinson's disease: Study protocol for a randomized controlled trial. *Trials*, *18*(1), 1–13. https://trialsjournal.biomedcentral.com/articles/10.1186/s13063-017-2223-x. doi:10.118613063-017-2223-x PMID:28049491

Lee, J., Kim, K. H., Webster, C., & Henning, M. A. (2021). The evolution of mindfulness from 1916 to 2019. *Mindfulness*, *12*(8), 1849–1859. doi:10.100712671-021-01603-x

Lengacher, C. A., Gruss, L. F., Kip, K. E., Reich, R. R., Chauca, K. G., Moscoso, M. S., Joshi, A., Tinsley, S., Shani, B., Cousin, L., Khan, C. P., Goodman, M., & Park, J. Y. (2021). Mindfulness-based stress reduction for breast cancer survivors: Evaluating mediators of psychological and physical outcomes in a large randomized controlled trial. *Journal of Behavioral Medicine*, *44*(5), 591–604. doi:10.100710865-021-00214-0 PMID:33963420

MacPherson, S. A., Grabovac, A. D., Collins, E. J., Heath, T., Rockman, P., & Winston, D. (2022). Transprofessional competencies across clinical, organizational, and educational professions: The case of mindfulness-based teaching and learning (MBTL). *Professional Development in Education*, 1–17. doi:10.1080/19415257.2022.2143863

Marques, J. (2022). Treading the noble eightfold path: A leadership development strategy in a VUCA world. In Developing Leaders for Real: Proven Approaches That Deliver Impact (pp. 163–173). Emerald Publishing. doi:10.1108/978-1-80071-364-220221024

Miller, J. (2003). Daoism and nature. *Nature across cultures: Views of nature and the environment in non-western cultures*, (pp. 393–409). Springer. https://link.springer.com/chapter/10.1007/978-94-017-0149-5_20

Ong, J. C., & Smith, C. E. (2017). Using mindfulness for the treatment of insomnia. *Current Sleep Medicine Reports, 3*, 57–65. https://link.springer.com/article/10.1007/s40675-017-0068-1

Penberthy, J. K., König, A., Gioia, C. J., Rodríguez, V. M., Starr, J., Meese, W., Worthington-Stoneman, D., Kersting, K., & Natanya, E. (2013). Mindfulness-based relapse prevention: History, mechanisms of action, and effects. *Mindfulness*, *6*(2), 151–158. doi:10.100712671-013-0239-1

Piparaiya, R. K. (2003). *Ten Upanishads of Four Vedas*. Motilal Banarsidass Publishing House. https://www.mlbd.in/products/ten-upanishads-of-four-vedas-ram-k-piparaiya-9788178221595-8178221594

Pyles, L. (2018). *Healing justice: Holistic self-care for change makers*. Oxford University Press., https://global.oup.com/academic/product/healing-justice-9780190663087

Querstret, D., Morison, L., Dickinson, S., Cropley, M., & John, M. (2020). Mindfulness-based stress reduction and cognitive therapy for psychological health and well-being in nonclinical samples: A systematic review and meta-analysis. *International Journal of Stress Management*, *27*(4), 394–411. doi:10.1037tr0000165

Salmon, P., & Loo, J. L. (2023). Mindfulness-based cognitive therapy. In Springer eBooks (pp. 1–19). doi:10.1007/978-3-030-42825-9_75-1

Sathiyaseelan, A., Balasundaram, S., & Zirkler, M. (2022). Indian perspectives on mindful leadership. In *Proceedings of the International Research Conference on Mindfulness 2022 (IRCM 2022)*. Research Gate. https://www.researchgate.net/profile/Sathiyaseelan-Balasundaram/publication/359199972_Indian_Perspectives_on_Mindful_Leadership/links/622da88797401151d216376b/Indian-Perspectives-on-Mindful-Leadership.pdf

Sharma, A., Sabharwal, P., & Dada, R. (2021). Herbal medicine—An introduction to its history. In *Herbal Medicine in Andrology* (pp. 1–8). Academic Press. doi:10.1016/B978-0-12-815565-3.00001-1

Singha, R., & Kanna, S. Y. (2022). Women's empowerment, mindfulness, and role of women in eradicating alcohol and drug addiction from Indian society. *Journal of International Women's Studies*, *24*(7), 7. https://vc.bridgew.edu/jiws/vol24/iss7/7/

Sipe, W. E., & Eisendrath, S. J. (2012). Mindfulness-based cognitive therapy: Theory and practice. *Canadian Journal of Psychiatry*, *57*(2), 63–69. https://journals.sagepub.com/doi/pdf/10.1177/070674371205700202. doi:10.1177/070674371205700202 PMID:22340145

Soumya, R. R., & Sathiyaseelan, A. (2021). Mindfulness: An emotional aid to the glass ceiling experiences. *Cogent Psychology*, *8*(1), 1907911. doi:10.1080/23311908.2021.1907911

Sun, S., Nardi, W., Loucks, E. B., & Operario, D. (2021). Mindfulness-based interventions for sexual and gender minorities: A systematic review and evidence evaluation. *Mindfulness*, *12*(10), 2439–2459. https://link.springer.com/article/10.1007/s12671-021-01710-9. doi:10.100712671-021-01710-9

Tan, M. Y. L., McConnell, B. L., & Barlas, J. (2022). Application of dialectical behaviour therapy in treating common psychiatric disorders: Study protocol for a scoping review. *BMJ Open*, *12*(9), e058565. doi:10.1136/bmjopen-2021-058565 PMID:36167385

Tatta, J., Willgens, A. M., & Palombaro, K. M. (2022). Mindfulness and acceptance–based interventions in physical therapist practice: The time is now. *Physical Therapy*, *102*(3), pzab293. doi:10.1093/ptj/pzab293 PMID:35079796

Vadivale, A. M., & Sathiyaseelan, A. (2019). Mindfulness-based relapse prevention–A meta-analysis. *Cogent Psychology*, *6*(1), 1567090. doi:10.1080/23311908.2019.1567090

Vadivale, A. M., & Sathiyaseelan, A. (2022). Need for mindfulness-based relapse prevention strategies for postpartum smoking relapse prevention. *Indian Journal of Public Health*, *66*(3), 334–336. https://journals.lww.com/IJPH/Fulltext/2022/66030/Need_for_Mindfulness_based_Relapse_Prevention.20.aspx. doi:10.4103/ijph.ijph_1494_21 PMID:36149116

Webster, M. (2011). Introduction to acceptance and commitment therapy. *Advances in Psychiatric Treatment*, *17*(4), 309–316. doi:10.1192/apt.bp.107.005256

Whitfield, T., Barnhofer, T., Acabchuk, R. L., Cohen, A., Lee, M., Schlosser, M., Arenaza-Urquijo, E. M., Böttcher, A., Britton, W. B., Coll-Padrós, N., Collette, F., Chételat, G., Dautricourt, S., Demnitz-King, H., Dumais, T., Klimecki, O., Meiberth, D., Moulinet, I., Müller, T., & Marchant, N. L. (2021). The Effect of mindfulness-based programs on Cognitive Function in Adults: A systematic review and meta-analysis. *Neuropsychology Review*, *32*(3), 677–702. doi:10.100711065-021-09519-y PMID:34350544

Williams, J. M. G., & Kuyken, W. (2012). Mindfulness-based cognitive therapy: A promising new approach to preventing depressive relapse. *The British Journal of Psychiatry, 200*(5), 359–360. doi:10.1192/bjp.bp.111.104745 PMID:22550328

Woods, S. L., & Rockman, P. (2021). *Mindfulness-based stress reduction: Protocol, practice, and teaching skills.* New Harbinger Publications. https://www.newharbinger.com/9781684035601/mindfulness-based-stress-reduction

Xu, R. (2020). Analysis of the concept of self between Brahmanism and Buddhism. *In 5th International Conference on Contemporary Education, Social Sciences and Humanities-Philosophy of Being Human as the Core of Interdisciplinary Research (ICCESSH 2020)* (pp. 103–106). Atlantis Press. 10.2991/assehr.k.200901.021

Zhang, D., Lee, K., Mák, E., Ho, C. Y., & Wong, S. Y. S. (2021). Mindfulness-based interventions: An overall review. *British Medical Bulletin, 138*(1), 41–57. doi:10.1093/bmb/ldab005 PMID:33884400

Chapter 12
Spiritual Intelligence and Srimad Bhagavad Gita

Srividya Subramaniam
Avinashilingam Institute for Home Science and Higher Education for Women, India

ABSTRACT

Most explanations of human behaviour as we know today come from the foundations of philosophers and mystics of Western traditions. In spite of any number of explanations, human miseries and sufferings continue to increase and there is an exponential growth of mental health issues. The present chapter has tried to understand how Vedic philosophy, especially Srimad Bhagavad Gita, offers a panoramic view on the functioning of human mind and its sufferings. Among the eighteen chapters of Srimad Bhagavad Gita, the author has chosen chapter two, consisting of 72 verses, which in detail talks about the Sankhya Yoga or dualistic realism. The reason for choosing the same has also been explained. A thematic analysis of the seventy-two verses and its commentaries resulted in six themes. The chapter concludes with the concept called "Sthitaprajñasamādhistha" or, "state of steady intelligence situated in a trance," which is a practice every human being should strive to relief themselves of all miseries and sufferings of human life and attain a state of permanent happiness.

INTRODUCTION

sarva-dharmānparityajyamāmekaṁśaraṇaṁvraja

*ahaṁtvāṁsarva-pāpebhyomokṣayiṣyāmi***māśucaḥ**

"Abandon all varieties of religion and just surrender unto Me. I shall deliver you from all sinful reactions. **Do not fear**.*" (Srimad Srimad Bhagavad Gita(18.66)*

The World Health Organization estimates the burden of mental health problems in India as 2443 disability-adjusted life years (DALYs) and the suicide rate as 21.1%. As a result the economic loss due to mental

DOI: 10.4018/978-1-6684-9778-4.ch012

health problems in future would be around 1.03 trillions. The National Crimes Report Bureau (NCRB) estimates that in 2021 the national suicide rate was 12 per lakh people.

Mental health problems are raising and its affecting millions of lives in terms of their disability in day-to-day activities as well as personal growth and development. The subject matter of Psychology which primarily deals with mental health is faced with the challenge of how to cope with raising number of mental health issues. The mental health professionals are working like emergency healthcare professionals to handle thought and behavioral distresses. How does the subject matter of psychology cope up with these challenges?

Psychology, like any other discipline, is evolving continuously. The scope of the subject matter of Psychology remains in explaining and understanding human behavior in several spheres of life and how human nature can maximize its full potential. The discipline tries to explain a range of phenomena using several methods of science and nuances of art. Originally, the term psychology comes from two Greek words "psyche" which means soul, and "logos" meaning a science. However, readers interested in the subject matter of Psychology would agree that the subject matter has gone a long way to understand Psyche, and has rather focused on more experimentation, finding evidence, and validating facts. In the name of science, the subject matter of psychology has become a scientific discipline to explain "processes" underlying "human experience and behavior". The science of "soul" has become almost become a science of "human behavior." The scope of the present-day psychology lies in using the scientific study of behavior to addresses variety of issues pertaining to the mechanics of behavior. It also prescribes ways and methods by which individuals can effectively face social and personal challenges. However, with increasing research interest in human growth and development and explaining the intricacies of human behaviors in a variety of settings, the quest never seems to be comprehensive. The quest seems to be more perplexed with the modern psychology offering various disciplinary perspectives. Although, the goal of a subject matter is to offer various dimensions of phenomenon, explaining human psyche is complicated.

A student of psychology begins to understand psychology as the science of soul explained by Western Philosophy using philosophical thought, epistemological, metaphysical methods about human nature and behavior (Cycleback,2020). When the methods of physiological investigations were applied to the study of mental phenomena, the subject matter took a leap and began to explain allied basic topics related to physiology such as sensation, perception, memory, and forgetting. Thus, over a period, the history of psychology started denying the concept of soul, altered the approach, to emerge as a separate, primarily scientific, field of study (Schultz and Schultz, 2011, p 2).

This led to growth of various schools of Psychology viz., Psychoanalytic, Adlerian, Behaviorism, Gestalt, and Cognitive and so on. With more emphasis on science, the present-day Western Psychology accepts the physical body the cortical structures as responsible for thinking and other higher order functions. The human psyche is thus explained in terms of a system approach beginning from birth to death. Each aspect of life is explained more in terms of developmental goals individually as well as socially. Thus, any discrepancies or mismatch between the systems leads to incongruence. This leads to problems in human life. Western psychology is still trying to figure out the reasons behind human problems (Osho, 2015). New therapeutic techniques are devised but not even one of them prescribes a comprehensive solution for anxieties, anguishes, fears, paranoia and other mental disturbances. In this perspective, the subject matter continues to evolve and offers a variety of theoretical and pragmatic solutions to human issues. The quest seems to be never ending with issues of human psyche becoming more and more intriguing as it caught in the vicious cycle of problem arising and solutions (Cycleback,

2020). This has led to several mental health issues and a greater number of psychological disorders being added in a human life.

INTELLIGENCE, AND ITS FACETS IN WESTERN PSYCHOLOGY

In the due course of time, in the history of Psychology, there were developments of understanding of human mind functioning in terms of the development of intelligence. Concepts such as meta-cognitive abilities, the "hypercognitive system" (Adey, Csapó, Demetriou, Hautamäki, and Shayer, 2007) were seen as building block of intelligence which led to development of intelligence. One such construct that has gained prominence is the facets of intelligence is "the search for meaning for life" (Emmons, 1999) which is conceptualized in adaptive, cognitive–motivational terms. Zohar (1997) introduced a concept called spiritual intelligence (SI) which is defined as the capacity and problem-solving ability and attain goals in difficulties of everyday lives. Previous works in the concept of Spiritual Intelligence (Emmons (1999, 2000a, b), lay emphasis on theoretical foundations of Spiritual Intelligence leading to models and workable hypothesis. Further research works by Gardner (2000) on Existential Intelligence (ExI), King (2008) on Spiritual Intelligence and Grifths (2017), overlap each other, and are ambiguous in establishing how SI approaches the process for the meaning of life. Grifths (2017) points out that Spiritual Intelligence results when intellectual and emotional intelligence act in the state of presence. The state of presence is further defined as more than simply being aware of your immediate surroundings with greater clarity than usual. Moreover, most of the discussions around the concept of Spiritual Intelligence center around the Intelligence which is defined as adaptive or reactive ability system and are stable. Whereas the "presence" which is involves immediate surroundings are fluid, conditioned by other external forces and exercised as a reaction to these conditioned system. Thus, intelligence is awareness of the existing conditioning system and limits the scope of psyche.

Comparison of Western and Eastern Concept of Spiritual Intelligence

The intelligence (either Existential Intelligence or Spiritual Intelligence) concept proposed by Emmons (1999), Zohar (1997), Gardner (2000) and Grifths (2017) in yet another type of intelligence relies on human capacity to problem-solving ability and attain goals in difficulties of everyday lives and as a search for the meaning of life. The models and hypotheses presented by the Western concept of Spiritual or Existential Intelligence looks human psyche in terms as a reactive organism to external environmental stimuli and ability to perceive clarity of his or her role. However, it has not considered the "psyche" itself is a part of the environment and it cannot be delineated from the system in which it works. Besides, the constructs in Western Psychology takes into consideration the human perception, cognitive, emotional and motivational systems interaction and its dynamics to define the concept. However, Eastern Psychology differs to explain the concept of Spiritual Intelligence.It points out how theses systems are limited in nature and does not offer scope beyond a point towards awareness of Self and rather constricts the panoramic view that human psyche should comprehend.

Eastern Psychology primarily the based-on Taoism, Buddhism, Vedanta and yoga revolves mainly around the philosophical roots and works on individual psyche as a part of comprehensive system of the Universe, connect to nature and improvement towards inner self and growth (Gordon,2015). Eastern Psychology remained within the realm of "Consciousness" (looking inward)to explain human soul and did not advance to explain the concept of mind in which the mental faculties such as sensations, perceptions, thoughts emotions, motivations revolve(Osho, 2015). Thus, Consciousness in Eastern Psychology is the purely awareness of one's existence (Prabhu and Bhat, 2015). The Eastern Psychological approach did not try to understand the problems of the mind, their roots, and the problems arising in the mind. Rather, theapproach is founded on the state of no-mind -- that silence, that purity, that serenity. It detaches itself from the problems, with all its roots and its functions. This is analogous to Mushin no shin, (a Zen expression for state of "no-mindness") (Mukherjee,2019).

The present article has tried to discuss briefly on how human psyche is perceived in Eastern tradition, in particular, in Vedic philosophy. The Vedic scriptures are divided into PrasthānTrayī- Upanishads, the Brahma Sutras, and the Srimad Bhagavad Gita. The Upanishads deal with philosophical knowledge and Brahma Sutras are synopsis of the Upanishads. The former two are difficulty to comprehend, whereas Srimad Bhagavad Gita is very simple and offers a very practical approach to understanding of the concept of Consciousness. Srimad Bhagavad Gita which literally means "Song of God" is a compilation of dialogue between Supreme Bhagwan Shri Krishna and His devotee Arjun, on the verge of the Mahabharat war. Srimad Bhagavad Gita is a 700-verses and a part of the epic Mahabharata divided into eighteen chapters. There are innumerable commentaries written on this scripture. However, the views presented in this chapter are based on the writer's reading of the few commentaries. Hence, the writer humbly submits to the limited understanding of Srimad Bhagavad Gita presented here.

Srimad Bhagavad Gita gives a summary of the Vedic philosophy and is also called as Smritiprasthāna the remembered tradition and foundation of Vedanta. Most of the commentaries on Srimad Bhagavad Gita states that Srimad Bhagavadgita espouses Brahmavidyā (theory), Yogaśāstra(practice) Srīkṛṣṇārjunasaṁvāde (realization).

Brahma-vidya is the science of the Absolute—that system of thinking which is enabled to comprehend within itself at any time the total structure of things. Brahmavidya teaches how to conceive the Absolute by considering the processes of thought, the inner constituents of the object and its relations to other objects. Brahma-vidya is the art and the science of educating oneself in the manner of correctly perceiving the world as such, including one's own self, in the totality of relations, in spite of being a part of the whole. Thus, the theoretical constructs proposed by Srimad Bhagavad Gita looks at the holistic nature of process of thought, its metaphysical aspect and its totality. Thus the psyche is not seen in isolation but as a part of the Universal capaciousness and retains its individuality.

The theoretical aspects of Brahma-vidya when applied is termed as the Yoga Shastra, or also called as the art of living, which is the practical application of the consciousness in our daily life. Based on Yoga sastra, Srimad Bhagavad Gita offers thumb rule suggestions to all human endeavors and sufferings and preaches simple solutions to understanding of the miseries.

SRIMAD BHAGAVAD GITA AND YOGA SASTRA

According to Swami Vireshananda (2023) the eighteen chapters of Srimad Bhagavad Gita explains eighteen schools of Yoga namely (1) Visada yoga (the cause of the origin of sorrow, delusion),(2)Sankhya yoga-annihilation of the cause of grief and delusion, (3) Karma yoga -doing work with a detached state of mind, controlling the senses, (4) Jnana yoga- ideal state of complete detachment and renunciation, (5) Karma Vairagya Yoga about renunciation, (6) Abhyasa yoga adept in meditation,(7) ParamahamsaVijnana yoga -personal realisation or experience, (8)Aksara-Parabrahman yoga- constant practice of contemplation on the Supreme consciousness,(9) Raja-Vidya-Guhya yoga on spiritual practice,(10) Vibhuti-Vistara-Yoga - divine manifestations, (11) Visvarupa-Darsana yogaessence of the whole Gita which is meant for liberation, (12) Bhakti yogathe characteristics of an ideal devotee, (13)Ksetra- KsetranjaVibhaga yoga – explains the whole creation, (14)Gunatraya-Vibhaga yoga transcending the *triguṇas*,sattva, rajas, and tamas, born out of *prakriti*.(15) Purusottama yoga- on how detachment leads to supreme knowledge, (16)Daivasura-Sampada-Vibhaga yoga- the nature of all beings (17)Sraddhatraya-Vibhaga yoga- the importance of developing *sattva* quality and (18)Moksa-Opadesa yoga- attain the state of knowledge through which one finds one's union with God.

From the above passages it may be inferred that all the eighteen chapters explains the whole creation, dynamics of human nature, and ways by which human nature can be transcended to superior creation. It does not attach tags or labels of any ascribed qualities in terms of genetics or racial demography. Rather, the yoga paths describe "human elevation" as a process through knowledge and practice. In addition, the yogic explanations offered in Srimad Bhagavad Gita also quite practical and applicable to human life issues in all spheres.

The purpose of Brahma vidya and Yoga Sastra leads to what is terms as the conversation of the soul with Ultimate Consciousness which is termed as Srīkṛṣṇārjunasaṁvāde or realization. The goal of human life is to transcend the limitations of bodily systems, limitations of the psychodynamics which are conditioned by society and realize the its realisation of the perfection that it has to achieve finally. Thus Srimad Bhagavad Gita give a complete view of what we are, what we have to do and what are its ultimate benefits. The most interesting aspect is that Srimad Bhagavad Gita begins with a conversation with between the human psychewho is in state of misery similar to anyone of us and looks for guidance. Shri Bhagwan Krisna offers the what, how and where does the psyche remains and also how to transcend. Thus the "intelligence" of the psyche remains not only about "quest for the meaning of life" or "being in the state of presence" as earlier discussed in its Western connotation. It is rather transcend life through Brahma Vidya or the knowledge of the psyche and practice of Yoga Sastra or the art of living

Srimad Bhagavad Gita, Its Context, and Its Relevance to Psychology

The context of Srimad Bhagavad Gita can be seen as a perfect setting of human psyche wherein, Arjuna in a state of confusion, seeks guidance from, Lord Krishna of approximately two hours, from a state of suffering of anxiety and depression to the path of enlightenment. The premise of the Srimad Bhagavad Gita is to address Arjuna who is in a distressed mental state as He was facing his own dearly people in a battlefield against him. It must be understood that the context that which Arjuna faces is no lesser to what every human being faces in almost every aspect of life, surrounded by anxieties and delusions.

In Chapter 1.28 Arjuna says "My dear Kṛṣṇa, seeing my friends and relatives present before me in such a fighting spirit, I feel the limbs of my body quivering and my mouth drying up." Arjuna, upon facing his own blood relatives and friends on the battlefield becomes emotional. He was sympathetic towards the warriors of enemies foreseeing their imminent death. His started shivering and his mouth became dry (Bhaktivedanta Swami, 1972). The state of mind of Arjuna is comparable to a state of neurosis (Srimad Bhagavad Gita, Chapter 1, verse 30 and -31) and of emotional suffering with guilt (Chapter 1 verse 35-39). It is pertinent to note that the character of Arjuna was a highly learned person and had spent most of his life with the Supreme (Bhagwan Shree Krishna). If such a learned person himself when faced with such difficult situations in addition to a teacher like Bhagwan Shri Krishna, undergoes anxiety and psychological turbulence, a common man would be much more handicapped to face the difficulties of life in terms of moral decision making. Srimad Bhagavad Gita adopts the teacher-student relationship to address the mental state of the Arjuna and with importance exercise of free-will, state of surrender, and devotion (Angiras, 2020).

The entire Srimad Bhagavad Gita is a compilation in which Shri Krishna explains in detail the cause of suffering, nature and functioning of the mind, the experience of consciousness, and attaining enlightenment. That is why, Srimad Bhagavadgita explains the characteristics and the dynamics of consciousness (that's why it is traditionally as termed *Brahmavidyā or the* knowledge of Brahman), and also the *method* to be adopted to reach the goal as taught in the Gita *(Yogaśāstra*, the scripture of Yoga).

The present paper has tried to understand how Chapter 2 of Srimad Bhagavad Gita views human suffering and miseries experienced in daily life and what should a common or rather should do. Chapter 2 has been chosen for the following reasons. (a) Chapter 2 is often deemed as the summary of the entire Srimad Bhagavad Gita (Markballi, 2013) (b) Chapter 2 explains in detail the causes and reasons for suffering. Probably, it explains how humans suffer and explain the causes and gives a prescription of what a human should strive in life. The conversation between the characters in Chapter is almost straight forward and is directive in nature. (b) The Chapter 2 explains how the concept of "I or Ego" as understood in the Western tradition is different from the concept of "Self" or "Atman". Thus it proceeds from the individual of the "Self" towards the "Universe" or "Supreme Consciousness". Most theories of psychology discuss the term "consciousness" in the context of awareness of internal and external objects (Bajpai, Yadav, and Tripathi, 2019). However, Srimad Bhagavad Gita explains consciousness as that remains which throughout the lifetime and to understand consciousness, "knowledge of the field",or "ksetrajna" is essential. Chapter 2 of Srimad Bhagavad Gita explains how an individual can become "Kshetrajna" (Verse 17).

Based on the verse-by-verse commentators of various authors, the paper has tried to use thematic analysis to understand the second chapter of the Srimad Bhagavad Gita that deals with what is known as Sankhya Yoga.

Several verses in Srimad Bhagavad Gita exemplify human mind and its functioning throughout eighteen chapters in various verses. But the beginning of the conversation between Bhagwan Shri Krishna and Arjuna begins in Chapter 2 in which Arjuna in a pitiable state of anxiety and depression. The Chapter 2 consists of 72 verses and the conversation between Arjuna and Krishna goes on till Verses 1-10 in which Lord Krishna asks Arjuna by questioning. Upon seeing a sad and crying Arjun, Shri Krishna says

Your cowardly behaviour is neither going to take you to heaven nor will bring you fame, and nor is the act of great men. They are not at all befitting a man who is intelligent. They do not lead to higher planets, but to infamy. Therefore, Oh Arjun, don't be a eunuch, give up inertness and get ready for the battle

In Verse 4-6, Arjun says

how can I counterattack with arrows in battle men like Bhīshma and Drona, who are worthy of my worship? It would be better to live in this world by begging than to live at the cost of the lives of great souls who are my teachers. Even though desiring worldly gain, they are superiors. If they are killed, everything we enjoy will be tainted with blood

The difficulty face by Arjuna was due to attachment resulting in an emotional state. As a consequence the mind and the emotional state is not under one's control. The attachment also leads to loss of freewill thereby control of the entire life. Thus the life was indirectly dependent on the emotional state.

In Verse 7-9, Arjun says,

"I am your disciple and am in your refuge. My mind has stopped working. Advise me whatever is in my interest."

CONCEPT OF PURUSHA, PRAKRITI, AND SANKHYA YOGA

It is in the context of answering the dialogue Shri Krishna propounds Chapter 2, Verses 11 to 39 contain the elements of Samkhya yoga. The word Samkhya has been given two meanings. The first meaning is "wisdom of Life". Shri Arjuna is said to have lack of wisdom of life and Shree Krishna in Chapter 2 preachers the art of wisdom of life or Samkhya Yoga.

Samkhya also means as dualistic realism- the realism of two ultimate sources: Prakriti, matter and Purusha, self (spirit). Purusha is the spirit and consciousness, and Prakriti refers to the manifested material world - nature, matter, physical and psychological character, constitution, temper and disposition. Together they create the flow of the universe. While Purusha is eternal, passive, pure and indestructible, Prakriti is dynamic, infinite, causative and active (Jayaram,2019). It has the desire to manifest and it is the primal material behind the universe. It is the first and foremost cause of all the gross and subtle objects in physical form (Meuller, 2021).

In the following pages, an attempt has been made to analyze the verses of in terms of the themes that seem to emerge and how Sankhya Yoga or the dualistic realism is connected and understanding of the connect between the two leads to a state of steady intelligence or "spiritual intelligence.

METHOD

Following Braun & Clarke (2006), and Caulfield (2023) every verse of the Chapter 2 was read thoroughly along with commentaries of various authors and the implicit meaning of the verses were coded in the analysis. Then the semantic and latent themes were identified. This resulted in six themes. The following pages deals in detail with the verses, commentaries, analysis and the emerging themes.

KNOW THY SELF

Every life born strives for eternal happiness. The concept of eternal happiness is synonymous with the concept of self realization (complete realization of one's potential, and the full development of one's abilities and appreciation for life) as proposed by need theories of psychology. He propounds yoga as the pursuit of self-knowledge and knowing who I am (my real nature). Sankya Yoga is explained as a prelude in verses 12(The "self" or the Purusha is the soul is eternal, not the material bodyPrakriti that consists of the 24 elements. Thus the soul does not follow the logic of life after death of the material body).

Table 1. Analysis of the verses and commentaries and analysis of the theme "know thy self"

Verse and Commentary	Analysis	Theme
V12. The "self" is really the soul, not the material body, and is eternal, just as God himself is eternal.	Impermanence of the world	Know Thy Self
V14The human body houses five senses—the senses of sight, smell, taste, touch, and hearing—and these, in contact with their objects of perception, give rise to sensations of happiness and distress both the perceptions of happiness and distress experienced through the senses are transitory. A person of discrimination should practice to tolerate both the feelings of happiness and distress without being disturbed by them.	Sensory perceptions and emotional state nonpermanent appearance of happiness and distress	
Verse 62. While contemplating the objects of the senses, a person develops attachment for them, and from such attachment lust develops, and from lust anger arises.	Interconnect between the emotion- memory and sensual pleasure	
Verse 63. From anger, delusion arises, and from delusion bewilderment of memory. When memory is bewildered, intelligence is lost, and when intelligence is lost, one falls down again into the material pool.	Flimsiness nature of mind	
V15 Rise above these dualities through discrimination. This would result in Infinite happiness. The material happiness that we perceive through the body can never satisfy the divine soul.With this discrimination, we must practice to tolerate the perception of material happiness. Similarly, we must tolerate the sensation of material distress	Sensory perceptions and emotional state nonpermanent appearance of happiness and distress Neutrality of Emotions	
V16. seers of the truth concluded the nonexistent the material body there is no endurance and of the eternal [the soul] there is no change.	nonpermanent appearance of happiness and distress	

Impermanence of the World

In Verse 14, Shri Krishna explains the state and nature of the five senses and how perception forms in connection to sense organs (mātrā-sparśhās). This leads to rise to sensations of happiness and distress (śhītoṣhṇa-sukha-duḥkha-dāḥ). These are transitory (apāyinaḥ and anityāḥnon-permanent). Thus when someone affects by the five senses, they will be swayed between happiness and unhappiness.

Sensory Perceptions and Emotional State

In Verse 62, contemplating the objects of the senses, a person develops attachment for them, and from such attachment lust develops, and from lust anger arises. In continuation, Verse 63, from anger, delusion arises, and from delusion bewilderment of memory. When memory is bewildered, intelligence is lost, and when intelligence is lost, one falls down again into the material pool (dhyāyatoviṣhayānpuṁs aḥsaṅgasteṣhūpajāyate)

Nonpermanent Appearance of Happiness and Distress

Verse 15 explains as to how the material happiness perceive through the body can never satisfy the soul. It also explains how it is pertinent to practice tolerance of material happiness and tolerate the sensation of material distressalike (sama-duḥkha-sukhaṁdhīraṁ). V16 explains how a person seeking the truth focuses on nonexistent of the material body and realizes that there is no cessation of this happiness and distress.(nasatovidyatebhavonabhavovidyatesatah)

Figure 1. The cycle of human psyche

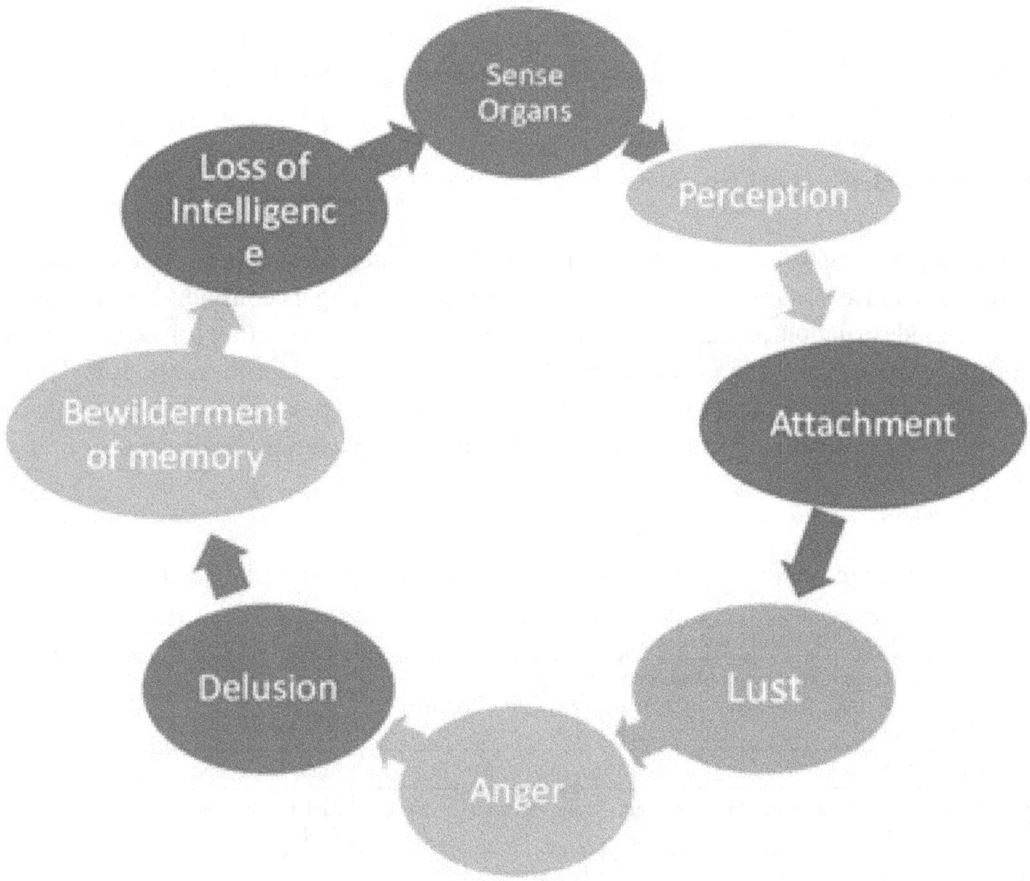

The theme on "Know Thy Self" is based on the Sankhya Philosophy explicitly speaks on the main theme of Chapter 2 which is the concept of Prakriti. It gives a vivid picture in three sub themes that describe (a) Impermanence of the world which is based on the human limitations set by sensory organs, (b) Sensory perceptions and emotional state which are galvanized and distorted through our perceptual processes conditioned by societal norms and instinctive fears and (c) nonpermanent appearance of happiness and distress leads to vicious cycle of sensory fulfillment. Thus the human consciousness charges the mind with an intelligence that peeps through the sense organs and locates objects, the world in front, in a particular juxtaposed manner (Swami Krishnananda, 2023). Thus the knowledge of the basic understanding of our own sensory and perceptual process and how it leads to loss of intelligence should be first considered as the first step towards "Spiritual Intelligence".

CHARACTERISTICS OF SOUL AND BODY

As mentioned earlier, the Chapter 2 of Srimad Bhagavad Gita in detail discusses the nature and components of the body as well as the soul. Verses 13 to 30 explains in the detail the nature of the soul and its connect to body.

Impermanence of Body

Verse 13 explains how the body is constantly changing, in one lifetime itself, from childhood to youth the soul passes through many bodies(kaumāraṁyauvanaṁjarā tathā) and passes into another body at the time of death (tathadehantara-praptir).

Link Between Body and Soul

As the V17, body is made from insentient matter, devoid of consciousness, whereas the soul is sentient, i.e. it possesses consciousness. The soul pervades the body by spreading its consciousness everywhere in it. Thus the soul is indestructible (avināśhi). The soul is neither born nor does it dies (nityasyoktāḥśharīriṇaḥ). It is unborn, eternal, ever-existing and primeval. Hence one is not slain when the the body is slain (anāśhino 'prameyasya) i.e., indestructible. As the soul remains unchanged, it discards its worn-out body and takes birth in a new body elsewhere (Verse 22) (vihāyajīrṇānyanyānisanyātinavānidehī)

Table 2. Analysis of the verses and commentaries and analysis of the theme "characteristics of soul"

Verse and Commentary	Analysis	Theme
V26 soul [or the symptoms of life] is always born and dies forever V 30, he who dwells in the body can never be slain. Therefore you need not grieve for any living being.	immortality of the self, and its distinction from the body.	
V19. The illusion of death is created because we identify ourselves with the body	Link between the body and soul	
V18. The material body of the indestructible, immeasurable and eternal living entity is sure to come to an end	Link between the body and Soul	
V20. The soul is transcendental to material existence. mere intellectual prowess is not enough to comprehend the soul, since the existence and nature of the soul are difficult to grasp.	Soul or the individual consciousness and its connect with the Divine Consciousness	
V22In the same manner, the soul remains unchanged, when it discards its worn-out body and takes birth in a new body elsewhere.		
V23 The soul can never be cut to pieces by any weapon, nor burned by fire, nor moistened by water, nor withered by the wind. Consciousness, which is the symptom of the soul, can be perceived by material instruments, but the soul itself cannot be contacted by any material object. This is so only because the soul is divine, and hence beyond the interactions of material objects. Vs. 24This individual soul is unbreakable and insoluble, and can be neither burned nor dried. He is everlasting, present everywhere, unchangeable, immovable and eternally the same.	The seat of the soul is in Consciousness, its non-connectivity with body	Characteristics of a soul
V25 It is said that the soul is invisible, inconceivable and immutable. Knowing this, you should not grieve for the body.		
V26 soul [or the symptoms of life] is always born and dies forever V 30, he who dwells in the body can never be slain. Therefore you need not grieve for any living being.	immortality of the self, and its distinction from the body.	
V19. The illusion of death is created because we identify ourselves with the body	Link between the body and soul	
V18. The material body of the indestructible, immeasurable and eternal living entity is sure to come to an end	Link between the body and Soul	
27 One who has taken his birth is sure to die, and after death one is sure to take birth again. Therefore, in the unavoidable discharge of your duty, you should not lament. 28. All created beings are unmanifest in their beginning, manifest in their interim state, and unmanifest again when annihilated. So what need is there for lamentation?	Lamentation	

Consciousness, which is the symptom of the soul cannot be contacted by any material object. The soul is transcendental to material existence and cannot be comprehended by intelligence. The nature of the soul are difficult to grasp. It cannot be cut to pieces by any weapon, nor burned by fire, nor moistened by water, nor withered by the wind. (V20, 23 and V24). It is invisible (avikāryaḥ), inconceivable (achintyaḥ) and immutable (avyaktaḥ).

Theme 2 on " Characteristics of Soul and Body" may be seen as an extension of the previous theme that extends to explain how human body which is an amalgamation of the sensory and perceptual organization is not the human life (which is coded as "impermanenece of Body" as the subtheme)should strive for but rather understand the " true Self" (which details the link between the soul and body") This theme exactly rests on the Samkhya Philosophy of dualistic realism.

SCIENCE OF WORK

Having explained the nature of body and soul the verses 38- 48 proposes how does one work amidst the dynamics of body and soul towards eternal happiness. This is explained as a science which is termed as Buddhiyog, or "Yog of the Intellect." The analysis of the verses led to codes such as Detachment from the consequences of action and ways to gain detachment.

Buddhi Yog, or "Yog of the Intellect"

Buddhi yog refers to detaching the mind from the consequences of actions cultivating single-minded focus on the goal which is termed as Yoga.

One should strive without considering the consequences (Verse 38) of the dichotomous results of actions. This would lead to detachment of the consequences of actions. The knowledge to act in such as way leads to discriminative intellect (Verse 39). This would further help to protect from fear.

The further verses also give a direct prescription as how to "practice intelligence". Unlike the other intelligence proposed by earlier theories, Bhagavad Gita rather recommends that intelligence should be practiced and is not a product of genetics or upbringing. By prescribing so, it rather considers the human

Table 3. Analysis of the verses and emergence of the theme "buddhi yog"

Verse and Commentary	Analysis	Theme
38. Fight for the sake of duty, treating alike happiness and distress, loss and gain, victory and defeat.	Detachment with the consequences of actions	**Buddhi yog, or "Yog of the Intellect."**
39. Actions resulting from such knowledge frees from the chains of bondage	detachment comes by practicing discrimination with the intellect.	
40. Such state of consciousness does not lead to adversities or anxieties and releases from great danger.	Ways to gain Intelligence	
48. Yogic state occurs when you are free from attachment to success or failure.	steadfast in yoga	
41. The one who practices such yoga cultivates single-minded focus on the goal	humans control mind with the intellect.	
42.-43 Lesser mortals aim at fruitive activities and desirous of sense gratification 44. In the minds of those resolute determination of devotional service to the Supreme Consciousness does not take place.	Men of lesser intelligent look for desirous of the sensory gratification	

psyche and intelligence as a systems approach and totally undermining the role of individual limitations in terms of physical or psychological metrics. It also allows the individual to liberty to gain intelligence by practice freedom using intellect (Buddhi). The verses clearly explain as to how humans can practice the Buddhi Yog and develop themselves an intelligent person. By ignoring the dichotomies of success and failure and performing one's duty, the individual becomes steadfast and develops evenness in all in actions which is termed as Buddhi Yoga (Verse 48). The life of such individual becomes more focused and they are free from the bewilderment of the sensual pleasures (Verse 41).

Further verses also explains how people get into the vicious cycle of sensuous pleasures leading to either gratification, opulent life, and sense enjoyment which leads to more and more seeking and an endless continuum of gratification (Verse 42-44). When the individual is free from dualities, he would be established in the understanding of "Self"(Verse 45). Then how would an individual perform his actions? Verse 47 clearly prescribes that a spiritually intelligent person should never consider the fruits of his actions nor considers himself as the doer. He needs to practice detachment from his actions which he is entitled to do (Verse 47). This theme which is named as "Budhi Yog" or the "Science of Work" may be considered as the crux of the concept of Spiritual Intelligence. This may also be considered as The Yoga or the practical aspect of living which is detailed in eight verses.

CHARACTERISTICS OF SPIRITUAL INTELLIGENCE

Analytical Knowledge of Sankhya

(i) The analysis of the verses 21, 49 to 53 clearly describes the characteristics of spiritual intelligence. The person develops the analytical knowledge of the immortal (Sankhya) (Verse 21) discards the ego that make him feel as the doer and able to understand that the soul actually does nothing. (ii) He moves away from the sensual pleasure of the materialistic world (Verse 49) to get rid of the benefits of his actions and does not work for Self-enjoyment in terms of either intrinsic or extrinsic motivation. (iii) Rather, he detaches himself for the expectations of rewards and reinforcements and commits towards higher consciousness. His action are devoid of any temporal gratifications and hence does not adversely affect performance (verse 50).

Table 4. Analysis of the verses and commentaries and analysis of the theme "characteristics of spiritual intelligent"

Verse and Commentary	Analysis	Theme
V21. A spiritually elevated soul dispels responsibility of the actions upon oneself and realize that the soul seated within actually does nothing.	the analytical knowledge of the immortal (Sankhya)	**Characteristics of a Spiritual Intelligent**
49. Do not attach to the results of the activities and surrender fully to that consciousness.	Move away from sensual pleasure produced by material energy	
50. A man engaged in devotional service rids himself of both good and bad actions even in this life.	giving up attachment to the fruits does not adversely affect performance	
51- 53. The intelligent free themselves from the karmic cycle (cycle of birth and death) bydetaching themselves from the fruits of action in the material world and attain a state beyond all miseries. They are free of delusions and in such yogic state the mind remains fixed in the trance of self-realization.	State of no suffering	

State of No Suffering

The verses 51 to 53 clearly state how humans can attain a state of no suffering by practicing spiritual intelligence and thereby understanding the delusional worldly attachments and its aftermath. The Spiritually intelligent person would engage in meditating on higher consciousness thereby relieving himself with the continuum of pain and pleasure (verse 51). Spiritually intelligent crosses delusion, and becomes indifferent to all sensations and its aftereffects. Thereby the Spiritually intelligent person remains fixed in the ultimate state of Self realization with the higher consciousness (Verse 53).

Thus, the characteristics of spiritual intelligence is not on mastery of skills but rather on attaining a state of mind that detaches itself from all the illusions and set a resolute determination towards a higher plane of consciousness.

GOALS AND CHALLENGES IN PRACTICING SPIRITUAL INTELLIGENCE

The Chapter 2 of Srimad Bhagavad Gita not only describes and prescribes means of Spiritual intelligence but also explains through 59 -72 the various challenges that a person may find in practicing Spiritual Intelligence but also ways to tackle the challenges to remain in "Steady Intelligence" and thereby attain transcendental consciousness in which the human life can be away from anxieties and sufferings. Probably, this is one of the scriptures in the world that has clearly spell out how any humans at any point of time in their lives can start "practicing steady intelligence" and how by practicing may achieve higher goals in life and that which is not contingent on genetic, racial, or handicaps of any circumstantial advantages. Rather, it is purely a human endeavor to remain "Intelligent".

However, the verses also explains some of the challenges which a person who tries to becomes" Spiritually Intelligence may face in the process. Intelligence is rather a state to be maintained rather some

Table 5. Analysis of the verses and commentaries of the theme "goals and challenges of challenges of spiritual intelligent"

<table>
<tr><th>Verses and Commentary</th><th>Analysis</th><th>Theme</th></tr>
<tr><td>59,68,65,66When the individual restrain from senses, it reaches a state of steady intelligence. However, an undisciplined person, who does not control the mind and senses, can neither have a resolute intellect nor steady mind nor steady intelligence</td><td>Development of attachment leads to lower psychological processes</td><td rowspan="8">Goals and Challenges of Challenges of Spiritual Intelligent</td></tr>
<tr><td>62.While contemplating the objects of the senses, a person develops attachment for them, and from such attachment lust develops, and from lust anger arises</td><td rowspan="2">Cycle of Human Psychological processes</td></tr>
<tr><td>67. When the mind focuses on senses, it carries away a man's intelligence.</td></tr>
<tr><td>69. For such as steadfast intelligent, night and day becomes viceversa for the state of awakening.</td><td>Dichotomy is of no relevance</td></tr>
<tr><td>70. A person who is not disturbed by the incessant flow of desirescan alone achieve peace, and not the man who strives to satisfy such desires</td><td>State of Contentment</td></tr>
<tr><td>60.The power of senses are so strong and impetuous that it can carry away the mind even of the learned man though he is striving to control them.The fickle mind can make even powerful personages to lose their spiritual powers.</td><td></td></tr>
<tr><td>64, 72. The one who has controlled the senses becomes free from attachment and aversion. The practitioner realizes the the Supreme Conscious and is always in a state of happiness</td><td>Road-map to happiness</td></tr>
</table>

that is not attained at one time and remains so. It is neither a quality or personality that is contingent on situational factors. It is rather a state that every human being should strive throughout their lifespan.

Verse 59 clearly states that the senses would act every point of time and human faculties continue to lean towards sensual enjoyment. It is rather a challenge for one who is practicing Spiritual Intelligence. The effort should be towards ceasing such sensual engagements and fixed in consciousness. Verse 60 also explains the nature of the senses as strong and impetuous and it also tests a man of discrimination who is endeavoring to control them. The one who has mastered the art of practicing this detachment from sensual faculties, and the processes that arise out of sensations becomes free from attachments and aversions.

STATE OF SPIRITUAL INTELLIGENCE (*STHITAPRAJÑASAMĀDHI-STHA*)

Probably no theories in psychology explains how the beginning point of sensation could begin the point of suffering and realization of this would lead to development of intelligence that would help the individual to attain a state of no suffering or anxiety. The goal of an "intelligent person" would be to restrain his sensory gratification and fix his consciousness upon "transcendental consciousness" (Verse 61). Verses 66 and 67 states that without transcendental consciousness, there cannot be steady intelligence and any one sensory process can carry away a man's intelligence. Thus he loses his intelligence and therefore require a focused practice on "Divine Consciousness"

The verses further also explain the concept of "Divine Consciousness" which is a state of no misery, a happy state without bewilderment, a state not of a seeker but of fulfillment. Thus "Divine Consciousness "is a state which needs to be attained at every moment and not that an attribute that is ascribed or achieved. The state is steady intelligence and can be practiced at any point of time. Thus for Spiritually Intelligent person "dichotomy is of no relevance"

CONCLUSION

Chapter 2 of Srimad Bhagavad Gita which deals in detail with the Sankya Philosophy discuss the concept of "Sthitaprajñasamādhistha" or "Steady Intellect"as the ultimate "state of intelligence" that which every individual should strive. The "Steady Intelligence" allows to understand existence in terms of objects that are outside our influence and the need to realize the concept of "Absolute". The "Steady Intelligence" also recognizes the total structure as a part of the Universe that exists even in the atomic structure. This

Table 6. Verses, codes, and theme emerged on "sthitaprajñasamādhistha (steady intellect situated in trance)

Verse and Commentary	Analysis	*Theme*
55. When an individual gives up desires and finds satisfaction in the self alone, he is said to be in pure transcendental consciousness.	How to practice Spiritual Intelligence	*Sthitaprajña*(steady intellect) and *Samādhi-stha* (situated in trance)
56-57 and 71 . One who is not disturbed in spite of the threefold miseries, craving for pleasure, free from fear and devoid of anger. is called a sage of steady mind.	Life of an Spiritual Intelligent person	
58. One who is able to withdraw his senses from sense objects, as the tortoise draws his limbs within the shell, is to be understood as truly situated in knowledge.	Goal of Human Life	

is real intelligence which an individual should try to cultivate in his lifetime as a skill to be practiced in all aspects of life. The narratives of the verses cleanly indicate that "steady intellect" is rather a state that can be practiced and sustained throughout one's life. The intelligence proposed by the Srimad Bhagavad Gita is different from the Existential and Spiritual Intelligence prescribed which takes into account all the psychodynamics where as the Intelligence prescribed by the Srimad Bhagavad Gita which state that devoid of the psycho-dynamics results in Steady Intellect. The analysis of the verses explains that (a) knowledge of 24 attributes of Sankhya upon the human creation is built upon (b) how sensory processes leads to further psychological phenomena and leads to anxieties and other delusionary processes (c) characteristics of soul (d) analytical knowledge of the Sankhya which leads to development of Buddhi Yog (d) what a person with steadfast intelligent should strive for and how a person without the insight gets in myriad trap of illness of the body and mind. The chapter 2 also contributes to understanding of "intelligence" is a much more comprehensive manner unlike other theoretical propositions and models proposed by Western psychologist in the context of Spiritual Intelligence. Chapter 2 of Shrimad Bhagavd Gita also provides epistemological foundations as well as prescriptive guidelines for understanding human suffering and reaches a state of "realization" by practicing it in day to day lives.

Sarvam Krishnaparnam

All Glories to Bhagwan Shri Krishna

REFERENCES

Adey, P., Csapó, B., Demetriou, A., Hautamäki, J., & Shayer, M. (2007). Can we be intel-ligent about intelligence? Why education needs the concept of plastic general ability. *Educational Research Review*, *2*(2), 75–97. doi:10.1016/j.edurev.2007.05.001

Aditya, A. (2020). Counselling in an Ancient Hindu text: A case for CBT in the Sri MadSrimad Bhagavad Gita Focusing on Arjuna's Distress. The European Journal of Social &Behavioural Sciences, *XXVIII*, 2301–2218.

Bajpai, P., Yadav, R., & Tripathi, M. (2019). Srimad Bhagavad Gita: A path leading to Consciousness andSelf Realization. *Journal of Emerging Technologies and Innovative Research*, *6*(3), 351–356.

Braun, V., & Clarke, V. (2006). Using thematic analysis in psychology. *Qualitative Research in Psychology*, *3*(2), 77–101. doi:10.1191/1478088706qp063oa

Caulfield, J. (2023). *How to Do Thematic Analysis | Step-by-Step Guide & Examples*. Scribbr. https://www.scribbr.com/methodology/thematic-analysis/

Emmons, R. (2000b). Spirituality and intelligence: Problems and prospects. *The International Journal for the Psychology of Religion*, *10*(1), 57–64. doi:10.1207/S15327582IJPR1001_6

Emmons, R. A. (1999). *The psychology of ultimate concerns*. Guilford Press.

Emmons, R. A. (2000a). Is spirituality an intelligence? Motivation, cognition, and the psychology of ultimate concern. *The International Journal for the Psychology of Religion, 10*(1), 3–26. doi:10.1207/S15327582IJPR1001_2

Jayaram, V. (2019). The Samkhya Yoga of the Bhagavadgita, An Analysis. *Hindu Website.* https://www.hinduwebsite.com/samkhya.asp

King, D. B. (2008). Brighter paths to wellbeing: An integrative model of human intelligence and health. Trent University Centre for Health Studies Showcase 2008, pp. 12–13. King, D. B. (2010). Personal meaning production as a component of spiritual intelligence. *International Journal of Existential Psychology & Psychotherapy, 3*(1), 1–5.

Marballi., G.K (2013). *Journey Through The Srimad Bhagavad Gita - A Modern Commentary With Word-To-Word Sanskrit-English Translation.* Lulu.

Meuller. (2021). *Aspects of Purusha (Consciousness) and Prakriti(Nature).* LinkedIn. .https://www.linkedin.com/pulse/aspects-purusha-consciousness-prakritinature-erica-mueller

Osho International. (2015). *Being Free in an Unfree Society: Different Approaches of Western Psychology and the Eastern Concept of Meditation.* The Concept of No-Mind. https://pragyata.com/the-concept-of-no-mind/

Prabhu, H. R., & Bhat, P. S. (2013). Mind and consciousness in yoga — Vedanta: A comparative analysis with western psychological concepts. *Indian Journal of Psychiatry, 55*(6, Suppl S2), 182–186. doi:10.4103/0019-5545.105524 PMID:23858252

Schultz, P. D., & Schultz, E. (2011). A History of Modern Psychology (10th ed.). Cengage Learning.

Swami Krishnananda. (2023). *The Teachings of the Bhagavadgita.* Swami Krishnananda. https://www.swami-krishnananda.org/bhagavad/bhagavad_pub.html

Swami Vireshananda. (2023) *How Each Chapter of the Bhagavadgita is a Yoga?* Swami Krishnananda. https://advaitaashrama.org/how-each-chapter-of-the-bhagavadgita-is-a-yoga/

Zohar, D., & Marshall, I. (2000). *SQ: Spiritual intelligence, the ultimate intelligence.* Bloomsbury Publishing.

Chapter 13
The Concept of Mindfulness:
Perspectives From Major Religions Practiced in India

Ayush Gupta
Indian Institute of Management, Bodhgaya, India

Cheena Agrawal
Indian Institute of Management, Bodhgaya, India

ABSTRACT

This chapter will give the reader a broad overview of mindfulness through the lens of various religions which are practiced in India. Religion provides a framework for their beliefs, customs, and social behavior. So, this chapter will guide religious people in taking insights from their scriptures about mindfulness and try to implement them in their professional and personal lives to deal with various psychological issues. Additionally, the chapter will serve key managerial position holders in organizations and therapists with extremely religious patients and researchers whose interest lies in the field of Indian Psychology to understand how to help different religious clients with these practices. The authors opted for an integrative literature review approach in order to combine existing secondary data and establish novel views.

INTRODUCTION

India is a country with diverse religions, cultures, and languages. With globalization, urbanization, and technological advancement, there is a series of social changes at an accelerated pace, which has led to a rise in mental health problems (Bhargava et al., 2017).

The Indian population firmly adheres to *karma* (actions) and *dharma* (responsibilities) while displaying deep confidence in superstitions, rituals, and mythology. Additionally, there is a propensity among Indians to attribute the causes of issues to external factors rather than introspecting within oneself. In the Indian cultural context, it has been conventionally understood that the act of vocal expression and overt manifestation of emotions is generally perceived as unfavorable, as it is commonly associated with vulnerability and potential harm to interpersonal connections.

DOI: 10.4018/978-1-6684-9778-4.ch013

Consequently, individuals may encounter difficulty in engaging in the process of emotional inquiry. The phenomenon observed by Indian therapists in their clients during earlier times was called a "cultural defense." In instances of this nature, using mythical narratives or fables facilitates a deep-seated transformation of challenging emotions while in the company of a sympathetic spectator (Bhargava et al., 2017). Therefore, this chapter, via perspectives of religion, explains mindfulness.

According to Clothey's (2007) research, Hinduism is considered the earliest religion to have arisen in India. It is followed by Jainism, Buddhism, Islamism, Sikhism, Christianity, and finally Zoroastrianism. As per the Cambridge Dictionary, mindfulness refers to the deliberate practice of cultivating an attentive awareness of one's physical sensations, mental processes, and emotional states in the immediate present, with the aim of fostering a sense of tranquility. Throughout the composition of the entire chapter, a diverse range of sources has been referenced in order to present readers with a multitude of opinions.

PERSPECTIVES FROM MAJOR RELIGIONS PRACTICED IN INDIA

Perspectives From Hinduism

Hinduism, a religion of Indian origin that comprises the beliefs and practises of Hinduism, is one of the world's earliest religious traditions (Verma, 2009). Hindu is derived from the Sindhu or Indus rivers. Hindu adherents support using the Sanskrit term *Sanatana Dharma* to define their religious practices. *Sanatan Dharma* means "endless custom" or "endless religion" in English. Hindu tradition encourages its adherents to voice spiritual and moral truth wherever it may be discovered. Our experience, our knowledge, and our interactions with others offer numerous opportunities to test our understanding of religion and moral truth. The Hindu scriptures, which are founded on the insights and visions of Hindu sages, serve as a guide for the same. But in the end, we attain the truth through direct awareness of the divine or ultimate reality, which is known as *Brahma* (Verma, 2009). The Hindus believe the *Gitā* to be an essence of the *Upanishads* (texts that form the core of Hindu philosophy), because of which it becomes the basis for our analysis (Panda, 2017). Briefly explaining about the Bhagavad Gita, it is part of Mahabharata, and is included in *Prasthanatreya*, the three foundation of classical Indian thought. The Gita gives a detailed study of the human mind from the point of view of an active living philosophy. The philosophies stated in the Gita are told with respect to Kurukshetra, the battle field. It explains the mental conflict that every human faces between what is right and what is duty. Gita is psychologically important as Krishna's intervention with the potential to change Arjuna gives him a new, long-lasting personality that goes beyond his body and society. (Menon, 2008, p. 163)

Mindfulness

According to the *Gita*, mindfulness is a means of detachment from the assault of the senses in order to achieve *Sthitaprajna* (i.e. a state of calmness). The *Gita* uses a variety of metaphors to describe this state, including "one should be tranquil like an ocean that is unaffected by rivers flowing into it," "one should withdraw from the senses as a tortoise withdraws its limbs," and "one should be like a water drop on a lotus leaf that has no attachment to the leaf." The above mentioned metaphors can be helpful for guiding patients toward mindfulness. *Shri Krishna* advises achieving the "mindful state" through meditation and preserving a calm and tranquil disposition. [See Appendix 1 for shlokas for mindfulness in Hinduism]

Lord Krishna, in the Gita, provides essential insights into the relationship between mindfulness, work and knowledge. According to him work can either bind the person or release the person. Krishna therefore gives two fold discipline for two class of the people "the discipline of knowledge for the Samkhyas and that of work for the Yogins" (3:3). Krishna says that an unintegrated mind dont know about the true nature of the Self and is not fit for meditation. Any attempt to control your senses without also controlling your thoughts can only be called hypocritical.

A mind that is pure is an alert mind. An alert mind is calm and is sensitive to small things. By *abhyasa* (practice) and *vairagya* (detachment) alertness can be gained. *Abhyasa* implies the practicing of evenness of mind and *vairagya* denotes "freedom from desire for covetable experiences in the plane of the seen and the unseen" (Samkarabhdsya, 6:35).

A mind is truly integrated if it is receptive rather than selective. Mind is the only reason for a person's bondage and his release. When a work is done as a sacrifice it will not leave any binding effect "wisdom fire reduces all actions to ashes" (4:37). "Of the man whose attachment is gone, who is liberated, whose mind is established in knowledge, who acts for the sake of sacrifice - his whole action melts away" (4:23). (Menon, 2008, p. 173-174)

Bhagavad-gita contains profound teachings on the significance of controlling one's mind and beliefs. It emphasizes that if we cannot control the garbage in our minds, it will manifest in our lives as uncontrollable refuse.

According to the *Bhagavad-gita*, our contemplation can progressively lead us down a path of infatuation, obsession, and delusion, resulting in degradation and destruction in the end. The comparison of the mind to ice for truth and fire for falsehoods highlights the need for spiritualized intelligence to overcome self-destructive desires. Everything enters our lives through the mind, making it crucial to reshape and elevate our thinking.

By being aware of our mental state, we can determine when it is in order, borderline, or out of order. Instead of permitting our mind to become our enemy, the *Bhagavad-gita* urges us to cultivate a relationship with it. It urges us to honor both our dark and light aspects, restraining the negative and cultivating the positive. In many ways, the media reflects the qualities of the mind, which are multiplied, amplified, and magnetized. (Charan, 2020)

Consciousness and Identity

According to the Gita the Self is pure awareness. The Self is only one and eternal as described by the verse, "Just as in this body the embodied (self) passes into childhood and youth and old age, so does He pass into another body..." (2:13). The Self "is not born, nor does it ever die, after having been, it again ceases not to be; nor the reverse. Unborn, eternal, unchangeable and primeval, it is not slain when the body is slain" (2:20).This verse says that the Self is not subject to any of the six changes of conditions, or vikara, that all things in the world are. The birth and death for the imperishable can be understood as "Just as a man casts off worn-out clothes and puts on new ones, so too the embodied (Self) casts off worn-out bodies and enters others which are new" (2:22). (Menon, 2008, p. 165-167)

All our experiences have two kinds of cognition 'cognition of the real and the unreal'. "The real is whose cognition is immutable and the unreal is whose cognition is mutable'' {Samkarabhasya 2:16). Real will always be existent and non real will never be existent. Krishna describes imperishable as *avinasi* and *nitya*. The eternality of consciousness is hence not misunderstood "to be like that of clay or other material objects" (Samkarabhasya, 2:18). "*Moksa* consists in the realization of the immutability of one's own Inner Self {Samkarabhasya, 18:55) (Menon, 2008, p. 167)

Conflict and Wisdom

In the Gita, Krishna places various alternatives before Arjuna and describes the full implication of each alternative, but never gives a conclusive answer. Heidegger compares an open mind to a meditative mind. He stipulates that conclusive thinking which is centered upon an answer, "... constructs a world of objects, understands these objects; but meditative thinking begins with awareness of the field within which these objects are.... Meditative thinking is thinking which is open to its content, open to what is given" (Heidegger, 1966, p. 24). Reflecting the Gita view he adds (p. 25), "...releasement involves openness. (Menon, 2008, p. 168-169)

Mindfulness and Yoga

According to the translation of Sir Edwin Arnold, Mindfulness Practice as per *Gita*: Chapter 6.11-6.19, when a person has learned to eat, sleep, and act in a balanced way, yoga becomes a way to get rid of pain. Research has shown that this is true. Yoga as well as mindfulness both are being used more and more in hospitals and offices to help people deal with pain. When your mind is on one thing, you can say no to distractions and pressures. It's like a lamb that is protected from the wind and stays lit without flickering. At this point, the mind goes beyond itself and reaches a higher state of awareness. There are a lot of similarities within the *Bhagavad Gita* and the Stoics' ideas. Both said that the mind is more important than the body. (Paul, 2015)

Yoga helped Mr. Vernon Kenny to get rid of smoking and alcohol within six months. The story of Vernon Kenny is:

Despite language barriers, he accompanied his wife in a yoga class in the United Kingdom despite his initial reluctance. Yoga altered his lifestyle of daily drinking and excessive smoking. Within six months, he gave up both vices and became happier and more compassionate as a result. His relationship with his wife improved, their disputes ceased, and he discovered solace in yoga's capacity to satisfy his need for happiness. The mental and spiritual space created by physical relaxation during practice taught him that enduring happiness could not be found externally. He now practices daily yoga, meditates, attends courses, and teaches. If embraced with an open mind, he believes yoga has transformative potential, despite not being universal.

In addition to Vernon, yoga helped a lot of other people get their lives back on track or saved them. Examples include Emily, a 17-year-old who had anorexia, she learned to have a better relationship with her body through yoga. Yoga assisted Che Marville, 45, in overcoming her condition and helped her fall asleep at night.

Perspectives From Jainism

Jainism originated centuries before Buddhism in Northern India. Jainas are the disciples of the conquering 'Jinas'. They are followers of certain great ascetics who attained omniscience and who propagate a doctrine said to have promised them the supramundane bliss of eternal salvation from the agony of metapsychosis. (Von Glasenapp, 1999) According to Jaina Psychology, the *jiva* (self), a living and aware being, is at the heart of Jaina psychology. Jaina Psychology is an attempt to present a psychological perspective from the exhaustive study of Jainist religious writings (Diggory,1959). As a whole, an organism is made up of two parts: *jiva* and *pudgal* (matter), also called mind and body. Both of the things are different in different ways. *Jiva* is an aware entity with subjective qualities like knowing and feeling. Body, or matter, on the other hand, is an insentient entity with sensory qualities like touch, smell, and taste. (Jain, 2008, p.55)

Jainism and Mindfulness

Mindfulness is an inherent capacity of the soul, which is endowed with *caitanya, sukha,* and *vrya* (infinite consciousness, bliss, and vigor), according to Jain doctrine. Since the mind works in tandem with the soul, it has also been affected in the same fashion, according to Jain principles. Thus, when humans strive for mindfulness, they attempt to connect their minds with the innate nature of their souls — the conscious essence that is the source of power and pleasure — thus harmonizing the mind and soul towards honorable living. (Jain, 2020)

Upayoga (Consciousness and Conscious Attentiveness)

Although several characteristics, such as existence, substantiality or functionality, changeability, knowability, etc., are shared by jiva with physical objects or matter, consciousness is the distinguishing feature that differentiates jiva or soul from inanimate, inanimate matter.

Conscious entity is described as *svaparaprakasham* (Kundakunda, Niyamsar, verse 161) or *svaparavabhaskam* (Samantabhadra, Svayambhu Stotra, verse 63) in religious texts. It refers to something that illuminates itself and other objects. Consciousness can therefore be defined as awareness of oneself and awareness of the objects in the universe. (Jagdish prasad Jain). *Samyag-critra* (right conduct), accompanied by vows such as *ahis* (nonviolence), leads to the essential inner peace for attaining mindfulness. (Jain, 2008, p. 57)

Jaina Concept of Self

When consciousness shows up as the psychic activity of apprehending or understanding, i.e., perceiving and knowing of objects, this is called conscious attentiveness or cognition. When it reacts to things or events based on likes and dislikes, it's called a feeling or emotion. When it leads to action, it's called a will or conation. These three forms of *psychic activity* are recognized as three functions of the psyche by modern psychology. (Jain, 2008, 61-62)

According to Jainism, the *self* is the basic force or force that stays the same behind *psychic events* that happen at different times (Jain, 2005a, pp. 19-52; Jain, 2005b, pp. 1-67). However, in Buddhism and Hume, the concept of self varies. According to them consciousness is made up of only single impressions, thoughts, or experiences and "the bundle of perceptions''.

Some characteristics of *jiva*:

- Consists of bio-energies or external manifestations of life
- Endowed with consciousness
- *Upayoga* is a feature of *jiva* which distinguishes living from non-living

- Lord or architect of his own destiny
- *Karta* (active agent) meaning being responsible for all his actions

Jaina Concept of Mind

According to Jainism, the mind coordinates the work of all the senses which is experienced by the body. It is not similar to consciousness. The function of the brain is not limited to only a particular field. The distinction of mind is made as psychic mind and physical mind. Psychic mind signifies structural and mental aspects while physical mind signifies structural and material aspect. As the psychic attention changes with it the location of the psychic mind changes in the body and according to modern psychology the physical mind is our brain and nervous system.(Jain, 2008, p.66)

The mind acts as a vehicle or tool for carrying out or putting into action the decisions of consciousness, such as the intention to act, the preparation for act, and the act itself. There are three types of acts: ones that you do yourself, ones that you convince others to do, and ones that you approve of that others have done. This kind of mental activity is done buddhi-purvaka, which means with conscious awareness and a sense of responsibility. This is different from mental functions done abuddhi-purvak, which means without conscious attention, such as when driven by instinctive urges, drives, or propensions. (Jain,2008, p. 67-68)

Dhyana (Meditation)

Dhyana is the process of focusing the mind on a single subject without allowing it to wander. If our concentration is motivated by intense passion or negative emotions such as attachment, aversion, hostility, or enmity, it is wrong, impure, and unworthy of us. If, on the other hand, our concentration stems from positive emotions, the pursuit of the truth, and a detachment from worldly concerns, then it is right, noble, and beneficial for us. This type of meditation promotes spiritual development and liberation. (Jainism: Know It, Understand It & Internalize It: Yoga and Meditation in Jainism)

Perspectives From Buddhism

Buddhism, a form of Eastern spirituality, is part of the shared human heritage of wisdom that has helped people get through this world and find a way to live forever without dying (Conze,2012) . The philosophy of Buddhism can be described as “dialectical pragmatism” with “psychological turn”. They believe that suffering is the basic essence of life. According to them we can judge the quality of thought by knowing what we can do with that thought and the quality of life which is the result of the thought.To have control of our mental processes Buddhist prefers meditation, which is the chief means of salvation in Buddhism.

Buddhist Psychology has evolved over 2500 years of duration because of some of the Asian minds (Komito et al., 1987). The fundamentals of Buddhist psychology are based on three terms: *citta* (thought), *mano* (mind) and *vinnana* (consciousness). The *Brahmajala-suttanta* says that one of the most important things about *citta* is that it helped create many of the *adhivutti-pada* (metaphysical views). Mind is called faculties, faculties are very important because they give us a way to keep our thoughts from wandering too far from the things we can see and touch. The moral life of a person is based on the nature of the human mind. The fact that the mind is at the centre of all the senses shows how important it is to Buddha’s theory of mind. Consciousness is an important part of personality. Human personality is analysed into five factors - material form, feeling, perception, disposition and consciousness. These five factors work together. Function of consciousness is as memory and it can even bring back information from past existence. (Kalupahana, 2008, p.73)

Mindfulness

In *Pāli*, *sati* means Mindfulness. Not only does the phrase "attention" refer to paying attention, but it also refers to memory and remembering things. The cultivation of present-centered, non-elaborative, and nonjudgmental attention may be only one aspect of what is included in the practice of mindfulness meditation. Additionally, it may include recalling the objectives of the practice based on previous experiences and knowledge. (Kirmayer, 2015)

The *Eightfold Path* is a framework that acts as a guiding principle for the practice of Buddhism. Within this framework, right mindfulness and right concentration are essential components that make up the Eightfold Path. A profound condition of non-reactive self-consciousness, which enables an individual to acquire conscious presence and emancipation from the afflictions caused by self-centeredness, is the defining characteristic of the idea of right mindfulness. Right Concentration is a term that is usually used to refer to the act of meditating with the intention of achieving enlightenment through its practice. Though different Buddhist sects practice mindfulness and meditation in slightly different ways, the end result is the same: detachment from oneself and suffering. (Timbers & Hollenberger, 2022)

According to Theravada vipassana literature, mindfulness is practiced through walking and sitting meditation. Vipassana meditation is also known as Insight meditation as earlier it was said that mindfulness practices lead to a form of insight called prajna (in Sanskrit) (Panna in Pali). Prajna means an immediately felt intuitive insight. Prajna-based knowing is different from knowing through one's senses or through your mind, though mental knowing is involved when you think about it later. In order to practise Prajna, you have to look deeply and mindfully into the core of things in a way that changes you. This is the final goal of meditation in basic Buddhism. For example, a deep understanding of how things change leads to less holding. Mindfulness was practiced and recommended by Buddha and his disciples to control stress and pain (Rao et al., 2008). Roberta A Szekeres and Eleanor H Wertheim in 2014 conducted a study on the post-course outcomes of the residential vipassana meditation courses. It was found that there was reduction in level of stress, increase in wellbeing, self kindness and overall mindfulness.

The verses that supports mindfulness the sacred text of Buddhism are: [See Appendix 2 for verses]

Verse 23, **Samavati Vatthu**

Buddha says, The wise, by constantly cultivating Tranquilly and Insight Development Practise, by being ever mindful and steadfastly endeavouring, realise Nibbana: Nibbana, which is liberated from the bonds of yoga; Nibbana, the Unrivalled! (The Dhammapada: Verses and Stories,n.d.)

Dhammapada Verse 24, **Kumbhaghosakasetthi Vatthu**

Buddha says that if a person is energetic, mindful, and pure in thought, word, and deed, and if he does everything with care and consideration, restrains his senses, earns a living in accordance with the Law (Dhamma), and is not careless, then that person's fame and fortune will increase steadily. (The Dhammapada: Verses and Stories,n.d.)

Dhammapada Verse 25, **Culapanthaka Vatthu**

Buddha says, "Let the wise man, through diligence, mindfulness, discipline (with regard to moral precepts), and control of his senses, become an island that no flood can submerge." (The Dhammapada: Verses and Stories,n.d.)

Vinnana (Consciousness)

Vinnana (Consciousness) is an essential component of human personality. In the discourses, the human personality is broken down into five components. They are *rupa* (physical form), *vedana* (emotion), *safina* (perception), *sarikhara* (traits), and *vinnana* (consciousness). *Vinnana* is not only a cognitive process, but it is also responsible for the continuity of the human personality. This is due to the fact that consciousness operates in the wake of *satanusart* (memory) and is capable of retrieving information from previous existences.

According to Buddha, the material form is contingent upon the four great elements, sensation, perception, and disposition are contingent upon *phassa* (contact), but consciousness is contingent upon the entire *nama-rupa* (psychophysical personality).

Consciousness is important because its:

- Relevance to human knowledge - There would be no knowledge or comprehension if the sense faculties and their objects did not direct their respective modes of consciousness. Thus, it is found the six modes of consciousness, including visual, auditory, olfactory, gustatory, tactile, and mental consciousness, corresponding to the six sense organs and the six sense objects.
- Relationship to the survival of the human personality after death - Consciousness is the factor that determines the continuation of the human personality. When continuity is felt not only during a single life term, but also from some previous existences to the present, it is very simple for an unenlightened person to conclude that it is the same consciousness that runs from the past to the present.

According to Buddhist thought conscious awareness arises in two different formulation that are major components of Yogacara model of mind:

- Visual conscious awareness depends upon eye and visible form. (S II73)
- Conscious awareness depends upon karmic functions. (S II2)

Early Buddhist noticed consciousness as continuously arising and flowing. The flow of consciousness will continue and will complete with the end of *samsara* (empirical existence) itself, that is *nirvana* (becoming extinguished). This uninterrupted stream of vijnana was in fact the only aspect of individual existence that was explicitly said to continue from one lifetime to the next.

Consciousness can't happen without the long-lasting *samskaras* (mental dispositions) that support it, like a person's senses, cognitive patterns, and emotional tendencies. But these samskaras didn't come fully formed from Zeus's head. They were made by people, one's karma is made up of the results of all the things he or she has done in the past.

"This body is not yours, nor does it belong to others," the Buddha declared, "it should be seen as [the product of] past karma, generated and fashioned by volition, and something to be felt" (SII64).

Alaya-Vijnana Model of Mind

The Alaya-Vijnana model is described as a systematic approach to solving the Abhidharma problem. It progressively reworked the entire Buddhist model of mind around the issues that had become problematic in *Abhidharma* - the continuities of latent dispositions and karmic potential - and incorporated them into the larger framework and terminology of dharmic analysis.

What was merely implicit in the early *Pali texts* is now made explicit in the *Yogacara texts*: a distinction between discrete, discontinuous modes of cognitive awareness and an underlying continuous sentience.

In the fifth chapter of *Samdhinirmocana Sutra,* a new model which is centered on 'alaya' awareness is found. Also, unlike previous models, it is now thought that all types of vijnana, both alaya and the six "functioning" consciousnesses, happen at the same time.

The Sutra compares this to waves coming up in a stream:

"If the conditions for two or more waves to come up are present, then many waves come up, but the flow of water is neither stopped nor slowed down" (V. 5).

This model adds some important new ideas to Buddhist ideas about the mind and how it works. Now, it's clear that perception is based on construction, which it couldn't be in early Buddhism. Because the contents of perception are now shaped not only by the specific sense faculties that serve them, as they were in early Buddhism, but also by alaya-vijnana, a layer of mental processes that is itself shaped by cognitive schemas that come from past sensory and conceptual experience. Not only do these complicated building processes happen all the time and at the same time, but they also happen mostly unknowingly. (Waldron, 2008, 105-106)

Perspectives From Islamism

Islam is the fastest growing and second largest religion in the world (Strindberg,2011). The Islamic creed is the hallmark of all belief systems inspired by the heavens. It is supported and clarified by the Holy Qur'an, as well as the actions and examples of the Prophet of Allah (Qaradawi,2010).

Muslims' basic beliefs lies in a basic statement: "*La ilaha illa Allah, Muhammadu Rasool Allah*", It means there is no diety except Allah and Muhammed is the messenger of Allah. From this expression of faith in the unity and uniqueness of Allah and the prophethood of Muhammed derive all of Islam's concepts, attitudes, moral values, and rules for human behaviour and interpersonal relationships (Haneef,1999).

Muraqabah (Mindfulness)

Muraqabah in Islamism is referred to as Mindfulness, whose root means "to watch, observe, or regard attentively." It can be observed how closely "mindfulness" and "*muraqabah*" are related linguistically and etymologically. The precise definition of this spiritual concept is "the constant knowledge of the servant and conviction in the supervision of the Truth, glory be to Him, over one's outward and inward states."

In other words, a Muslim who is in the state of *muraqabah* is always conscious of Allah's internal and outward protection. It's a state of being fully conscious of one's emotional, intellectual, and physical connections to Allah. The concept of *muraqabah* rests on the idea that Allah is ever-present. (Parott, 2017).

According to *Surah An-Nahl*, Verse 108:

Those are the ones over whose hearts and hearing and vision Allah has sealed, and it is those who are the heedless

The above verse teaches us that although Allah urges us to watch, think critically, and extend our perspectives, some of His creations will develop the predisposition to observe their own desires rather than Allah's signs. If such a practice is not stopped, one will completely become consumed by gratifying their own desires, or consumed by themselves. By doing this, one drifts further from surrendering oneself to Allah's Will. Instead of using these resources mindfully to maintain a state of being aware of God and find happiness in this life, people tend to use them for instant gratification rather than spending them on connecting with The Divine. (Quranic, 2022).

When he got distracted and forgot about Allah for a second, the Prophet (SallAllahu Alayhi Wa Sallam) would ask Allah to forgive him. This helped him stay focused and remember Allah.

Al-Aghar al-Muzani narrated that The Messenger of Allah, SallAllahu Alayhi Wa Sallam, said:

Occasionally, a haze envelops my heart, so I seek Allah's forgiveness a hundred times a day

Source: Ṣaḥīḥ Muslim 2702, Grade: *Sahih* [See Appendix 3]

According to Al-Nawawi:

قِيلَ الْمُرَادُ الْفَتَرَاتُ وَالْغَفَلَاتُ عَنِ الذِّكْرِ الَّذِي كَانَ شَأْنُهُ الدَّوَامَ عَلَيْهِ فَإِذَا فَتَرَ عَنْهُ أَوْ غَفَلَ عَدَّ ذَلِكَ ذَنْبًا وَاسْتَغْفَرَ مِنْهُ

According to some, this indicates that the Prophet (SallAllahu Alayhi Wa Sallam), who made remembering Allah a habit, occasionally became distracted from it. He would consider moments of distraction or inattention as sins, and he would ask for pardon.

Source: Sharḥ al-Nawawī 'alá Ṣaḥīḥ Muslim 2702

While practicing mindfulness meditation, a person might employ similar Sunnah expressions like the name of Allah or a supplication to bring one's focus back to Allah as soon as one becomes aware of one's mind restlessness. Because over time, one's mind will start to link these words with the experience of mindfulness, this is referred to as anchoring one's mindfulness.

Ibn al-Qayyim compared the wandering ideas to pedestrians who, if ignored, will ultimately move on: [See Appendix 4]

Understand that transient thoughts are harmless. These are hazardous if these are sought for and used. Because if you don't pay attention to a notion, it will pass you by and move on.

Source: al-Jawāb al-Kāfī 1/157

The above-mentioned realization is referred to as cognitive defusion by psychologists, is that one's thoughts do not define one and one should not associate oneself with them. Naturally, thoughts come to mind. Sometimes they are inspired by *Satan* (angels), while other times they come from the depths of the *nafs* (ego).

Based on this realization, mindfulness meditation teaches one to maintain a mental distance from one's thoughts so that one may more easily see them and regulate one's response to them. This is referred to as finding the reaction space. One can explore an idea on one's own terms if it is useful. One can block out negative thoughts by bringing one's focus back to Allah through anchoring. Being able to use the reaction space is a gift from Allah, while being unable to use it gives Satan the upper hand.

Anas ibn Malik, RadhiAllahu Anhu, narrated that The Prophet, SallAllahu Alayhi Wa Sallam, said: [See Appendix 5]

"Allah possesses deliberateness, while Satan possesses recklessness."

Source: al-Sunan al-Kubrá 18651, Grade: *Hasan*

Ta'anni (Deliberation) refers to being cautious and taking your time to react. *Ajalah* (recklessness) is the Arabic word for a hasty, impulsive reaction. By practicing mindfulness meditation, one may train oneself to be aware of one's thoughts, which will allow one to widen the reaction gap and, as a result, exercise the proper amount of thought before action. It will stop one from reacting violently to intense emotions like rage or grief. (Ahmed, 2020)

Perspectives From Sikhism

Sikhism derives from Guru Nanak, the first guru or teacher believed to have been divinely inspired (Singh, 2004). Sikhism is the largest religion in India and the fifth largest religion worldwide (Singh and Smith, 2007). Its adherents are known as "Sikhs". The fundamental principle of Sikhism is '*Ikk oan kar sat nam'* - 'There is only one being and truth is his name'. Sikhs believe in the divine one, the greatest ultimate reality that created and sustains the universe. The Supreme Ultimate Reality, according to Sikhs, cannot be seen or formed in a statue; it can assume any space, form, time, or gender. As a result, the Sikh ideal includes people of various races, religions, and cultural backgrounds (Singh,2004).

Sikhism and Meditation

The primary objective of Sikh meditation is to move beyond the ego. This is done by gradually realising and accepting the holiness of oneself and, by extension, the sacredness of Existence. This union is felt as a connected, nondual, sovereign, sacred Oneness.

Simran (Mindfulness)

Man jeetai jag jeet

(Conquer your mind and Conquer the world)

This saying is one of Guru Nanak dev ji's most well-known and frequently repeated passages from Gurbani. It is pointing in the direction of overcoming the physical world. From a Sikh perspective, mastering the mind entails mastering *Haumai* (Ego).

In Sikhism, egoism, also known as *Hankar, or Haumai*, is a notion. Guru Nanak Dev Ji described this idea as the root of the five evils of lust, covetousness, wrath, pride, and attachment. The teachings of the Sikh Guru claim that *Haumai* is what turns a person into a *manmukh* and causes them to experience infinite cycles of reincarnation. They claim that in order to gain God's grace, one must reject *Haumai*, transform into a *gurmukh*, and walk in the footsteps of the Guru. According to Sikhism, the only ways to defeat the *Haumai* are through *Simran, Sewa,* and *Naam* meditation.

Nām Japna, Kirat Karo, and *Vand Chhako*

Naam Japo, alongside *Kirat Karo* and *Vand Chhako,* is one of the three pillars of Sikhism. Meditation is given significant weight in the Guru Granth Sahib as the means by which humans can overcome the Five Evils or Five Thieves (ego, avarice, attachment, wrath, and lust) and achieve mental peace and tranquility. *Naam Simran* and *Naam Jaap* are both practices among Sikhs. However, this is not a literal definition of these phrases.

Nām Japna requires remembering God or the *Akal Purkh*, the greatest formless power that has always existed and will always exist, by repeating and focusing on one of God's many names or qualities. When someone is initiated into the Sikh faith, they are typically given the *Mul Mantar*, a particular appellation or phrase repeated throughout the Guru Granth Sahib. In addition to the 950 names of God, the *Jaap Sahib* of Guru Gobind Singh includes numerous other names. In Guru Gobind Singh's *Rehat Maryada*, *Naam Simran* is mandated as a daily discipline for Sikhs. (Naam Japo, 2023).

Kirat Karo means to provide for oneself and loved ones and the community via the use of an individual's God-given abilities, skills, talents, and hard work. This means putting in effort till your forehead sweats, keeping your head down, and not wasting your life. (Kirat Karo, 2022).

Vand Chhako represents communal consumption and resource sharing. This could include wealth, sustenance, etc. Additionally, the term refers to sharing one's prosperity with others in the community, donating to charity, distributing in a Langar, and assisting those in need within the community. A Sikh is expected to give a portion of their fortune or income to those in need or to a worthy cause. (Vand Chhako, 2021).

If one is ignorant of the mind, then one is ignorant of meditation.

It is crucial to understand meditation in the perspective of Sikh philosophy's views on the mind, awareness, consciousness, ego, and egolessness. The term "mind" refers to the faculty within an individual that consists of *man* (cognition), *buddh/bodhi* (discrimination/intellect), *chit* (memory/intention), and ahamkara (I am-ness), which is the dynamic and ongoing activity of the ego. The source of all existence and the constant observer of all phenomena is consciousness. (Panesar, 2017) (Jas, 2022).

In meditation, if you lift your eyes to the spot between your eyebrows, also called the tenth gate, while you are in a deep state of relaxation and calmness, you will finally become fully aware of the highest part of yourself.

According to the Guru Granth Sahib,

"The Yogi draws the breath upwards and opens the Tenth Gate" (SGGS p905)

"In the Tenth Gate, the Primal Lord, the unknowable and infinite, resides; the unseen Lord reveals Himself" (SGGS p1033)

By being receptive to emotion and empathy in addition to thought, you will develop intuition, the defining characteristic of superconsciousness.

"Those who utter and hear the Name of the Lord find peace. Those who believe in it acquire the greatest treasure. (SGGS p798)

Guru Arjan Dev reminds us,

"Those who listen with their mind and ears to the Lord's meditative remembrance, O mortal, are blessed with peace at the Lord's Gate." (SGGS p200).

Therefore, if you want serenity in this life and the next, you must eliminate the randomness in your mind and replace it with love for God's name — listen to the advice of wiser people!

As Guru Nanak states in Japji sahib,

"Within the mind are gems, jewels, and rubies, if you listen to the Guru's Teachings even once" (SGGS p2), we must learn to listen to the deep voice within our "inner" mind. (All About Sikhs, 2017)

Similarity Between Religions (Islamism and Hinduism) with *Naam* (Sikhism)

Dr. Mcleod has attempted, on the one hand, to find a hint of sacrifice in Japuji, and, on the other, he has considered *Zikr, Muraqbat, Fana,* and *Bakaw* as alternatives to *Naam Simran*, recognizing that the concept of *Naam simran* is of Islamic origin. This form of unbalanced observation cannot be accepted as a 'perspective' because these Islamic practices cannot be accepted as a substitute for *Naam simran*.

The results indicate that the similarity of means cannot be acknowledged. It is widely accepted that *Naam* derives from Sanskrit 'Name' in the context of dictionary definitions. Its significance is described as gravitating toward its meaning. The Rig Veda describes *Naam* as form, actuality, and truth. *Naam* is described as a concealed form, concealed truth, concealed power, or fundamental nature in the Atharva Veda. According to the *Chandogya Upanishad, Naam* is the Name or Reality of Brahm. In other contexts, the concealed Name of God *'Sat'* is referred to as *Sat*. It has been stated that *Naam* is the basis of all visible phenomena in the universe. Guru Arjan Dev explains in Gurbani that *Naam* is the one and only Truth, and that this Truth is the focal point of spiritual pursuit (All About Sikhs, 2017).

Perspectives From Christianity

According to the Christian religion, it is possible to attain eternal life in the midst of time through the power of God's grace. There is no moral or social panacea for preserving or enhancing objects. Christianity cannot be limited to Jesus Christ's ideologies and teachings alone; his disciple's teachings must also be considered.(Harnack, 2006)

Mindfulness and God

From the beginning Christian tradition has something similar to mindfulness that is 'silent prayer' or 'contemplative prayer', 'the desert tradition' or 'mystical theology'. It is being practiced today as well.

Mindfulness in Gospels:
The Parable: 'Waking up'

When he came to senses, he said: 'How many of my father's hired servant have food to spare, and here I am starving to death!' (Luke 15.17 NIV)

The reader is familiar with the story, for them it is very obvious to them that what is happening to the extravagant, he on his way would have to think about travel, lodging, and how he will spend money on various entertainments. His brain was working effectively on the journey, but in reality, he was sleep-walking without being aware of what he was doing or where he would inevitably end up. Similarly, as in the story of the prodigal, we are often unaware of what we are doing at the moment and are lost in the thoughts of the future or past.

At every moment we are partly awake - partly aware. To know God and his will for us it is very important to know who we are, where we are and what we are doing. We could answer this only when we spent time practicing waking up. And this is what mindfulness practices do for us. (Stead, 2017)

For christians, their knowledge that God is present with them enhances their awareness of the present moment. Just like prayer, worship, Bible study, meditation is a biblical practice to connect to god. Being close to God brings peace to mind, heart and soul. According to the christian tradition, God is a thing that is always there, cares about everything, and helps people who are suffering. In Christian practices, this might mean sitting with and accepting God's mystery and the fact that we don't know everything about him (via negativa). Sometimes, this practice is meant to help people think about certain facts about God (via positiva). (Timbers & Hollenberger, 2022) (Grace, 2020) Christians believe that creating stillness, silence and solitude before God helps to remove distractions, allowing them to concentrate on God and commune with them. According to mindfulness research, spending time alone, in silence and stillness brings peace and calm to our mind and soul.

Verses that support this are:

- *Be still before the Lord and wait patiently for him. ~ Psalm 37:7 ESV*
- But when you pray, go into your room, close the door and pray to your Father, who is unseen. Then your Father, who sees what is done in secret, will reward you. ~ *Matthew 6:6 NIV*
- *But Jesus often withdrew to lonely places and prayed. ~ Luke 5:16 NIV*

In general, mindfulness emphasizes drawing our attention to the present moment by focusing on our sensations or breath and christians believe that God is always present near them and they enjoy the presence of God in the present moment.

Verses that support this are:

- *Surely I am with you always, to the very end of the age. ~ Matthew 28:20 NIV*
- Blessed are those who have learned to acclaim you, who walk in the light of your presence, Lord. They rejoice in your name all day long; they celebrate your righteousness. ~ *Psalm 89:15-16 NIV*
- *Even though I walk through the valley of the shadow of death, I will fear no evil, for you are with me; your rod and your staff, they comfort me. ~ Psalm 23:4 ESV*

While practicing mindfulness a person observes the thought to be aware about what they are thinking without thinking about it and letting go of the thoughts that are affecting them. When Christians become aware that their beliefs are in conflict with the Bible, they replace them with biblical truth. They let go of notions that are in opposition to God's will. In essence, we are concentrating on God, His Word, and what He is doing in the world, while "detaching" ourselves from the things that preoccupy the world.

Verses that support this are:

- *We destroy arguments and every lofty opinion raised against the knowledge of God, and take every thought captive to obey Christ. ~ 2 Corinthians 10:5 ESV*
- Do not conform to the pattern of this world, but be transformed by the renewing of your mind. … Do not think of yourself more highly than you ought, but rather think of yourself with sober judgment. ~ *Romans 12:2-3 NIV*
- *Forget the former things; do not dwell on the past. See, I am doing a new thing! Now it springs up; do you not perceive it? I am making a way in the wilderness and streams in the wasteland. ~ Isaiah 43:18-19 NIV*

The Bible encourages contemplating God, his word, and all he has done for us and the way to it is meditation.

Verses that support this are:

- For God alone, O my soul, wait in silence, for my hope is from him. ~ *Psalm 62:5 ESV*
- *Keep this Book of the Law always on your lips; meditate on it day and night, so that you may be careful to do everything written in it. ~ Joshua 1:8 NIV*
- *Within your temple, O God, we meditate on your unfailing love. ~ Psalm 48:9 NIV*

Perspectives From Zoroastrianism

The term "Zoroastrianism" is derived from *Zoroaster,* the Greek translation of the Persian name *"Zarathushtra"*. Zarathustra is regarded as the religion's founder and prophet who has direct communication with God (Kreyenbroek, 2013). The fundamental sacred text of Zoroastrianism is a collection of five poems called the Granthas. Zarathushtra argued in the Gathas that the single deity *Ahura Mazda* is superior, but that he is in constant pursuit of humanity and the world god created by his dimensions (Iyer, 2009).

Mindfulness

The holy book *Zend Avesta* defines mindfulness on the same lines of the Merriam-Webster definition which says that it is the practice of being fully or acutely aware of one's thoughts, emotions, and experiences. There is no mention of discrimination in the *Gathas* but rather the inclusivity of all human beings. The prophet only distinguished people who chose to follow the path of righteousness and those who chose to be deceitful. As we know, traditionally, the Turanis were enemies of Iran, and there have been several wars between these two countries for millennia. However, in *Yasna 46 verse 12 of the Gatha,* Zarathustra applauds the family of a Turani who chose to follow the path of righteousness.

This concept of togetherness amongst like-minded people, honest people, righteous people is highlighted in the opening lines of the *Airyaman Ishya Prayer Yasna 54 verse 1* which is translated by a professor in Iraq as follows:

"May the much-desired brotherhood come hither for our rejoicing for the men and for the maidens of zarathustra for the fulfillment of va humana."

Professor Tarapur Allah considers *va humana* to mean more than just a good mind; he says the one thing essential for the good mind is all-embracing love, the brotherhood mentioned here refers to the people who choose to follow the path of usher or righteousness.

According to the Merriam-Webster dictionary, another interpretation of mindfulness is that in order to love someone or something, one must be mindful of their needs. A prayer popularly known as the *Yatha Ahu Vairyo* teaches us to help the needy in a mindful manner. That is to say, we give help when the person needs it, not just when it is convenient.

The prophecy is defined as the divine essence in all creations of *Ahura Mazda*. This divine essence is sent down to earth to help us follow the path of *Asha*. Since preachers of zorastrianism share a part of *Ahura Mazda*, they share a bond of togetherness as human beings in the *Yasha Gatha 31 verse 145*, which is that we pray, we revere the prophecies of righteous men and women of all countries. (yazdi, 2022)

The figure below gives the flowchart of how Zoroastrian virtues which help in achieving a state of mindfulness lead to the attainment of positive business outcomes when applied in organizations.

(Bhattacharjee, 2021) According to Zarathustra, *Vohu Manah (*Good-Mind) is fundamental to the nurturing of virtues in an individual who can be a divine instrument of the creator *Ahura Mazda* for maintaining harmony in the overall Universal existence. Zarathustra preaches the importance of *Vohu Manah* for the nurturing of a spirit of benevolence in an individual which contributes towards the overall social and cosmic development towards the ideal state of existence which is termed as *Asha* as against *Daruj* which is a state of utmost confusion and frustrations. The Middle Persian version of the term, as evidenced in the Pahlavi script literature of the Zoroastrian tradition, is represented by the characters

Figure 1. The framework for Zoroastrian ethics in business

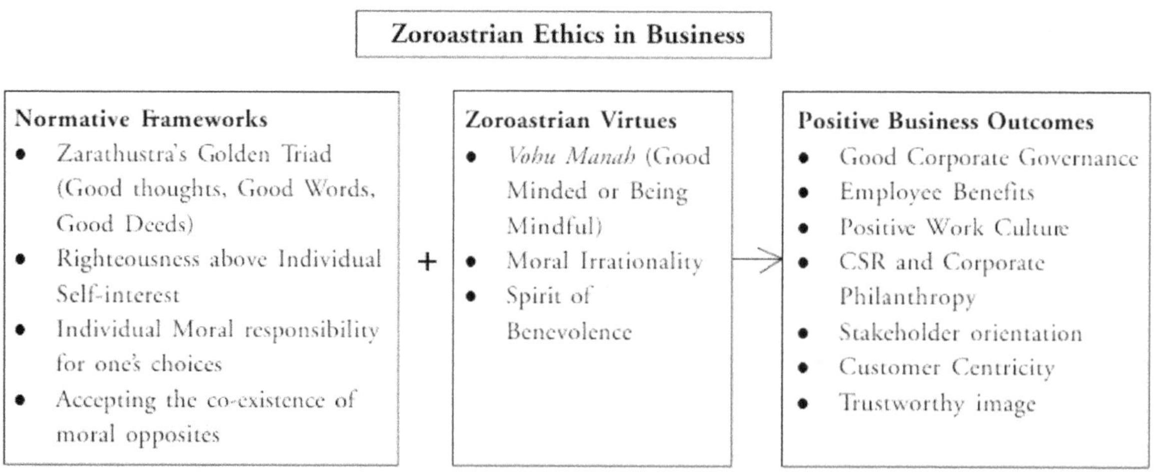

□□□□□ Wahman. This Middle Persian term is borrowed from the Avestan language expression and retains the same semantic significance. Furthermore, this term persists in the New Persian language as بهمن Bahman and its other forms. The term "Manah" exhibits a linguistic resemblance to the Sanskrit term "Manas," implying a potential shared conceptual framework between the Gathas and the Rigveda. The antithesis of Vohu Manah is akem manah, also known as Aka Manah, which denotes a malevolent intent or malevolent cognition.

Similarity Between Zoroastrianism and Hinduism

Tr*zetna's tr*anslation now in a similar vein the hindu greeting namaste has been commonly translated as we bow to each other, the spiritual interpretation of this is the divinity within me recognizes the divinity within you, it's a beautiful sentiment when you when you say namaste to each other. When the pandemic first hit during COVID-19, it brought out a remarkable degree of cooperation on all of us neighbor helping neighbor communities lending a helping hand to each other.

The Ma*nthra of Ahunavar,* also known as the Y*atha Ahu Vairyo,* is the primordial sound of Reality that transcends time and space. What the OM is to Hindus and Buddhists, the Ahunavar is to Zoroastrians: a means of concentrating and arousing forces that already exist within the human psyche. When spoken with feeling and concentration, the Manthra induces subtle vibrations that influence the body's various psychic centers or chakras.

Similarity Between Zoroastrianism and Buddhism

Dhammapada Verse 24, **Kumbhaghosakasetthi Vatthu** [See Appendix 2]

Buddha says, If a person is energetic, mindful, pure in his thought, word and deed, and if he does everything with care and consideration, restrains his senses, earns his living according to the Law (Dhamma) and is not unheedful, then, the fame and fortune of that mindful person steadily increase.

Professor Tarapur Allah considers *va humana* to mean more than just a good mind; he says the one thing essential for the good mind is all-embracing love, the brotherhood mentioned here refers to the people who choose to follow the path of usher or righteousness.

CONCLUSION

After extensive study of different religions, it becomes clear that their methods may be different, but their main goal is very similar. Most religions try to find inner peace, enlightenment, or a deeper connection with the divine as their final goal. Mindfulness also has a place in all of these beliefs because it stresses how important it is to be fully present and aware in the moment. Even though different faiths use different methods and rituals, they all have the same goal: to help people become more focused and attentive. Recognising this basic similarity can help people from different faith groups understand and appreciate each other better. This can lead to more harmony and unity in the beautiful tapestry of human spirituality.

Religions agree on the value of meditation as a way to achieve awareness, which is another thing they have in common. Even though each faith has its own rituals and practices, most of them recommend meditation as a powerful way to become more aware. By practicing different kinds of meditation, people learn to calm their minds, focus their attention, and reach a higher level of awareness. Also, righteous behavior or righteousness is often emphasized as a way to get to awareness. Religions emphasize the significance of living an ethical and moral life because it lays the foundation for the transformational journey towards mindfulness.So, meditation and doing the right thing are important parts that help followers get to awareness, which is the same goal for everyone.

IMPLICATIONS

This chapter will have several implications for the people working in different fields like psychologists, managers, organization and religious leaders.

Therapist - A therapist with expertise in addressing mental, emotional, or behavioral illnesses can utilize the strategies outlined in this chapter to effectively persuade patients to pursue treatment. Additionally, they can incorporate therapeutic approaches and techniques derived from religious texts to facilitate the healing process for these disorders. Various western psychotherapies have been practised throughout the world since their inception, but the therapies that developed in the South Asian region, known as eastern approaches to psychotherapy, are distinct and incorporate various parts of religion. Eastern approaches are primarily concerned with overall well-being and self-awareness. These practises, which will include practises from several religions, may assist therapists in better addressing the issue. For example Dharma therapy, a Buddhist counseling approach which is very effective in helping individuals dealing with psychological issues and was used to help Mr. Chan with anxiety and panic disorder. He was able to significantly reduce his pain as a result of his parent's passing with the aid of Dharma Therapy. (Hung, 2021)

The principles of Jainism can provide a valuable perspective for the treatment of neurological conditions. Mindfulness meditation is consistent with the Jainist principles of nonviolence, nonattachment, and self-control, which are emphasised in Jainism (Upadhyay,2023). Research demonstrates that mindfulness meditation can be an effective treatment for neurological disorders such as anxiety, depression, and chronic pain. The mindfulness-based stress reduction (MBSR) reduced anxiety and depression symptoms in patients with multiple sclerosis, as well as enhanced the quality of life in patients with Parkinson's disease (Goldin,2010). In continuation to the above research in Jainism, there has been research in Christianity as well. (Trammel, 2018) The Mindfulness Awareness Assessment Scale (MAAS) and the Perceived Stress Scale (PSS) can be used to measure how Christian frameworks for mindfulness based therapies can improve awareness states and decrease perceived stress. The study also backs the use of a therapy called "mindfulness," which is heavily affected by Christian spiritual practices. Using a Christian framework for mindfulness based treatments in clinical settings can be helpful, just like using a secular or Buddhist framework for mindfulness-based interventions can be helpful.

Organization or Institutions - Institutions, such as corporations in their entirety, often adopt basic values that draw inspiration from religious beliefs. For instance, Patanjali, an organization, aligns its vision and mission with the provision of ayurvedic products, which are derived from the principles of Hinduism. These firms have the potential to apply this knowledge in their routine activities or perhaps to enhance their market dominance. Institutions like non-governmental organizations for example Sir Dorabji Tata Trust, which was a well-known trust that has been established since 1932 by Dorabji Tata, who was a true zoroastrian believer has inculcated the mindfulness practices in the trust in the form of righteousness that celebrates togetherness. Hence, the money was intended to be utilised "without regard to place, nationality, or religion" for things like helping those in need, funding scientific endeavours, and expanding knowledge. His collection of paintings, sculptures, and other works of art were some of the things he gave to the Prince of Wales Museum in Mumbai. An educational institution also has been formed on the principles of Sir Dorabji Tata Trust which is Tata Institute of Social Sciences (TISS). (Tata Trusts, 2023).

Managerial implication - Managers can utilize the knowledge obtained from this chapter to gain a comprehensive understanding of the concept of mindfulness as interpreted by many religious traditions, and subsequently apply this understanding to support employees in a manner that aligns with their respective cultural backgrounds. According to a study conducted by IBR, the recognition of religious diversity by supervisors and managers has been found to result in a noteworthy enhancement in employee well-being and job satisfaction. Organizational leaders after reading through the chapter will better be able to understand the concept of mindfulness through various religions and would inculcate practices like no discrimination policy. (Güven, 2023) In Islamism, Shar al-Nawawi Ala Muslim 2702 states that those who recall Allah constantly and become occasionally disoriented should beg for forgiveness because he deems this to be sinful. For example, the manager at Maple Holistics noted that several employees left the office for prayer at various times, and that their productivity was suffering because during prayer, they were distracted by their workloads. As a result, the business sets aside spaces for special prayer, which boosts employee morale and productivity and eventually fosters a welcoming environment. (Guruchiek, 3 C.E.)

The main focus of the Jaina Theory of Business Ethics is on doing the right thing in business. The theory sets up a consistent set of business rules that seem to be obvious. Shyama Prasad (2010) says that it is fine for a business to try to make money. But it's unethical for a company to make goods that aren't up to par, use unfair means to get a bigger share of the market, ignore its duty to the environment, or try to wipe out its rivals.

Religious and Spiritual Leaders - Religious leaders are individuals who are held in high esteem due to their perceived authority within a religious organization. As previously mentioned, religious leaders will have the opportunity to gain insights from the chapter. It is worth noting that Indians possess a profound faith in religious beliefs, often seeking guidance from these leaders when faced with challenges. Thus, the practical applications and quotations of deities inside the chapter will aid individuals in implementing the therapeutic interventions for themselves. Religiousness and religious practices have been distinguished from spirituality, which places more of an emphasis on one's inner development and personal progress. According to Sperry, more and more people today are searching for deeper purpose and fulfillment in their lives, feeling that spirituality is fundamental to their development and to assisting them in overcoming obstacles in life. Therefore these practices of mindfulness can be linked with spirituality which would help individuals focus into knowing about themselves.

Here is a Sikhism example where following the sayings of a religious leader helped Ravi. Kirat Karo, one of the core Sikhism principles, refers to using one's abilities and labor-intensive work for the good of society. By focusing on this idea, Mr. Ravi Singh, Sikh Humane, has been making a lot of effort since 1999 to win over people's confidence in mankind. He was able to live a calm and contented life by working in accordance with Sikhism's guiding principles.

LIMITATIONS AND RECOMMENDATIONS

The present study has identified some constraints which require consideration and may guide future research endeavors. In light of these limitations, we propose the future potential researchers for their research ahead.

The chapter primarily examines the religious practices within the Indian setting, specifically focusing on the faiths observed in India. Nonetheless, the themes discussed can also be extended to other nations who have a collectivistic culture. in which these similar religions are practiced. Furthermore, for the countries which have individualistic culture, the above mentioned practices may differ. Additionally, the chapter is entirely based on Integrative literature review, however future researchers can take interviews of people from different religions and perform systematic review and meta analysis.

REFERENCES

TrustsT.AboutS. D. T. (2023, July 18), Retrieved from https://www.tatatrusts.org/about-tatatrusts/about-sir-dorabji-tata

Ahmed, I. (2020, February 17). How To Achieve Mindfulness In Islam. *The Siasat Daily*. https://www.siasat.com/how-achieve-mindfulness-islam-1828249/

Bhargava, R., Kumar, N., & Gupta, A. (2017). Indian perspective on psychotherapy: Cultural issues. *Journal of Contemporary Psychotherapy*, *47*(2), 95–103. doi:10.100710879-016-9348-1

Bhattacharjee, A., & Singh, S. (2021). Zoroastrian Ethics in Business. *IIMS Journal of Management Science, 3si*, 133–143. doi:10.5958/0976-173X.2021.00010.5

Charan, C. (2020). *Bhagavad Gita: 365 Reflections for Daily Mindfulness*. Wikas Printing & Carriers Pvt. Ltd.

Clothey, F. W. (2007). *Religion in India: A historical introduction*. Routledge. doi:10.4324/9780203967836

Conze, E. (2012). *Buddhism: Its essence and development*. Courier Corporation.

Diggory, J. C., & Mehta, M. L. (1959). Jaina Psychology: A Psychological Analysis of the Jaina Doctrine of Karma. *Journal of the American Oriental Society*, *79*(2), 136–138. doi:10.2307/595861

Goldin, P. R., & Gross, J. J. (2010). Effects of mindfulness-based stress reduction (MBSR) on emotion regulation in social anxiety disorder. *Emotion (Washington, D.C.)*, *10*(1), 83–91. doi:10.1037/a0018441 PMID:20141305

Grace, S. (2020, June 16). *65 Bible Verses That Show Mindfulness Was God's Idea*. Calming Grace. https://www.calminggrace.com/bible-verses-about-mindfulness/

Gurchiek, K. (3 C.E.). *Prayer and Meditation Rooms Can Increase Inclusion*. SHRM; SHRM. https://www.shrm.org/resourcesandtools/hr-topics/behavioral-competencies/global-and-cultural-effectiveness/pages/prayer-meditation-rooms-can-increase-inclusion.aspx

Güven, C. (2023, January 27). *Promoting religious diversity in the workplace - Ruul.* Ruul I Worktech Solutions for Modern and Global Work. https://ruul.io/blog/promoting-religious-diversity-in-the-workplace#:~:text=The%20importance%20of%20religious%20diversity%20in%20the%20workplace,-More%20than%2085&text=A%20diverse%20workforce%20is%20essential,come%20up%20with%20versatile%20solutions

Haneef, S. (1979, January 1). What Everyone Should Know about Islam and Muslims. (pp. 4-25).

Harnack, A. (2006). *What is Christianity?* Book Tree.

Parott (2017, November 21) How to be a Mindful Muslim: An Exercise in Islamic Meditation I Yaqeen Institute for Islamic Research. Retrieved from Yaqeen Institute for Islamic Research. https://yaqeeninstitute.org/read/paper/how-to-be-a-mindful-muslim-an-exercise-in-islamic-meditation

Hung, S. H., & Wa, J. Y. S. (2021). Dharma therapy: A Buddhist counselling approach to acknowledging and enhancing perspectives, attitudes and values. *International Perspectives in Values-based Mental Health Practice: Case Studies and Commentaries*, 305-311.

Iyer, M. (2009). *Faith & philosophy of Zoroastrianism* (Vol. 7). Gyan Publishing House.

Jain, P. (2021, May 25). Living with Mindfulness — Parveen Jain. Parveen Jain. Retrieved from https://www.parveenjain.com/blog/living-with-mindfulness

Jainism Says. (2020). Jainism: Know It, Understand It & Internalize It. *Jainism Says.* https://jainismsays.blogspot.com/2020/05/yoga-and-meditation-in-jainism.html

Jas (2022, May 7). Conquer your mind and Conquer the world - ReflectandRespond. ReflectandRespond. https://reflectandrespond.com/guru-nanak-conquer-your-mind-conquer-the-world/

KaroK. (2022, August 17). Wikipedia. Retrieved from https://en.wikipedia.org/wiki/Kirat_Karo

Kirmayer, L. J. (2015). Mindfulness in cultural context. *Transcultural Psychiatry*, *4*(4), 447–469. doi:10.1177/1363461515598949 PMID:26264787

Komito, D. R., Rinchen, G. S., & Dorjee, T. (1987). *Nagarjuna's Seventy Stanzas*. Snow Lion.

Kreyenbroek, P. G. (2013). *Living Zoroastrianism: urban Parsis speak about their religion*. Routledge. doi:10.4324/9780203037133

Lazaridou, A., & Pentaris, P. (2016). Mindfulness and spirituality: Therapeutic perspectives. *Person-Centered and Experiential Psychotherapies*, *15*(3), 235–244. doi:10.1080/14779757.2016.1180634

Mazumdar, D. A. (2021). Importance of Jain values in shaping. *Business Ethics (Oxford, England).*

JapoN. (2023, September 27). Wikipedia. Retrieved from https://en.wikipedia.org/wiki/Naam_Japo#:~:text=In%20Sikhism%2C%20N%C4%81m%20Jap%C5%8D%20

Panda, S. N. (2017). The bhagavad gitā and health management of psychotherapy. *Odisha journal of social science, 106.*

Panesar, D. S. (2017). Meditation (Sikhism). In Encyclopedia of Scientific Dating Methods (pp. 238–241). Springer Netherlands. doi:10.1007/978-94-024-0846-1_498

Paul, D. P. (2015, December 5). *Bhagvad Gita's Guide to Mindfulness*. Atlantadunia. https://www.atlantadunia.com/dunia/Features/F242.htm#:~:text=It's%20succinctly%20stated%20in%20Bhagvad,and%20his%20enemy%20as%20well

Qaradawi, Y. (2010). *Islam: an introduction*. The Other Press.

Quranic. (2022, November 29). *Mindfulness in Islam - Quranic Arabic For Busy People*. Quranic Arabic For Busy People. https://www.getquranic.com/mindfulness-in-islam/

Rao, K. R., Paranjpe, A. C., & Dalal, A. K. (2008). *Handbook of Indian Psychology*. Foundation Books. doi:10.1017/UPO9788175968448

Singh, K., & Smith, A. (2007). *Sikhism*. QED.

Singh, N. G. K. (2004). *Sikhism*. Infobase Publishing.

Stead, T. (2017). *Mindfulness and Christian Spirituality*. Presbyterian Publishing Corp.

Bhatia, S. C., Madabushi, J., Kolli, V., Bhatia, S. K., & Madaan, V. (2013, January). The Bhagavad Gita and contemporary psychotherapies. *Indian Journal of Psychiatry*, *55*(Suppl 2), S315–S321. doi:10.4103/0019-5545.105557

The Dhammapada. Verses and Stories. (n.d.). Retrieved from https://www.tipitaka.net/tipitaka/dhp/

All About Sikhs. (2017, February 12). The Sikh Perspective Of Meditation. *Gateway to Sikhism*. https://www.allaboutsikhs.com/scriptures/guru-granth-sahib/the-sikh-perspective-of-meditation/

Timbers, V. L., & Hollenberger, J. C. (2022). Christian Mindfulness and Mental Health: Coping through Sacred Traditions and Embodied Awareness. *Religions*, *1*(1), 62. doi:10.3390/rel13010062

Trammel, R. (2018). Effectiveness of an MP3 Christian mindfulness intervention on mindfulness and perceived stress. *Mental Health, Religion &amp. Mental Health, Religion & Culture*, *5*(5), 500–514. doi:10.1080/13674676.2018.1505837

Upadhyay, N. (2023, April 4). *Managing Neurological Disorders with Mindfulness Meditation: A Jainism Philosophy Perspective*. LinkedIn.

ChhakoV. (2021, May 28). Wikipedia. Retrieved from https://en.wikipedia.org/wiki/Vand_Chhako

Verma, R. (2009). *Faith & philosophy of hinduism* (Vol. 1). Gyan Publishing House.

Von Glasenapp, H. (1999). *Jainism: An Indian religion of salvation, 14*.

APPENDIX

APPENDIX ONE

Chapter 2, Shloka 70:

"Even as all waters flow into the ocean, but the ocean never overflows, even so the sage feels desires, but he is ever one in his infinite peace."

Chapter 5, Shloka 10:

"Offer all thy works to god, throw off selfish bonds, and do thy work. No sin can then stain thee, even as waters do not stain the leaf of the lotus."

Chapter 2, Shloka 58:

"When in recollection he withdraws all his senses from the attraction of pleasures of sense, even as a tortoise withdraws all its limbs, then his is serine wisdom."

(The Bhagavad Gita and Contemporary Psychotherapies - PMC, n.d.)

APPENDIX TWO

Verse 23:

Te jhayino satatika

ni ccam dalhaparakkama

phusanti dhira nibbanam

yogakkhemam anuttaram.

Verse 24:

Utthanavato satimato

sucikammassa nisammakarino

sannatassa dhammajivino

appamattassa yaso bhivaddhati.

Verse 25:

Utthanena ppamadena

samyamena damena ca

dipam kayiratha medhavi[1]

yam ogho nabhikirati.

APPENDIX THREE

إِنَّهُ لَيُغَانُ عَلَى قَلْبِي وَإِنِّي لَأَسْتَغْفِرُ اللَّهَ فِي الْيَوْمِ مِائَةَ مَرَّةٍ\

APPENDIX FOUR

وَاعْلَمْ أَنَّ وُرُودَ الْخَاطِرِ لَا يَضُرُّ وَإِنَّمَا يَضُرُّ اسْتِدْعَاؤُهُ وَمُحَادَثَتُهُ فَالْخَاطِرُ كَالْمَارِّ عَلَى الطَّرِيقِ فَإِنْ تَرَكْتَهُ مَرَّ وَانْصَرَفَ عَنْكَ

APPENDIX FIVE

التَّأَنِّي مِنَ اللَّهِ وَالْعَجَلَةُ مِنَ الشَّيْطَانِ

Chapter 14
The Power of Words:
Daily Life Practices Incorporating Teachings From Indian Psychology

Sandhya Shankar
Chinmaya Vishwavidyapeeth, India

Vishaka Venkat
Chinmaya Vishwavidyapeeth, India

ABSTRACT

Language holds a multifaceted influence on our thoughts and culture, embodying the creative power of expression as recognized in Indian philosophies like Sabda Sakti. The Vedas highlight language's divine essence, linking it to cosmic energy and the profound connection between humanity and the divine. Chanting and linguistic vibrations serve as bridges to higher realities, exemplified by the concept of "Shabda Brahman" and the sacred syllable 'Om'. The transformative potential of language is evident in practices like "nadopasana," elevating individuals and reflecting divine revelation. Beyond communication, positive language engrains ethical values and gratitude in daily life, reflecting interconnectedness as emphasized in Hindu teachings. This interconnectedness extends to psychology, where language shapes cognitive processes, self-perception, and relationships, particularly within the Indian context. This chapter delves into the potency of positive words, exploring their therapeutic impact and integration into daily practices.

INTRODUCTION

Language shapes our thoughts in many ways, the extent though is debatable. Language is also cultural. It carries the traditions and thought process of a community in it. As per Sondhi (2021), "In the Indian notions about Sabda Sakti, meaning the 'Power of the Word', language is seen from the earliest times as creative power both at cosmic and human levels. Modern science sees energy as the ultimate form of reality. In India, language has been worshipped and used as a manifestation of the energy of the goddess Saraswati since the Rg Veda."

DOI: 10.4018/978-1-6684-9778-4.ch014

In Vedas language is seen as a creative and divine force. The act of chanting and medium of words is supposed to connect the atman with the divine and ultimate reality. The vibrations produced by these sounds are considered to be impactful. The concept of "Shabda Brahman" and the sacred syllable of Om shows how sound itself can make a sense of reality and identity. The "nadopasana" done by musicians like Tyagaraja Swami and Muthuswami Dikshithar also portray that the sadhana of sound, language and rhythm in itself can elevate an individual to the higher reality. Language, therefore, was considered to be part of divine revelation.

Language was not just a means of communication, it enlightened human experience. One might have heard in India to always say the positive words. Positive language is not about using words in a specific context to encourage or motivate someone to do something. It was a part of the everyday language people spoke. Most religions have a prayer before eating, before sleeping, which indicates gratefulness and humbleness at the same time. They kept us rooted and allowed one to always follow the righteous path.

The power of language also reiterates the sense of oneness in an Indian mind. Among the eastern perspective on psychology, the main teachings of Hindu traditions emphasize the interconnectedness of all things. The idea of harmonious union among all individuals is woven throughout the teachings" Cornelissen (2011). The use of positive words, thereby, enhances a positive psychology. In *Positive Psychology in Practice* (2004) edited by P. Alex Linley and Stephen Joseph, they give an overview of a set of practices which can help one in building a positive outlook. Ranging from the act of gratitude to physical activity and routine, language (verbal/non-verbal) constitutes a significant component in these practices. Sheldon Pollock in *The Language of the Gods in the World of Men: Sanskrit, Culture, and Power in Premodern India* (2006) examines how a language can build a powerful culture. Kamlesh Singh, Mahima Raina and Doug Oman in "Positive Psychology and Hinduism" discuss how "Hindu thought has always deliberated on the process, nature, conditions, and practices that lead to a fulfilled life" (2023). They delve deep into how "Hinduism's core beliefs and tenets…guide daily living". In *Mantras: Words of Power* (2005) Swami Sivananda Radha explores how mantra becomes a tool to train as well as liberate the mind. Language thus becomes a macrospace through which positive culture can be reaffirmed. Andrew Newberg and Mark Robert Waldman in *Words can Change your Brain* examine the power of words in shaping reality. They detail out how negative words can affect reality as well as the genes (2012). Words, thus, positive or negative have equal impact. Language, therefore, can be used for constructing and destructing reality.

Positive words have a hermetic and therapeutic impact on human psychology, shaping our thoughts, emotions and behaviours. Within the field of psychology, language plays a crucial role in shaping our cognitive processes, self-perception and interpersonal relationships. This paper explores the power of positive words, with a specific focus on the Indian psychological perspective and looking into practices that incorporate these into our daily life.

THE CULTURE OF SPEAKING WELL

A solitary and imperishable syllable, known as an "Akshara," is perceived as the minuscule and formless core of the Absolute Reality. Understanding this eternal essence empowers an individual to attain all their aspirations and goals in life. (Sondhi 2021) Akshara refers to the imperishable, eternal and indestructible reality in contrast to Kshara which would mean that 32which changes. In Bhagavad Gita, Chapter 8, Lord says:

अक्षरं ब्रह्म परमं स्वभावोऽध्यात्ममुच्यते ।

भूतभावोद्भवकरो विसर्ग: कर्मसञ्ज्ञित: ॥ 3॥

(akṣaraṁ brahma paraṁ svabhāvo'dhyātmamucyate |

bhūtabhāvodbhavakaro visargaḥ karmasañjñitaḥ || *3* ||*")*

Lord Krishna defines Brahman as Akshara, one which is the supreme indestructible entity. As language constitutes the reality,it is also evident that language and words play a significant role in constructing the reality. In this context positive words and affirmations are important.

Indian culture has long recognized the significance of positive words and their impact on mental well-being. Ancient Indian texts, such as the Vedas and Upanishads, emphasize the power of spoken and written words, stating they have the potential to heal, uplift and transform individuals.

वाक्भुषणं वाक्पतुता परमं वाक्प्रपञ्चःसतां अधिराजति

शिष्या वत्सरस्य पदानि शिरसि क्षिपन्ति छाया तदनन्तरुपमा॥

(vākbhuṣaṇaṁ vākpatutā paramaṁ vākprapañcaḥ satāṁ adhirājati,

śiṣyā vatsarasya padāni śirasi kṣipanti chāyā tad-anantarupamā.)

Ornament of speech surpasses all ornaments; the multitude of words adorns those wise. Disciples' feet are placed on the head of the teacher, like the reflection beneath the sun.

(Bhartrihari's Vairagya Shatakam)

This verse beautifully conveys the idea that the greatest ornament a person can possess is the art of eloquent speech. It emphasizes that the use of words and the ability to communicate effectively are superior to all other forms of adornment.

The word Sanskrit itself derives from the word that means cultured. Language had the power to civilize humanity, one that distinguished it from other forms of life. Language in Indian culture is not just a medium to communicate thoughts. At the time of creation, speech emerged as a cosmic power or Sakti, which could be accessed through a structured language to reach the higher goal of life (Sondhi, 2021). As with other forms of power, it could be used for the upliftment or destruction of the self, which is also why it is revered as Goddess, Vak devi or Saraswati.

The Sanskrit Subhashitas are a great example of the power of words in daily life with simple aphorisms and maxims, which are often lyrical so that they are easily remembered, to be quoted as life mantras on a regular basis.

Some famous examples of Sanskrit subhashitas include:

Table 1. Sanskrit subhashitas

Sanskrit Subhashita	Transliteration	Meaning	Message
अहसिा परमो धर्मः	Ahimsa Paramo Dharmaḥ	Non-violence is the highest virtue	Practicing non-violence and avoiding harm to others is the most important moral duty.
यत्र नार्यस्तु पूज्यन्ते, रमन्ते तत्र देवताः	Yatra Nāryastu Pūjyante, Ramaṇte Tatra Devatāḥ	Where women are honored, there the deities are pleased	Respecting and valuing women leads to blessings and harmony.
धर्मो रक्षतरिक्षतिः	Dharmo Rakṣati Rakṣitaḥ	Duty protects the one who protects it.	Uphold your responsibilities and obligations; they will safeguard you in return.
आपदामपहर्तारं दातारं सर्वसंपदाम्	Āpadāmapahartāraṁ Dātāraṁ Sarvasaṁpadām	Adversity takes away, but it also gives the gift of true wealth	Difficult situations can lead to personal growth and valuable experiences.
सत्यं ब्रूयात् प्रयिं ब्रूयात्, न ब्रूयात् सत्यं अप्रयिम्	Satyaṁ Brūyāt Priyaṁ Brūyāt, Na Brūyāt Satyaṁ Aprīyam	Speak the truth, speak what is pleasant; do not speak the truth that is unpleasant.	While truth is important, delivering it in a considerate manner is also essential.

POSITIVE PSYCHOLOGY AND LANGUAGE USE

This also aligns with the research findings in positive psychology, which highlight the positive influence of language on human psychology. Positive psychology emphasizes well-being, happiness, and optimal functioning, focusing on positive aspects of human experience. Language plays a vital role in this, enabling positive self-talk, gratitude expression, strengths-based communication, optimism, and effective social connections. Language helps amplify positive emotions, foster mindfulness, and shape a growth-oriented mindset. It aids in setting and articulating positive goals, facilitating positive communication patterns, and cultivating optimistic outlooks. Through linguistic practices, positive psychology encourages personal growth, resilience, and supportive relationships, contributing to an overall sense of flourishing and positivity.

Positive psychology encourages individuals to engage in positive self-talk. This involves using affirming, encouraging, and self-compassionate language when addressing oneself. By using positive language, individuals can boost their self-esteem, self-efficacy, and overall sense of well-being. (Seligman, 2002). Expressing gratitude through language is a core practice in positive psychology. Regularly acknowledging and verbalizing gratitude for the positive aspects of life can enhance feelings of happiness and life satisfaction. (Lyubomirsky & Layous, 2013). Language plays a role in framing situations positively, even in the face of challenges. By reframing negative experiences in a more optimistic light, individuals can reduce stress and increase resilience. (Duckworth, 2016).

Language is integral to mindfulness and self-awareness practices. By using language to describe thoughts, emotions, and sensations, individuals can develop a deeper understanding of themselves and their experiences, leading to personal growth and well-being. Language shapes thoughts and beliefs. By consistently using positive language, individuals can cultivate a more optimistic and growth-oriented mindset, leading to increased resilience and well-being. (Fredrickson, 2013).

Sanskrit is a sacred language and the use of this language in mindfulness practices evokes a sense of connection, reverence and thus, creates a conducive ambience for meditation and mental wellbeing. The vibration theory words carry energy and frequency, and these vibrations can influence our thoughts, emotions, and overall well-being. In Bhartṛhari's Vākyapadīya he details about the vibrations (spanda) of consciousness through language.

DINACHARYA AND LANGUAGE

The above western positive psychology works, show that there are various ways in which positive words can influence our behaviour and that one of the main ways is through shaping our cognitive processes. In her book, Boroditsky elaborates how the language shapes the way people think. When we use positive language, our attention is drawn towards favourable aspects, leading to more optimistic outlook. There are instances when one leaves the house, there are no goodbyes. The person is taught to say, /poi varām/ (Malayalam) or /lauṭta hũn/ (Hindi) which mean 'I'll go and come back'. Those are the words with which one parts. Similarly, whenever there is negative news, one says /śubh śubh/, indicating that let there be positive words. The attitude of welcoming guests or visitors which often sees the process of reduplication, as in /vʌru-vʌru' or /āije āije/ or even the English form, 'come come', signalling the aspect of respect one has to offer and insistence of welcoming them. Most of the Indian languages have a third form of respect which is used to mark when addressing a person elder to us or a complete stranger. The gender-neuter honorific -ji is also a respect marker that is prevalent in most of the languages spoken in India.

Reciting mantra, chanting hymns, and reading religious scriptures are daily practices for many Indians. The words and sounds used in these practices are believed to have spiritual significance as well as physical benefits, with research being conducted in how they reduce stress. (Agarwal, 2013) At the same time there are several studies that also show how positive thinking can bring about physical healings as well. The great placebo effect is just one example of that. (Colaguiri et.al. 2015) Though these things had often had a religious touch to them, they were practices by people from all walks of life in their daily routines. Politeness and respect were highly valued in the Indian Culture. They conveyed a sense of respect and connection.

These are some of the daily practices that are followed throughout the nation of India, irrespective of the different languages that are spoken here. This reflects the intimate relationship between language and its contribution to well-being.

As per the dinacharya recommended in our texts it begins with the recitation of "karāgre vasatē lakṣhmī"

करागे्र वसते लक्ष्मी, करमध्ये सरस्वती। *Karāgrē vasatē Lakṣhmī, karamadhyē Saraswati*

करमूले तु गोविन्दि; प्रभाते करदर्शनम्॥. *Kara-mūlē tu Govindah, prābhatē kara-darśanam.*

At the tip of your hand (fingertips) resides Goddess Lakshmi,

In the middle of your hand resides Goddess Saraswati,

At the base of your hand (palm) resides Lord Govinda (Krishna),

Therefore, in the morning, one should have the darshan (sight/view) of the hand.

This particular mantra is recited as a way to start the day with gratitude and is a reminder of the presence of auspicious energies and deities associated with different aspects of life. It also acknowledges the importance of using one's hands for various tasks. It gives positive affirmation as it says lakshmi, goddess of wealth, Saraswati goddess of knowledge and Krishna who shows to perform our action are all within one's hands. With the belief that "I am enough" the mind is tuned positively.

After this, as one steps on the floor the mantra the following mantra is stated:

समुद्रवसने देवि पर्वतस्तनमण्डले। *(Samudra-vasane devi parvata-stāna-maṇḍale)*

वष्णिुपत्निमिस्तुभ्यं पादस्पर्शं क्षमस्व मे॥ *(Vişhṇu-patni namastubhyaṁ pāda-sparśam kṣhamasva me)*

O Goddess, whose garments are the oceans, and whose bosom is adorned with mountains,

O Consort of Vishnu (Lord Narayana), I bow to you, please forgive me for touching your feet.

This sloka in turn asks for forgiveness as one steps on mother earth. While taking a bath one evokes all the sacred rivers in the water. These practices show how the language reiterates the feeling of oneness. This feeling of oneness can create a harmonious thought. Even the Tulsi Pooja, sun worship, making of kolam or rangoli are all parts of building a positive psychology.

Most of the poojas end with the slokas like:

पूर्णमदः पूर्णमिदं पूर्णात् पूर्णमुदच्यते पूर्णस्य पूर्णमादाय पूर्णमेवावशिष्यते

(Pūrṇamadaḥ Pūrṇamidaṁ Pūrṇāt Pūrṇamudachyate Pūrṇasya Pūrṇamādāya Pūrṇamevāvaśiṣhyate)

That is full; this is full. From fullness, fullness arises. When fullness is taken from fullness, fullness remains.

This verse is often interpreted philosophically to convey the idea of completeness, unity, and the interconnectedness of all things in the universe. It is frequently used to contemplate the nature of reality and the relationship between the individual and the universe.

The phrase "Loka Samasthā Sukhino Bhavantu" reflects a sentiment of compassion, well-wishing, and a desire for the well-being and happiness of all living beings, not just within one's immediate surroundings but across the entire universe. It's a call for universal harmony and peace. The reiterations of such aphorisms automatically creates a sense of gratitude and gratification, ultimately leading to a formation of positive psychology.

As one becomes grateful for the part, this realisation makes one whole and hence helps move towards satisfaction and contentment. This is where the Self-perception aspect comes in. By incorporating positive words into our self-talk and self-affirmations, we cultivate a healthier self-image and promote self-acceptance. Positive self-perception contributes to improved mental health and a greater sense of self-worth. Gratitude is an integral part of Indian philosophy, emphasising the appreciation of life's blessings. Practising gratitude involves acknowledging and expressing thankfulness for the positive aspects of life, no matter how small. Positive psychology suggests maintaining a gratitude journal as a form of practising it regularly, whereas in Indian Tradition this was inculcated into the above-mentioned daily life practices. Regularly expressing gratitude to others can shift focus from negativity to positivity, promoting psychological well-being.

TRIGUNAS AND LANGUAGE USE

The concept of Trigunas, derived from ancient Indian philosophy, provides a unique perspective on human psychology and its connection to positive well-being. Trigunas, also known as the three Gunas, are Sattva, Rajas, and Tamas. These Gunas represent different qualities or modes of existence that influence human behavior, emotions, and thought patterns. By understanding the Trigunas and their implications, we can explore the relationship between Indian Trigunas and positive psychology.

The gunas that were considered important for a child can be seen to be complementary to the positive psychology character traits. Atharva Veda provides information on inner workings of personality. These structures include the gunas and the doshas. A human is a combination of trigunas, which determine their personality based on which guna is dominant to what extent. The language that is used has the power to influence these gunas and thereby the consciousness.

Every human being will be a combination of these different gunas. Understanding the dominant Guna within ourselves can promote self-awareness and help identify areas for personal growth. By recognizing our tendencies and working towards cultivating Sattva qualities, we can foster positive emotions, thoughts, and behaviours. Positive psychology encourages individuals to strike a balance among the three Gunas.

While Rajas and Tamas have their place, excessive dominance of either can hinder overall well-being. Cultivating Sattva qualities through practices such as mindfulness, meditation, and self-reflection can help restore balance. It also emphasises the importance of a positive mindset in enhancing well-being. By nurturing positive emotions, engaging in gratitude practices, and cultivating a growth mindset, individuals can experience increased life satisfaction, resilience, and overall psychological well-being. Finally, exploring one's purpose and aligning it with positive psychology principles can lead to a more fulfilling life. By connecting with one's core values, strengths, and passions, one can cultivate a sense of purpose and meaning, which are fundamental to human flourishing.

As mentioned before, it's important to note that the Trigunas are not fixed; they can influence us differently in various situations. By being mindful of our language choices, we can consciously shift our mental and emotional states toward sattva, promoting well-being and fostering a positive and harmonious environment. Integrating positive language into our communication contributes to a healthier and more balanced lifestyle, aligning us with the higher qualities of consciousness.

MANTRA JAPA AND WELL-BEING

Mantra Vijnana is the science about the hidden and big powers of sound. Mantras are made up of specific sounds that are put together in a certain way. When these mantras are said in a particular tone, loudness, strength, and rhythm, they spread out really fast, even faster than laser beams. They spread out into the world as energy waves and in people's minds. Since sound can travel through space like radio waves, when many people chant Vedic mantras together, it can have a big impact on the universe. (Acharya, 2003).

The ancient Vedic scriptures, detailing the universe's origin, state that the existence of Brahmam finds expression and realisation through the profound vibrations of śabda and nāda. Sabdaitavada, an ancient

Vedic idea about sound, tells us that sound (sabda) is like a super powerful force that's everywhere. It's like a never-ending source that made the whole universe. This idea says that everything in the world comes from the big sound boom, like a cosmic explosion of sound. This sound is like the energy and movement that started everything and japa is a part of it. (Acharya, 2003).

Every mantra and metre it is sung in holds importance in Vedas. Among these, the Gayatri mantra is honoured as the distinguished one in the Mantra Vignjana. The Gayatri Mantra is a sacred chant from Hindu scriptures, invoking the divine energy of the Sun to illuminate our minds with wisdom and guide our intellects toward truth. It acknowledges the interconnectedness of the physical, mental and spiritual realms. Its essence lies in acknowledging the interconnectedness of the physical, mental, and spiritual realms.

Emphasis on pronunciation (Uccarna shuddhi) is another crucial aspect of language in India. The power of words and intonation are also evident in the way the shlokas, mantras and stotras are performed. Especially the vedic mantras are bound to intonation. In " Brain Waves, Sanskrit Chanting And Sacred Silence " yogi Andri Richl talks about the effect of vibrational syllables on brain waves. In their study on the effect of Gayathri mantra meditation on naive subjects, Thomas and Rao (2016) showcased a positive impact on the personality of the subjects. Studies show that sound definitely has an impact on the brain and the personality. Bhavna and Hiwale (2018) in their paper on EEG spectral analysis on OM mantra meditation, also study the impact of the om sound on the brain.

In a study conducted by Sudha (2020) on students aged 10-17 to test the intervention of Gayatri Mantra and social skill training for two months found a significant reduction in the social anxiety and stress levels and significant improvement in self concept and wellbeing in the experimental group showcasing the power of words in ones dinacharya. A similar result was found in a study conducted by Sharma and Singh (2014) on educational stress among students. Around 200 students who practised Om and Gayatri mantra chanting had significant reduction in educational stress in the intervention group.

An increasing volume of methodical and observational studies suggests that meditation is effective in assisting with stress reduction and enhancing psychological wellness among both clinical and non-clinical groups (Lynch et.al., 2018). .However, In various studies conducted, it has been found that the reciting mantras daily have a profound impact on the psychological well-being of people (Susan and Rao, 2016; Lolla, 2018; Rastogi et.al., 2020; Sharma & Soni, 2022). Interestingly, that mantra can be any positive affirmation the person believes in, thereby showing that it is primarily the words which bring that positive impact just like the rhythmic tone that is often used in Sanskrit mantras.

Chanting Mantras can be integrated with mindfulness. The focus on sound, breathing awareness, vibrations, bodily sensations and the transition to silence shows how mantras can heal and create a positive personality. Even the gestural language which includes mudras and asanas reaffirm the fact that language plays a crucial part in developing a positive psychology.

CONCLUSION

Incorporating Sanskrit mantras or other positive affirmations or maxims in daily life and embracing aspects of the Indian lifestyle can offer a comprehensive solution to enhancing overall well-being for human beings. The profound wisdom encapsulated within Sanskrit mantras serves as a transformative tool, promoting mental clarity, inner peace, and spiritual growth. These mantras, with their positive language and resonance, create a harmonious vibration that resonates within individuals, fostering a sense of connection to the universe and promoting a balanced and fulfilling life. The Indian lifestyle, rooted in ancient traditions and holistic practices, especially one that is rooted in humility and harmony, through its stress on positive words, complements the efficacy of mantras.

REFERENCES

Acharya, P. S. S. (2003). *Eternity of Sound and the Science of Mantras*. Shri Vedmata Gayatri Trust-Uttarakhand.

Agarwal, A., & Agarwal, A. (2013). Impact of mantra chanting on stress coping. *Indian Journal of Positive Psychology*, *4*(1), 96.

Atwal, S. (2010). *Indian psychology: The connection between mind, body, and the universe*. Pepperdine University.

Colagiuri, B., Schenk, L. A., Kessler, M. D., Dorsey, S. G., & Colloca, L. (2015). The placebo effect: From concepts to genes. *Neuroscience*, *307*, 171–190. doi:10.1016/j.neuroscience.2015.08.017 PMID:26272535

Cornelissen, M. (2011). *Foundations of Indian Psychology Volume 2: Practical Applications*. Pearson Education India.

Duckworth, A. (2016). *Grit: The power of passion and perseverance* (Vol. 234). Scribner.

Fredrickson, B. L. (2013). Positive emotions broaden and build. In Vol. 47, pp. 1–53). Advances in experimental social psychology. Academic Press.

Gupta, S. K. (2019). Meditation, Yoga and Health. *Think India Journal*, *23*(3), 188–191.

Harne, B. P., & Hiwale, A. S. (2018). EEG spectral analysis on OM mantra meditation: A pilot study. *Applied Psychophysiology and Biofeedback*, *43*(2), 123–129. doi:10.100710484-018-9391-7 PMID:29752573

Linley, P. A., & Joseph, S. (Eds.). (2004). *Positive Psychology in Practice*. Wiley. doi:10.1002/9780470939338

Lolla, A. (2018). Mantras help the general psychological well-being of college students: A pilot study. *Journal of Religion and Health*, *57*(1), 110–119. doi:10.100710943-017-0371-7 PMID:28271341

Lynch, J., Prihodova, L., Dunne, P. J., O'Leary, C., Breen, R., Carroll, Á., Walsh, C., McMahon, G., & White, B. (2018). Mantra meditation programme for emergency department staff: A qualitative study. *BMJ Open*, *8*(9), e020685. doi:10.1136/bmjopen-2017-020685 PMID:30249626

Lyubomirsky, S., & Layous, K. (2013). How do simple positive activities increase well-being? *Current Directions in Psychological Science*, *22*(1), 57–62. doi:10.1177/0963721412469809

Menon, S. (2005). What is Indian psychology: Transcendence in and while thinking. *Journal of Transpersonal Psychology*, *37*, 2.

Newberg, A. & Waldman, M. (2012). *Words can Change your Brain*. A Plume Book.

Pollock, S. (2006). *The Language of the Gods in the World of Men: Sanskrit, Culture, and Power in Premodern India*. University of California Press. doi:10.1525/9780520932029

Rastogi, R., Saxena, M., Maheshwari, M., Garg, P., Gupta, M., Shrivastava, R., & Gupta, H. (2020). Yajna and mantra science bringing health and comfort to the Indo-Asian public: a healthcare 4.0 approach and computational study. *Machine Learning with Health Care Perspective: Machine Learning and Healthcare*, 357-390.

Seligman, M. E. (2002). Positive psychology, positive prevention, and positive therapy. Handbook of positive psychology, 2(2002), 3-12.

Sharma, A., & Singh, R. (2014). Combating educational stress in adolescents: The miraculous role of chanting mantras. *Indian Journal of Psychological Science*, *5*(1), 25–37.

Sharma, N., & Soni, D. (2022). *Effect of Gayatri Mantra on Health: A Narrative Review*. OSF.

Singh, K., Raina, M., & Oman, D. (2023). Positive Psychology and Hinduism. In E. B. Davis, E. L. Worthington Jr, & S. A. Schnitker (Eds.), *Handbook of Positive Psychology, Religion, and Spirituality*. Springer. doi:10.1007/978-3-031-10274-5_13

Sivananda Radha, S. (2005). *Mantras: Words of Power*. Timeless Books.

Sondhi, S., & Sakti, S. (2021). Power of Words in India's Linguistic Tradition. *Kalakalpa IGNCA Journal for Arts, 6*(1). https://ssrn.com/abstract=3874909

Srivastava, K. (2012). Concept of personality: Indian perspective. *Industrial Psychiatry Journal, 21*(2), 89.

Sudha, R. (2020). Gayathri Mantra and Social Skills Training for Social Anxiety, Stress, Self Concept, and Well Being among School Students with Learning Difficulties. *International Journal of Psychosocial Rehabilitation*, *24*(3), 1983–2004. doi:10.37200/IJPR/V24I3/PR200946

Thomas, S., & Rao, S. L. (2016). Effect of Gayatri mantra meditation on naive subjects: An EEG and fMRI pilot study. *International Journal of Indian Psychology*, *3*(7), 14–18.

Chapter 15
Therapeutic Potential of Ayurvedic Practices for the Mental Health of the Geriatric Population:
A Personalized Ayurvedic Protocol

E. Remya
Central Council for Research in Ayurvedic Sciences, Ministry of Ayush, Cheruthuruthy, India

ABSTRACT

Drastic population ageing points to increased prevalence of physical and mental disorders in the elderly. Mental illnesses of the elderly are often related to biological and psychosocial risk elements which can be predicted and prevented using Ayurvedic diagnostic tools such as Dosha and Prakriti. This chapter presents a hypothetical personalised model to preserve the mental health of geriatric population w.s.r to dietary and lifestyle modifications. This section also explores the translational research outlook and evidence-based perspectives of Rasayana drugs, and Panchakarma procedures in most prevalent and distressing psychological disorders such as anxiety, post-traumatic stress disorders, insomnia, psychological imbalances inherent to mood disorders, psychotic diseases, neuro-degenerative disorders, etc.

INTRODUCTION

Fast-paced population ageing both in size and proportion of the elderly is experienced by every country in the world. This demographic transition is occurring more drastically in low- and middle-income countries like India. It is estimated that the proportion of world's elderly population will nearly double from 12% to 22% between 2015 and 2050. The United Nations (UN) General Assembly declared 2021–2030 as the UN Decade of Healthy Ageing (World Health Organization: WHO, 2022). Ageing is a complex mixture of biological ageing resulting from the accumulation of molecular and cellular changes and social ageing occurs from life transitions such as retirements, relocations and death of nearest ones. Premature

DOI: 10.4018/978-1-6684-9778-4.ch015

ageing is a condition in which biological ageing is more intense irrespective of chronological age due to the effect of dietary habits, lifestyle, disease states, medications, mental make-up, familial, social and other environmental factors (Samarakoon et al., 2011). Increase in life expectancy points to increased prevalence of physical and mental disorders in the elderly.

Mental illnesses in the elderly population are often related to cerebral neurodegeneration, cerebral vascular disease and psychosocial risk elements and generally end up with social deprivation, poor quality of life, cognitive decline and disability, increased risk for somatic disorders, suicide and non-suicidal formality (Skoog, 2011). National Mental Health Survey of India (NMHS) 2015-16 points out that mental health is of low priority in Indian public health sector. Based on NMHS 2015-16, Preeti Sinha et al., states that older adults had a higher lifetime (6.93%) prevalence of depressive disorders as compared to younger adults (4.96%) and specific phobias (1.72%) was the most prevalent anxiety disorders in the elderly. The most prone individuals for mental disorders in the older population were females, urbans, unemployed, single relationship status and those with lower income (Sinha et al., 2021). Provision of supportive physical and social environment with person centred integrative health care system for elderly is the need of the hour.

In India, the contributions in geriatric research are less than 1% in the world scientific literature and budget allocation for geriatric health research and care is less than 0.1% of the GDP (Tiwari & Pandey, 2012). Focused epidemiological studies and scientifically designed community trials are indispensable for the establishment of psychogeriatrics in India. This is especially challenging for the Ayurvedic system of medicine as geriatrics is one of its core strengths. Ayurveda, the traditional medical system of India, is the sole medical science which can proclaim preventive or retarding potential of age-related changes and also can offer customised solutions for physical, physiological, psychological and emotional illnesses. This chapter highlights the Ayurvedic methodology for the assessment of *Dosha, Prakriti* and other homologous parameters to evaluate physical, physiological and psychological imbalances and also to propose customised preventive and therapeutic solutions.

DOCTRINES OF AYURVEDA IN DIAGNOSIS AND TREATMENT

Ayurvedic Medicine is popularly known as Holistic Medicine as it addresses biological, psychological and spiritual dimensions of health and illness (Gordon, 1982). Ayurveda is one of the world's most authoritative mind-body-spirit medicinal systems and it relies on a comprehensive programme that includes dietary, lifestyle, behavioural, psychological and pharmacological interventions for a prolonged and successful health-span (Rao, 2018). Basic foundation of Ayurveda lies on the principles of *Tridosha* – the biological energy systems - *Vata, Pitta* and *Kapha.* Health and disease are the direct reflection of the status and interaction of the *Doshas* in the body that in turn provokes or delays the aging process (*Ashtangahridaya*, 2014) (*A Comprehensive Guide to Traditional Indian Medicine for the West-anatomy*, 2010). Physical and psychological states have a bidirectional impact on body and mind. This interaction can be explained on the basis of stimulation of hypothalamic-pituitary-adrenal axis (HPA) through stress response (Montiel-Castro et al., 2013). As the physiology and pathology of both body and mind are interlinked, healing of physical and mental illnesses demand bidirectional approach. Physical illnesses can create a negative impact on mind. The mental status of an individual has great role in the curing process of every disease. This justifies the rationale of physical treatments in mental illnesses and vice versa. *Ayurvedic* mental health promoting factors can be identified as healthy regimen (day, night and seasonal regimens), periodical detoxification, purification and rejuvenation therapies (*Panchakarma* and *Rasayana Chikitsa)* and behavioural etiquette (*Sadvritta* and *Achara Rasayana*).

PRAKRITI AND P4 MEDICINE

Prakriti, the constitutional phenotype or psycho-somato typing, is an *Ayurvedic* concept which refers to inherent balance of unique combinations of *Tridoshas* which show up as predictable patterns in mind-body system within an individual(Mills et al., 2019). *Prakriti* is a specific individualistic trait which reflects the baseline characteristics such as metabolism, mental make-up, immunity, inherent strength and weakness and proclivities and it determines the individual response to internal and external stimuli and susceptibility to different diseases. This is the age-old concept of the newly developed health care model – P4 (predictive, preventive, personalized and participatory) medicine (Boffetta & Collatuzzo, 2022) and this concept can be successfully utilized in the prevention and management of ageing related pathologies including mental illnesses. *Prakriti* based drug discovery and development of personalised medicine has been evolved as a new field of Ayurgenomics which integrates the concepts of Ayurveda, such as Prakriti, with modern genetic research and this resulted in the discovery of the molecular and genomic basis of *Doshaj Prakriti.* Genomic studies have shown that main *Prakriti* types differ significantly in gene expression levels especially in immunity, blood coagulation, cell division and so on (Chatterjee & Pancholi, 2011).

Genetics, ethnicity, geoclimatic regions, familial characteristics, milieu throughout foetal development determine the phenotypic variability and this constitutional phenotype which is established at the moment of birth cannot be fully altered during one's lifetime (Huang et al., 2022). According to *Ayurvedic* classics, based on the predominance of *Dosha* in the phenotype, persons can be categorized into seven *Prakriti* ie. *Vataj, Pittaj, Kaphaj, Vatapittaj, Pittakaphaj, Vatakaphaj and Samadoshaj* (three *Doshas* in equal state) (*Charaka Samhita*, 1998). *Samadoshaj Prakriti* is considered as homeostatic state and others as defective constitutions. A similar stressful situation precipitates different types of stress disorders in persons of different *Prakriti*. This can be supported by the evidence of incidences of certain diseases in certain *Prakriti*. For eg: *Vataj* individuals are more prone to develop anxiety neurosis and dementia while *Kaphaj* individuals are more prone to depression. Hence interaction between the environmental factors and *Doshaj Prakriti* determines the final outcome – illness or wellness. Here comes the original contribution of *Ayurveda* to bring about epigenetic changes through *Doshaj Prakriti* oriented practices for the restoration of physical and mental health (Tripathi & Singh, 1994).

Purvya MC et al., states that predominance of *Pitta* in the constitution causes increase in the metabolic level of biotransformation, energy consumption and it results in various types of tissue destruction and premature manifestation of ageing (Purvya & Meena, 2011). *Kapha* predominant *Prakriti* shows tendency for delayed manifestation of ageing due to its specific synthetic properties and inherent prolonged healthspan (*Charak Samhita*, 1998). Various studies have been published in high impact journals on the link between biological and genome wide levels of expression of participants in the three main *Prakriti* groups. The researches reveal that there was overexpression of genes in the immune response pathways and haemoglobin pathways in *Pitta* dominants and inflammatory pathways in *Kapha* dominants. *Kapha Prakriti* demonstrates higher lipid profile values, higher levels of natural killer cells and activated B cells, upregulation of genes involved in ATP and cofactor production and downregulation of genes for fibrinolysis (Prasher et al., 2008) (Rotti et al., 2014). Ghodke et al., exposed that genes associated with drug metabolism and detoxification were downregulated in *Kapha* and upregulated in *Pitta* dominants (Ghodke-Puranik et al., 2011). Inflammatory genes were upregulated in *Vata Prakriti*, and protein sequence involved in oxidative stress pathway were upregulated in *Pitta* and *Kapha Prakriti* (Juyal et al., 2012). These finding points to the preponderance of specific psychiatric illnesses in *Doshaja Prakriti* **(Table No.1)** In a cohort study published by Ruth Ann Marrie et al., in 2017, Immune Mediated Inflammatory Disease (IMID) population shows relatively higher incidence of depression, anxiety, bipolar disorders and schizophrenia (Marrie et al., 2017).

SCOPE OF AYURVEDIC METHODOLOGIES IN CLINICAL PSYCHOLOGY

Every person is born with a unique percentage of *Tridosha* which refers to *Doshaj Prakriti* and the onset of illnesses occur when *Tridosha* are increased past the individual's threshold. Systematically and scientifically designed phenotype based practice of fundamental *Ayurvedic* methodologies – *Ahara* (diet), *Achara* (healthy regimen and behavioral etiquette) and *Oushadha* (*Panchakarma* and *Rasayana Chikitsa)*– can accomplish quality of life with longevity. For preserving and restoring the mental health of geriatric population, personalized care should begin from the early adulthood in terms of these three pillars of *Prakriti* based healthcare (Huang et al., 2022b). Easy accessibility to time tested personalised prevention and lifestyle control suggestions will enable the individuals to engage in self – care effortlessly.

Table 1. Biochemical profiles, biological processes, pathways (Prasher et al., 2008b) and disease preponderance in Doshaja Prakriti

		Parameters	Vata	Pitta	Kapha
Biochemical Profile	Lipid Profile Haematological	TC, TG, VLDL, LDL HDL Hb, PCV, RBC, UA Zinc, Copper, Phosphurus	- + - -	- - + +	+ - - -
Biological process		Immune response Regulation of enzyme activity	- +	+ -	- -
Biological pathways	Immune System	Natural killer cell mediated cytotoxicity Antigen processing & presentation B cell & T cell receptor signalling pathway Cell cycle	-	+ +	- +
Disease preponderance	**Neurocognitive** **IMID** **Sleep – wake disorders** **Stress related disorder** **Hormone – mediated Mood disorder**	Dementia Delirium Depression, Schizophrenia, Anxiety, Bipolar disorder (Marrie et al., 2017b) Insomnia Anxiety PTSD Phobia Post Menopausal Depression	+ - + + + -	- + + + + -	+ - - - - +

* TC – Total Cholesterol, TG - Triglycerides, VLDL – Very Low Density Lipoprotein, LDL – Low Density Lipoprotein, HDL – High Density Lipoprotein, Hb - Hemoglobin, PCV – Packed Cell Volume, RBC – Red Blood Cell, UA – Uric Acid

AHARA (DIET), ACHARA (HEALTHY REGIMEN), AND SADVRITTA (BEHAVIOURAL ETIQUETTE)

Diet and lifestyle are the modifiable risk factors for preventing premature ageing, age related diseases and preserving physical and mental health. Ayurvedic classics reiterate that physique, mind and diseases are of dietary origin. Hence diet is considered as one among the three pillars (*Tristhuna*) of life. Effects of nutrition are not only limited to the individual, but can be passed on the next generations. Major factors which determine *Doshaj Prakriti* are quality of sperm and ova and environment (maternal diet and lifestyle) during development ("Pharmacogenetics, Pharmacogenomics and Ayurgenomics for Personalized Medicine: A Paradigm Shift," 2015). Quality and quantity of food and eating patterns can determine the health status and disease risk. Fernando Gomez Pinilla has studied the influences of dietary factors on neuronal function and synaptic plasticity and that revealed the vital mechanisms responsible for the action of diet on brain health and mental function which can influence mood and has psychiatric manifestations. This study has established the influence of visceral signals – vagal nerve stimulation and gut hormones – on mental function and the application of lifestyle factors such as diet and exercise as therapy to reduce depression, schizophrenia and bipolar disorders (Gómez-Pinilla, 2008). Irrespective of the psycho-somato typing, *Acharya Charaka* has instructed specific dietary and lifestyle guidelines for all to preserve healthy and harmonious life. Warm and unctuous food is recommended to be consumed in proper quantity and time after the complete digestion of previous food at favourite places with loyal companions without any kind of distractions (*Charaka Samhita*, 2011).

Achara refers to the healthy regimens laid down by Ayurvedic science to maintain the synchronicity of circadian rhythm for healthy life which prevents diseases and delays ageing. These set of operational guidelines include optimal timings and methods for sleeping, waking up, breathing, excretion, bath, massage, study, travel, prayer, diet and other pursuits which are collectively known as *Dinacharya* (daily regimen), *Ratricharya* (Night regimen) and *Ritucharya* (Seasonal regimen) (Approach Towards Life Style Modification Plan as per Ayurveda and Modern Technique for Prevention of Geriatrics, 2013), (Yogic Life Style and Geriatric Care- Review Article, 2017). Ayurvedic classics encourage the adoption of medium path in all deeds. *Sadvritta* or *Achara Rasayana* is the code of ethics required to maintain a balanced state of physical and mental life which influence the individual values, interpersonal relationships and social behaviour. This concept laid foundation for Ayurvedic psychotherapy – *Satvavajaya Chikitsa* which involves mind control method, replacement of emotions, psycho physical shock, moral and behavioural code and inhibiting stressors (Behere et al., 2013), (*Charak Samhita*, n.d.).

PHENOTYPIC VARIABILITIES AND CUSTOMIZED SOLUTIONS

Generally, *Vataj* phenotypes are talkative, sleepless, competitive, atheist individuals having inconsistent cognition, emotions and relationships. They will be lean, weak and cold body types with unhealthy bones, eyes and hair having unpredictable actions, swift mood changes, easy susceptibility to diseases and non-compliant senses. *Pittaj* phenotypes will have yellowish skin, lax joints, intense hunger, thirst and anger, possessiveness and leadership qualities. Though they are proud and brilliant, they will be obsessed with cleanliness and cosmetics and prefer cold items. Compared to other phenotypes, these individuals are more prone to addictions, sexual dysfunctions and premature ageing. *Kaphaj* phenotypes appear to be calm and composed with compact physique and mental power, and better tolerance. They will have patience, better sleep, consistent actions and relationships. Depends on the predominance of *Doshas* in constitution, mixed characteristics may be evident in individual's personality. Extensive researches have been carried out to correlate the determinants of Prakriti with the tools of contemporary science using AyuSoft Prakriti diagnostic software, developed by C-DAC (Centre for Development of Advanced Computing) with a vision to convert classical Ayurvedic texts into comprehensive and authentic knowledge repositories with complex analytical tools (Rotti, Raval, et al., 2014), (Bhargav et al., 2021). Adherence to constitution specific dietary pattern and lifestyle beneficial for preserving and restoring physical and psychological health irrespective of age are enlisted in **Table No.2**. It is also stated that dietary factors and life style opposite to the inherent characteristics of *Doshaja Prakriti* has to be adopted by the individuals (*Charaka Samhita*, 1998a).

TRANSLATIONAL RESEARCH OUTLOOK OF RASAYANA DRUGS IN PSYCHOLOGIC IMBALANCES

Rasayana is a comprehensive *Ayurvedic* discipline specifically devoted for the rejuvenation of body and psyche, immunomodulation and healthy ageing. This branch of medicine comprises of pharmacological and non-pharmacological approach which emphasizes on dietetics, lifestyle modification and self-discipline

Table 2. Constitution specific dietary and lifestyle suggestions as customized preventive strategies for physical and psychological wellbeing (Ashtangahridaya, 2014a)

Prakriti	*Pathya* **(Wholesome)**	*Apathya* **(Unwholesome)**
Vata	Warm food and climate	Cold food and beverages, exposure to cold climate, air, water etc.
	Tastes predominantly sweet, sour and salt, easily digestible unctuous foods	Dried and fried items
	Moderate exercises, Breathing exercises (*Anuloma Viloma, Bhramari*), Relaxing Yogic postures – *Savasana* (Corpse pose), *Makarasana* (Crocodile pose)	Heavy exercises, Workout in gym
	Visiting sacred places, reading holy books	Fasting
	Proper care for eyes, oil massage	
	Sleep hygiene	
Pitta	Lukewarm or cold dietary articles	Hot items and climate, exposure to sunlight
	Frequent snacks and liquids (in an interval of 2-3 hours)	Fasting
	Tastes predominantly of sweet, astringent, bitter	Pungent, salty, sour foods, pickles, pappadam, fried items
	Cold shower, well dressed, anointing with cosmetics and perfumes, spending leisure time with family members at enjoyable locations	Heavy exercise, all kinds of addictions including tobacco, alcohol, beetle
	Mental detachment, Pranayama and Yoga for anger Management	Overindulgence into others activities
Kapha	Warm food	Cold food and beverages, exposure to cold climate, air, water etc.
	Tastes predominantly bitter, astringent, pungent	Excessive sweet, salty, sour foods, oily, dried and fried articles
	Heavy exercises, Pranayama and Yoga, *Kapalabhati*	Sedentary lifestyle
	Reduce sleeping hours	Day sleep & excessive sleep

with social etiquette to achieve homeostasis and to retard the ageing process (Goyal, 2018). *Ayurvedic* system has been utilising the prophylactic and therapeutic potential of age-specific, tissue specific and disease specific *Rasayanas* in clinical and research settings. Though the ideal age for *Rasayana* therapy is early and middle adulthood for excellent action, *Dosha* and *Prakriti* based selection of *Rasayanas* will enable the elderly to enhance mental health, reduce the prevalence of psychological diseases and also to improve quality of life. Among the various domains of *Rasayana* therapy, the group of *Medhya Rasayanas* (neuro nutrients) were reported to enhance neuro-cognitive abilities and emotional well-being. *Ashwagandha (Withania somnifera), Brahmi (Bacopa monnieri), Mandukaparni (Centella asiatica), Sankhapushpi (Convolvulus pleuricaulis), Yashtimadhu (Glycyrrhiza glabra), Guduci (Tinospora cordifoloia)* etc. are identified as *Medhyarasayana*. Clinical trials, systematic reviews and experimental studies conducted on these drugs have established their effectiveness in the prevention and management of cognitive disabilities and psychiatric disorders of the elderly (Singh et al., 2008).

Aswagandha supplementation has beneficial effect in anxiety, stress (Akhgarjand et al., 2022), neuropsychiatric diseases (D'cruz & Andrade, 2022), depression and anxiety symptoms of Schizophrenia (Jm et al., 2019). These effects are attributed to its anti-inflammatory, antioxidant properties, modulation of neurotransmitters and induction of neuroplasticity. Internal administration of *B.monnieri* can significantly improve cognitive functions particularly memory, learning and attention in the elderly and also have tranquilizing and sedative properties (Morgan & Stevens, 2010) (Kongkeaw et al., 2014). Age associated memory improvement has been demonstrated in older adults taking *Brahmi* compared to placebo (Raghav et al., 2006). Aqueous extract of *G. glabra* has significantly improved learning and memory in dementia (Dhingra et al., 2004) and produced antidepressant like effect comparable to the standard antidepressants – imipramine and fluoxetine (Dhingra & Sharma, 2006). A handful of in vivo studies conducted on *T. cordifolia* have proven its learning and memory enhancing, anti-oxidant anti stress activities (Agarwal et al., 2002) (R. Singh et al., 2006) (Prince & Menon, 2001) ("Antistress Activity of Tinospora Cordifolia (Willd) Meirs," 1997). Major constituents of *Mandukaparni* juice are saponins which are neuro-protectives, learning and memory enhancers, brain growth promoters and acts on behavior also (*Database on Medicinal Plants Used in Ayurveda and Sidha*, 2005) ("Neuroprotective Evaluation of Standardized Extracts of Centella Asiatica in Monosodium Glutamate Treated Rats," 2007) ("Synergetic Effect of Vallarai and Brahmi on Learning Ability of Albino Mice and School Children," 1995) (K. G. M. Rao et al., 2006). Methanolic and water extract of *C. asiatica* has shown highest anti-oxidant activity due to the presence of polyphenols and flavonoids, which help to delay ageing (Anand et al., 2010). Menotab – a herbo-mineral preparation containing *C. asiatica* was proven to be effective for post-menopausal symptoms like vasomotor instability and psychological symptoms (Devi & Swarup, 2000).

Neuroprotective and intellect promoting activity of *C.pleuricaulis* is attributed to its free radical scavenging and anti-oxidant properties (Bhatnagar et al., 2005) and is reported to relieve the signs and symptoms of anxiety disorders by regulating the production of stress hormones, adrenaline and cortisol (Kumar, 2006) . Polyherbal formulations of *Sankhapushpi,* BR – 16A (Mentat) has stress relieving property (A. Kumar & Sk, 2006), and Ayushman – 8 is reported to be effective on mental retardation (*Seminar on Research in Ayurveda and Sidha*, 1995). *Kushmanda (Benincasa hispida)* has tissue protective and preventive effect on colchicine induced Alzheimer's disease ("Effects of Fractions of Benincasa Hispida on Antioxidant Status in Streptozotocin Induced Diabetic Rats," 2007) and significant relief for anxiety disorders (*Clinico-experimental Study of Kushmandadi Ghrita in Generalized Anxiety Disorder(DSM-IV) w.s.r.to Chittodvega*, 2005). Rhizomes of *Vaca (Acorus calamus)* have cognitive, sedative and anticonvulsant properties and has been specifically used to cure the diseases of central nervous system like speech disorders, epilepsy, schizophrenia etc. since centuries (Lai et al., 2002) (Shukla et al., 2006) (Koo et al., 2003) (Mukherjee et al., 2007) (Kulkarni et al., 2012b). *Jatamansi (Nardostachys jatamansi)* and *Tagara (Valeriana wallichii)* have antidepressant and sedative properties and their potential in the management of neuropsychiatric disorders like depression, insomnia, Post Traumatic Stress Disorder (PTSD) etc. is well established. Root decoction has shown protective effect on stress induced impairment of hippocampus dependant learning and memory behaviour (Karkada et al., 2012) (Panara et al., 2020) (Li et al., 2020) (Toolika et al., 2015) (Ayyathan et al., 2015). Herbo-mineral preparations like *Smriti Sagara Rasa, Unmada Gaja Kesari Rasa* have better results in depression, paranoid and catatonic varieties of Schizophrenia (Dubey et al., 2010) ("Clinical Evaluation of Smrtisagararasa in Cases of Residual Schizophrenia," 1994). Ghee preparations like *Kalyanaka, Panchagavya, Mahapanchagavya* etc. and *Arishta* (fermented liquids) formulations like *Aswagandharishta, Saraswatarishta* etc. have proven neuroprotective, cognitive, antidepressant and anti-psychotic effects in animal models and clinical trials (Prabhu et al., 2020) (P. Tiwari & Patel, 2013) (Kulamarva et al., n.d.). Customised *Rasayana* selection for different phenotypes and *Doshic* states are depicted in

Rasayanas enlisted in Table No.3 can be used as either prophylactic or therapeutic, but the consumption of poly herbal formulations and herbo-mineral preparations is restricted only for therapeutic purposes and should be administered under the strict supervision of a qualified Ayurvedic medical practitioner. Apart from these, there are many single drugs, poly herbal and herbo-mineral formulations which have proven clinical efficacies, but yet to explore the potential drug candidates through transdisciplinary exploratory studies.

PANCHAKARMA PROCEDURES FOR MENTAL WELL BEING

Ayurvedic Panchakarma (purificatory therapy), is a group of therapies, having the capacity to influence the relationship between psycho-neuro-endocrine-immune systems. Intimate relationship between immune, physical, emotional and psychological aspects enables bi-directional communications between body and psyche, which ultimately determines the states of health and disease. In general, all the external therapies like *Lepana* (Anointment), *Dhara* (Medicinal irrigation), *Shirotala* (application of medicine

Table 3. Customisation of Rasayanas for psychological imbalances on the basis of Dosha and Prakriti (Ayurvedic Pharmacoepia of India, 2016)

Dosha/Prakriti	**Single herbs**	**Poly herbal preparations**
Vata		All types of ghee
Vata Pitta	*Yashti*	*Kalyanakaghrita Panchagavya Ghrita*
Vata Kapha	*Aswagandha, Brahmi, Vaca*	*Aswagandharishta Sarasvatarishta*
Pitta		*Tiktaka Ghrita*
Pitta Kapha	*Sankhapushpi, Mandukaparni*	
Kapha		
Tridosha	*Amalaki, Guduci, Jatamansi, Tagara Kushmanda*	*Mahatiktaka Ghrita* *Mahapanchagavya Ghrita Mahakalyanaka Ghrita* *Chyavanaprasa*

over bregma), different types of fomentations; and in specific five body purificatory procedures ie. *Vamana* (Therapeutic emesis), *Virechana* (Purgation), *Nasya* (Errhine), *Vasti* (Therapeutic enema) and *Raktamoksha* (Blood letting therapy) refer to *Panchakarma*. The potential of *Panchakarma* to stabilize *Dosha* (regulatory functional factors), strengthen and nourish *Dhatu* (major structural components) and to pacify and retard age-related biological changes is well established. These therapies promote cerebral and peripheral blood and lymphatic circulation which enables the efflux of toxins (Bredesen & Rao, 2017) (Ouchi et al., 2006). These detoxification procedures can be practised as a part of healthy regimen to balance the lifestyle and biorhythms. The group of *Panchakarma* which can effectively address psychological imbalances and also enhance mental wellbeing in geriatric population include *Abhyanga* (oil massage), *Udvartana* (powder massage), *Shirotala, Shirodhara* (Therapeutic streaming of medicated liquids), *Nasya*, *Virechana* etc. Clinical trials and case reports have established the efficacy of the combinations of Ayurvedic formulations and Panchakarma therapies in the management of psychotic disorders, mood disorders, neuropsychiatric conditions and stress related disorders (Dubey et al., 2010b).

Oil and powder massage can produce significant brain functional activation changes, increased cerebral blood flow, reduced stress hormone levels, facilitate the passage of solutes through blood brain barrier and hence it is recommended as a preventive and therapeutic strategy for neurodegenerative disorders, dementia, anxiety, stress esp. of *Vatapitta* phenotype or *Doshic* presentation (Keir, 2010) (Basler, 2011). *Shirotala* is the application of medicated powders or oils over the vertex which enhances cerebral circulation and produce relaxation. *Shirotala* with *Ksheerabala* oil, *Chandanadi* oil, *Kachuradi Churna, Panchagandha Churna,* powders of *Amalaki (Emblica officinalis), Usheera (Vettivera zizanoides)* etc. are being recommended for insomnia, anxiety, stress, psychosis etc (Kulamarva et al., 2023). Sujata Rajan et al., has demonstrated the effect of *Sirodhara* in improving serum biomarkers of stress – S. Cortisol and Dehydroepiandrosterone (DHEA), reduction of systolic and diastolic blood pressure and its appropriate responsiveness to stress system in a case report (Rajan et al., 2021). Antidepressant and effective neuroendocrine modulatory influence of *Ayurvedic* intervention along with *Sirodhara* in Major Depressive Disorder was demonstrated by Kishor et al (Kishore et al., 2014). *Sirodhara* has psycho-neuro-immunological effects such as a decrease in noradrenaline level, sympatholytic effect, activation of peripheral skin circulation, and increase level of natural killer cells (Uebaba et al., 2008).

Therapeutic purgation and nasal instillation are the major purificatory procedures which can be utilised in all types of psychological imbalances irrespective of the phenotype or *Doshic* state. As per *Ayurvedic* classics, purificatory procedures like *Virechana* and *Nasya* are contra-indicated after the age of 70 years and hence the methodology and duration of these procedures should be modified as per the strength and tolerance of the patient. Variability in phenotype or *Doshic* state will determine the drug selection as depicted in **Table No.4.** Prospects of *Nasya* in psycho neuro endocrinology can be derived from its CNS targeted drug delivery and significant action on hypothalamo-pituitary axis (HPA). Clinical trials have established the efficacy of *Nasya* alone and in combination with other Ayurvedic practices in conditions like insomnia (Bansal et al., 2020), positive symptoms of schizophrenia ("Effect of Madhookasaradi Nasya in the Management of Positive Symptoms of Schizophrenia," 2013), depressive disorder ("A Clinical Study to Evaluate the Efficacy of Nasya With Sarshapataila in Vishada (Depression)," 2020), stress reduction and improvement in cognitive functions (Verma et al., n.d.). A comprehensive *Ayurvedic* package including *Virechana* has shown complete remission for the symptoms of Major Depressive Disorder in a case study published by Basavaraj R Tubaki et al. (Tubaki et al., 2021). Though the mode of action of *Virechana* in systemic disorders is validated scientifically, its mechanism of action in psychological imbalances of elderly need more clarity through neurobiologically informed clinical trials.

Table 4. Doshic and phenotype-based selection of Panchakarma procedures for the management of psychological distress

Procedure	*Vata*	*Pitta*	*Kapha*
Massage	Oils - *Dhanvantara, Ksheerabala*	Oils – *Ksheerabala, Chandanadi*	Powders – *Kolakulathadi, Triphala*
Shirotala	Oil – *Dhanvantara,* Castor oil Powder - *Kachuradi, Panchagandha*	Powders – *Usheera, Amalaki, Kachuradi, Panchagandha* Oils - *Nimbamruteranda*	Castor oil Powder - *Rasnadi*
Shirodhara		Oils – *Ksheerabala, Chandanadi*	Oils - *Triphaladi, Asaneladi*
Nasya	Oils - *Anutaila, Dhanvantara, Ksheerabala*	Oils – *Ksheerabala, Chandanadi*	Powder – *Rasnadi* Leaf juice of Tulsi, Moringa

CONCLUSION

Extensive network of molecular interactions involved in ageing process underlines the necessity of holistic approach, rather than the reductionistic or target-based methods for delaying and reversing ageing process. Being one of the world's most authoritative holistic medicinal system, doctrines and programmes put forward by *Ayurveda* can be vigorously utilized for the mental well-being of elderly. Customised hypothetical model proposed in this chapter signifies the assessment of *Doshas* and *Prakriti* in predicting and preventing the health and disease states of body and mind and this put forwards a novel individualised approach for preserving mental health and for reducing health care burden. Implementation of community health programmes incorporating comprehensive Ayurvedic programme including dietary, lifestyle, behavioural, psychological and pharmacological interventions w.s.r to *Rasayana* Drugs and *Panchakarma* techniques can prolong healthspan successfully. Though clinical trials, experimental studies, systematic reviews and meta-analyses conducted in this field objectively measures the mechanism of action of these treatments, there is a large scope for conducting neurobiologically informed clinical research in psychogeriatrics which can help us in formulating standardized protocols of integrative approach, exploring potential drug candidates through transdisciplinary studies and to provide better outcomes in the mental health of geriatric population.

REFERENCES

Agarwal, A., Malini, S., Bairy, L. K., & Rao, M. S. (2002). EFFECT OF TINOSPORA CORDIFOLIA ON LEARNING AND MEMORY IN NORMAL AND MEMORY DEFICIT RATS. *Indian Journal of Pharmacology, 34*(5), 339–349. https://www.researchgate.net/profile/Laxminarayana_Bairy/publication/228366221_Effect_of_Tinospora_cardifolia_on_learning_and_memory_in_normal_and_memory_deficit_rats/links/00463514b28a457b90000000.pdf

Ahir, Y. (2005). *Clinico-experimental study of Kushmandadi Ghrita in Generalized Anxiety Disorder(DSM-IV) w.s.r.to Chittodvega.* IPGT and RA, Gujarat Ayurveda University, Jamnaga.

Akhgarjand, C., Asoudeh, F., Bagheri, A., Kalantar, Z., Vahabi, Z., Shab-Bidar, S., Rezvani, H., & Djafarian, K. (2022). Does Ashwagandha supplementation have a beneficial effect on the management of anxiety and stress? A systematic review and meta-analysis of randomized controlled trials. *Phytotherapy Research, 36*(11), 4115–4124. doi:10.1002/ptr.7598 PMID:36017529

Anand, T., Naika, M., Phani, K. G., & Khanum, F. (2010). Antioxidant and DNA Damage Preventive Properties of Centella asiatica (L) Urb. *Pharmacognosy Journal, 2*(17), 53–58. doi:10.1016/S0975-3575(10)80010-0

Ayurvedic Pharmacoepia of India. (2016). Dept. of AYUSH, Ministry of Health and Family Welfare, Govt. of India.

Ayyathan, D. M., Chandrasekaran, R., & Kalaivani, T. (2015). Neuroprotective effect of Tagara, an Ayurvedic drug against methyl mercury induced oxidative stress using rat brain mitochondrial fractions. *BMC Complementary and Alternative Medicine, 15*(1), 268. doi:10.118612906-015-0793-2 PMID:26264039

Bansal, C., Upadhyay, A., & Shukla, U. (2020). Efficacy of Brimhana Nasya and Ashwagandha (Withania somnifera (L.) Dunal) root powder in primary insomnia in elderly male: A randomized open-label clinical study. *Ayu, 41*(3), 159. doi:10.4103/ayu.AYU_177_19 PMID:35370376

Basler, A. J. (2011). Pilot Study Investigating the Effects of Ayurvedic *Abhyanga* Massage on Subjective Stress Experience. *Journal of Alternative and Complementary Medicine (New York, N.Y.), 17*(5), 435–440. doi:10.1089/acm.2010.0281 PMID:21568717

Behere, P. B., Das, A., Yadav, R., & Behere, A. P. (2013). Ayurvedic concepts related to psychotherapy. *Indian Journal of Psychiatry, 55*(6), 310. doi:10.4103/0019-5545.105556 PMID:23858273

Bhargav, H., Jasti, N., More, P., Kumar, V., Chikkanna, U., Kumar, R. K., & Varambally, S. (2021). Correlation of prakriti diagnosis using AyuSoft prakriti diagnostic tool with clinician rating in patients with psychiatric disorders. *Journal of Ayurveda and Integrative Medicine, 12*(2), 365–368. doi:10.1016/j.jaim.2021.01.012 PMID:33750638

Bhatnagar, M., Sisodia, S. S., & Bhatnagar, R. (2005). Antiulcer and Antioxidant Activity of Asparagus racemosus WILLD and Withania somnifera DUNAL in Rats. *Annals of the New York Academy of Sciences, 1056*(1), 261–278. doi:10.1196/annals.1352.027 PMID:16387694

Bhovi, P., Hegde, R., K., S., & D'Souza, V. (2020). A Clinical Study To Evaluate The Efficacy Of Nasya With Sarshapataila In Vishada (Depression). *International Ayurvedic Medical Journal.*

Boffetta, P., & Collatuzzo, G. (2022). Application of P4 (Predictive, Preventive, Personalized, Participatory) approach to Occupational Medicine. *PubMed, 113*(1), e2022009. doi:10.23749/mdl.v113i1.12622 PMID:35226650

Bredesen, D. E., & Rao, R. V. (2017). Ayurvedic profiling of Alzheimer's disease. *PubMed, 23*(3), 46–50. https://pubmed.ncbi.nlm.nih.gov/28236613

Charak Samhita. (n.d.). SBP Nirnay Sagar.

Charak Samhita: Vol. Sutrasthana. (1998). Chaukhamba Bharti Academy. [Hindi]

Charaka Samhita. (1998a). Chaukhamba Bharti Academy.

Charaka Samhita: Vol. Sutrasthana. (1998b). Chaukhambha Bharati Academy. [Hindi]

Chatterjee, B., & Pancholi, J. (2011). Prakriti -based medicine: A step towards personalized medicine. *Ayu, 32*(2), 141. doi:10.4103/0974-8520.92539 PMID:22408293

Chavan, S. (2013). Approach towards life style modification plan as per ayurveda and modern technique for prevention of geriatrics. *Int Res J Pharm.*

D'cruz, M., & Andrade, C. (2022). Potential clinical applications of Ashwagandha (*Withania somnifera*) in medicine and neuropsychiatry. *Expert Review of Clinical Pharmacology, 15*(9), 1067–1080. doi:10.1080/17512433.2022.2121699 PMID:36062480

Devi, U. K., & Swarup, A. (2000). Evaluation of Clinical Efficacy of Menotab in Alleviating Symptoms of Menopausal Syndrome: Phase III Open Clinical Trial. *The Antiseptic, 98*. https://www.himalayawellness.com/pdf_files/menosan001.pdf

Dhingra, D., Parle, M., & Sk, K. (2004). Memory enhancing activity of Glycyrrhiza glabra in mice. *Journal of Ethnopharmacology, 91*(2–3), 361–365. doi:10.1016/j.jep.2004.01.016 PMID:15120462

Dhingra, D., & Sharma, A. (2006). Antidepressant-like activity of Glycyrrhiza glabra L. in mouse models of immobility tests. *Progress in Neuro-Psychopharmacology & Biological Psychiatry, 30*(3), 449–454. doi:10.1016/j.pnpbp.2005.11.019 PMID:16443316

Dubey, S., Tripathi, J. N., Gupta, S., & Reddy, K. R. C. (2010). A comparative clinical trial on the role of Panchakarma therapy and Unmada Gajankusha Rasa in the cases of major depressive disorder vis-à-vis kaphaja Unmada. *Ayu, 31*(2), 205. doi:10.4103/0974-8520.72396 PMID:22131711

Bhat, R. (2013). Effect of Madhookasaradi Nasya in the Management of Positive Symptoms of Schizophrenia. *Int. J. Ayu. Alt. Med, 1.*

Ghodke-Puranik, Y., Joshi, K., & Patwardhan, B. (2011). Traditional Medicine to Modern Pharmacogenomics: Ayurveda*Prakriti*Type and CYP2C19 Gene Polymorphism Associated with the Metabolic Variability. *Evidence-Based Complementary and Alternative Medicine, 1–5*, 1–5. doi:10.1093/ecam/nep206

Gómez-Pinilla, F. (2008). Brain foods: The effects of nutrients on brain function. *Nature Reviews. Neuroscience, 9*(7), 568–578. doi:10.1038/nrn2421 PMID:18568016

Gordon, J. S. (1982). Holistic medicine: advances and shortcomings. *PubMed, 136*(6), 546–551. https://pubmed.ncbi.nlm.nih.gov/7113200

Goyal, M. (2018). *Rasayana* in perspective of the present scenario. *Ayu, 39*(2), 63. doi:10.4103/ayu.AYU_300_18 PMID:30783358

Gupta, P. (2015). Pharmacogenetics, Pharmacogenomics and Ayurgenomics for Personalized Medicine: a Paradigm Shift. *Indian J. Pharm. Sci., 77*(2). doi:10.4103/0250-474X.156543

Huang, Z., Chavda, V. P., Bezbaruah, R., Uversky, V. N., Sucharitha, P., Patel, A., & Chen, Z. (2022a). An Ayurgenomics Approach: Prakriti-Based Drug Discovery and Development for Personalized care. *Frontiers in Pharmacology, 13*, 866827. doi:10.3389/fphar.2022.866827 PMID:35431922

Huang, Z., Chavda, V. P., Bezbaruah, R., Uversky, V. N., Sucharitha, P., Patel, A., & Chen, Z. (2022b). An Ayurgenomics Approach: Prakriti-Based Drug Discovery and Development for Personalized care. *Frontiers in Pharmacology, 13*, 866827. doi:10.3389/fphar.2022.866827 PMID:35431922

Jm, G., Brar, J. S., Rai, A., & Knr, C. (2019). Effects of a standardized extract of Withania somnifera (Ashwagandha) on depression and anxiety symptoms in persons with schizophrenia participating in a randomized, placebo-controlled clinical trial. *PubMed, 31*(2), 123–129. https://pubmed.ncbi.nlm.nih.gov/31046033

Juyal, R. C., Negi, S., Wakhode, P., Bhat, S., Bhat, B., & Thelma, B. (2012). Potential of Ayurgenomics Approach in Complex Trait Research: Leads from a Pilot Study on Rheumatoid Arthritis. *PLoS One, 7*(9), e45752. doi:10.1371/journal.pone.0045752 PMID:23049851

Karkada, G., Shenoy, K., Halahalli, H. N., & Karanth, K. S. (2012). Nardostachys jatamansi extract prevents chronic restraint stress-induced learning and memory deficits in a radial arm maze task. *Journal of Natural Science, Biology, and Medicine, 3*(2), 125. doi:10.4103/0976-9668.101879 PMID:23225973

Keir, S. T. (2010). Effect of massage therapy on stress levels and quality of life in brain tumor patients—Observations from a pilot study. *Supportive Care in Cancer, 19*(5), 711–715. doi:10.100700520-010-1032-5 PMID:21046417

Kilamarva, K. (1994). Clinical evaluation of Smrtisagararasa in cases of residual schizophrenia. *J Research Ayurveda Siddha, 15.*

Kishore, R. K., Ashok, A. H., Udupa, K., Thirthalli, J., Lavekar, G. S., Gangadhar, B. N., Raju, T., & Sathyaprabha, T. (2014). Evaluation of the influence of ayurvedic formulation (Ayushman-15) on psychopathology, heart rate variability and stress hormonal level in major depression (Vishada). *Asian Journal of Psychiatry, 12*, 100–107. doi:10.1016/j.ajp.2014.07.002 PMID:25219946

Kongkeaw, C., Dilokthornsakul, P., Thanarangsarit, P., Limpeanchob, N., & Scholfield, C. N. (2014). Meta-analysis of randomized controlled trials on cognitive effects of Bacopa monnieri extract. *Journal of Ethnopharmacology, 151*(1), 528–535. doi:10.1016/j.jep.2013.11.008 PMID:24252493

Koo, B., Park, K., Ha, J., Park, J. H., Lim, J., & Lee, D. (2003). Inhibitory Effects of the Fragrance Inhalation of Essential Oil from Acorus gramineus on Central Nervous System. *Biological & Pharmaceutical Bulletin, 26*(7), 978–982. doi:10.1248/bpb.26.978 PMID:12843622

Kulamarva, K., Shivakumar, V., Chikkanna, U., Ramakrishna, K. K., Bhargav, H., & Varambally, S. (2023, May). Role of Ayurveda in the management of psychotic disorders: A systematic review of clinical evidence. *Journal of Ayurveda and Integrative Medicine, 14*(3), 100720. doi:10.1016/j.jaim.2023.100720 PMID:37290315

Kulamarva, K., Shivakumar, V., Chikkanna, U., Ramakrishna, K. K., Bhargav, H., & Varambally, S. (2023). Role of Ayurveda in the management of psychotic disorders: A systematic review of clinical evidence. *Journal of Ayurveda and Integrative Medicine, 14*(3), 100720. doi:10.1016/j.jaim.2023.100720 PMID:37290315

Kulkarni, R., Girish, K., & Kumar, A. (2012a). Nootropic herbs (Medhya Rasayana) in Ayurveda: An update. *Pharmacognosy Reviews, 6*(12), 147. doi:10.4103/0973-7847.99949 PMID:23055641

Kulkarni, R., Girish, K., & Kumar, A. (2012b). Nootropic herbs (Medhya Rasayana) in Ayurveda: An update. *Pharmacognosy Reviews*, *6*(12), 147. doi:10.4103/0973-7847.99949 PMID:23055641

Kulkarni, R. (1995). Synergetic effect of Vallarai and Brahmi on learning ability of albino mice and school children. *International Seminar on Recent Trends in Pharmaceutical Sciences.*

Kumar, A., & Sk, K. (2006). Protective effect of BR-16A, a polyherbal preparation against social isolation stress: Possible GABAergic mechanism. *Phytotherapy Research*, *20*(7), 538–541. doi:10.1002/ptr.1873 PMID:16691632

Kumar, V. (2006). Potential medicinal plants for CNS disorders: An overview. *Phytotherapy Research*, *20*(12), 1023–1035. doi:10.1002/ptr.1970 PMID:16909441

Lai, X., Liang, H., & Zhao, Y. (2002). A survey of the studies on chemical constituents and pharmacological activities of Acorus plants. *PubMed*, *27*(3), 161–165, 198. https://pubmed.ncbi.nlm.nih.gov/12807142

Li, Y., Wu, L., Chang, C., Wang, L., Guo, C., Zhao, X., Zhao, T., Wang, X., Liu, A., & Zhang, Y. (2020). Serum Metabolic Profiling Reveals the Antidepressive Effects of the Total Iridoids of Valeriana jatamansi Jones on Chronic Unpredictable Mild Stress Mice. *Frontiers in Pharmacology*, *11*, 338. doi:10.3389/fphar.2020.00338 PMID:32265710

Lim, S. J. (2007). Effects of fractions of Benincasa hispida on antioxidant status in Streptozotocin induced Diabetic rats. *Korean J Nutr, 40.*

Marrie, R. A., Walld, R., Bolton, J. M., Sareen, J., Walker, J. R., Patten, S. B., Singer, A., Lix, L. M., Hitchon, C., El-Gabalawy, R., Katz, A., Fisk, J. D., & Bernstein, Ç. N. (2017a). Increased incidence of psychiatric disorders in immune-mediated inflammatory disease. *Journal of Psychosomatic Research*, *101*, 17–23. doi:10.1016/j.jpsychores.2017.07.015 PMID:28867419

Marrie, R. A., Walld, R., Bolton, J. M., Sareen, J., Walker, J. R., Patten, S. B., Singer, A., Lix, L. M., Hitchon, C., El-Gabalawy, R., Katz, A., Fisk, J. D., & Bernstein, Ç. N. (2017b). Increased incidence of psychiatric disorders in immune-mediated inflammatory disease. *Journal of Psychosomatic Research*, *101*, 17–23. doi:10.1016/j.jpsychores.2017.07.015 PMID:28867419

Mills, P. J., Peterson, C. T., Wilson, K., Pung, M. A., Patel, S. V., Weiss, L., Kshirsagar, S. G., Tanzi, R. E., & Chopra, D. (2019). Relationships among classifications of ayurvedic medicine diagnostics for imbalances and western measures of psychological states: An exploratory study. *Journal of Ayurveda and Integrative Medicine*, *10*(3), 198–202. doi:10.1016/j.jaim.2018.02.001 PMID:30385015

Montiel-Castro, A. J., González-Cervantes, R. M., Bravo-Ruiseco, G., & Pacheco-López, G. (2013). The microbiota-gut-brain axis: Neurobehavioral correlates, health and sociality. *Frontiers in Integrative Neuroscience*, *7*. doi:10.3389/fnint.2013.00070 PMID:24109440

Morgan, A. K., & Stevens, J. D. (2010). Does *Bacopa monnieri* Improve Memory Performance in Older Persons? Results of a Randomized, Placebo-Controlled, Double-Blind Trial. *Journal of Alternative and Complementary Medicine (New York, N.Y.)*, *16*(7), 753–759. doi:10.1089/acm.2009.0342 PMID:20590480

Mukherjee, P. K., Venkatesan, K., Mal, M., & Houghton, P. J. (2007). *In vitro* Acetylcholinesterase Inhibitory Activity of the Essential Oil from *Acorus calamus* and its Main Constituents. *Planta Medica, 73*(3), 283–285. doi:10.1055-2007-967114 PMID:17286241

Ninivaggi, F. (2010). *A comprehensive guide to traditional Indian medicine for the west-anatomy* (Vol. 3). Rowman & Littlefield Publishers.

Ouchi, Y., Kanno, T., Okada, H., Yoshikawa, E., Shinke, T., Nagasawa, S., Minoda, K., & Doi, H. (2006). Changes in cerebral blood flow under the prone condition with and without massage. *Neuroscience Letters, 407*(2), 131–135. doi:10.1016/j.neulet.2006.08.037 PMID:16973270

Panara, K., Nariya, M., & Nishteswar, K. (2020). Central nervous system depressant activity of Jatamansi (Nardostachys jatamansi DC.) rhizome. *Ayu, 41*(4), 250. doi:10.4103/ayu.AYU_251_20 PMID:35813358

Patil, M. & Patwardhan, B. (1997). Antistress activity of Tinospora cordifolia (Willd) Meirs. *Indian Drugs, 34*. https://api.semanticscholar.org/Corpus

Prabhu, J., Prabhu, K., Chaudhuri, A., Rao, M. R. K., Selvi, V., Balaji, T., & Dinakar, S. (2020). Neuroprotective effect of Ayurveda formulation, Saraswatharishtam, on scopolamine induced memory impairment in animal model. *Pharmacognosy Journal, 12*(1), 6–13. doi:10.5530/pj.2020.12.2

Prasher, B., Negi, S., Aggarwal, S., Mandal, A. K., Sethi, T., Deshmukh, S., Purohit, S. G., Sengupta, S., Khanna, S., Mohammad, F., Garg, G., Brahmachari, S. K., & Mukerji, M. (2008a). Whole genome expression and biochemical correlates of extreme constitutional types defined in Ayurveda. *Journal of Translational Medicine, 6*(1), 48. doi:10.1186/1479-5876-6-48 PMID:18782426

Prasher, B., Negi, S., Aggarwal, S., Mandal, A. K., Sethi, T., Deshmukh, S., Purohit, S. G., Sengupta, S., Khanna, S., Mohammad, F., Garg, G., Brahmachari, S. K., & Mukerji, M. (2008b). Whole genome expression and biochemical correlates of extreme constitutional types defined in Ayurveda. *Journal of Translational Medicine, 6*(1), 48. doi:10.1186/1479-5876-6-48 PMID:18782426

Prince, P. S. M., & Menon, V. P. (2001). Antioxidant action ofTinospora cordifolia root extract in alloxan diabetic rats. *Phytotherapy Research, 15*(3), 213–218. doi:10.1002/ptr.707 PMID:11351355

Purvya, M. C., & Meena, M. (2011). A review on role of prakriti in aging. *Ayu, 32*(1), 20. doi:10.4103/0974-8520.85719 PMID:22131753

Raghav, S., Singh, H., Dalal, P. K., Srivastava, J. S., & Asthana, O. P. (2006). Randomized controlled trial of standardized Bacopa monniera extract in age-associated memory impairment. *Indian Journal of Psychiatry, 48*(4), 238. doi:10.4103/0019-5545.31555 PMID:20703343

Rajan, S., Shamkuwar, M. K., & Tanwar, A. K. (2021). Impact of Shirodhara on biological markers of stress: A case study. *Journal of Ayurveda and Integrative Medicine, 12*(1), 178–181. doi:10.1016/j.jaim.2021.01.008 PMID:33637424

Ramanathan, M. (2007). Neuroprotective evaluation of standardized extracts of Centella asiatica in monosodium glutamate treated rats. *Indian J Exp Biol., 45*.

Rao, K. G. M., Rao, S., & Rao, S. (2006). Centella asiatica (L.) Leaf Extract Treatment During the Growth Spurt Period Enhances Hippocampal CA3 Neuronal Dendritic Arborization in Rats. *Evidence-Based Complementary and Alternative Medicine*, *3*(3), 349–357. doi:10.1093/ecam/nel024 PMID:16951719

Rao, R. V. (2018). Ayurveda and the science of aging. *Journal of Ayurveda and Integrative Medicine*, *9*(3), 225–232. doi:10.1016/j.jaim.2017.10.002 PMID:29276113

Rotti, H., Guruprasad, K. P., Nayak, J., Kabekkodu, S. P., Kukreja, H., Mallya, S., Nayak, J. N., Bhradwaj, R. C., Gangadharan, G. G., Prasanna, B. V., Raval, R., Kamath, A., Gopinath, P. M., Kondaiah, P., & Satyamoorthy, K. (2014). Immunophenotyping of normal individuals classified on the basis of human dosha prakriti. *Journal of Ayurveda and Integrative Medicine*, *5*(1), 43. doi:10.4103/0975-9476.128857 PMID:24812475

Rotti, H., Raval, R., Anchan, S., Bellampalli, R., Bhale, S., Bharadwaj, R., Bhat, B. K., Dedge, A. P., Dhumal, V. R., Gangadharan, G. G., Girijakumari, T. K., Gopinath, P. M., Govindaraj, P., Halder, S., Joshi, K., Kabekkodu, S. P., Kamath, A., Kondaiah, P., Kukreja, H., & Valiathan, M. V. S. (2014). Determinants of Prakriti, the Human Constitution Types of Indian Traditional Medicine and its Correlation with Contemporary Science. *Journal of Ayurveda and Integrative Medicine*, *5*(3), 166. doi:10.4103/0975-9476.140478 PMID:25336848

Samarakoon, S., Chandola, H., & Ravishankar, B. (2011). Effect of dietary, social, and lifestyle determinants of accelerated aging and its common clinical presentation: A survey study. *Ayu*, *32*(3), 315. doi:10.4103/0974-8520.93906 PMID:22529643

Seminar on research in Ayurveda and Sidha. (1995). CCRAS.

Sharma, P. (2005). *Database on Medicinal plants used in Ayurveda and Sidha* (Vol. 1). CCRAS, Dept. of AYUSH, Ministry of Health and Family Welfare, Govt. of India.

Shukla, P. K., Khanna, V. K., Ali, M. M., Maurya, R., Khan, M. Y., & Srimal, R. C. (2006). Neuroprotective effect of Acorus calamus against middle cerebral artery occlusion–induced ischaemia in rat. *Human and Experimental Toxicology*, *25*(4), 187–194. doi:10.1191/0960327106ht613oa PMID:16696294

Singh, R., Banerjee, S., Kumar, P., Raveesha, K. A., & Rao, A. (2006). Tinospora cordifolia induces enzymes of carcinogen/drug metabolism and antioxidant system, and inhibits lipid peroxidation in mice. *Phytomedicine*, *13*(1–2), 74–84. doi:10.1016/j.phymed.2004.02.013 PMID:16360936

Singh, R. P., Narsimhamurthy, K., & Singh, G. (2008). Neuronutrient impact of Ayurvedic Rasayana therapy in brain aging. *Biogerontology*, *9*(6), 369–374. doi:10.100710522-008-9185-z PMID:18931935

Sinha, P., Hussain, T., Boora, N. K., Rao, G. N., Varghese, M., Gururaj, G., & Benegal, V. (2021). Prevalence of Common mental disorders in older adults: Results from the National Mental Health Survey of India. *Asian Journal of Psychiatry*, *55*, 102463. doi:10.1016/j.ajp.2020.102463 PMID:33212298

Skoog, I. (2011). Psychiatric disorders in the elderly. *Canadian Journal of Psychiatry*, *56*(7), 387–397. doi:10.1177/070674371105600702 PMID:21835102

Tiwari, P., & Patel, R. (2013). Estimation of total phenolics and flavonoids and antioxidant potential of ashwagandharishta prepared by traditional and modern methods. *Asian Journal of Pharmaceutical Analysis*, *3*(4), 147–152. https://www.indianjournals.com/ijor.aspx?target=ijor:ajpa&volume=3&issue=4&article=009&type=pdf

Tiwari, S. K., & Pandey, N. M. (2012). Status and requirements of geriatric mental health services in India: An evidence-based commentary. *Indian Journal of Psychiatry*, *54*(1), 8. doi:10.4103/0019-5545.94639 PMID:22556431

Toolika, E., Bhat, N. P., & Shetty, S. K. (2015). A comparative clinical study on the effect of Tagara (Valeriana wallichii DC.) and Jatamansi (Nardostachys jatamansi DC.) in the management of Anidra (primary insomnia). *Ayu*, *36*(1), 46. doi:10.4103/0974-8520.169008 PMID:26730138

Tripathi, J., & Singh, R. (1994). Concept of deha prakriti vis-à-vis human constitution in ayurveda. *PubMed*. https://pubmed.ncbi.nlm.nih.gov/22556666

Tubaki, B. R., Chandake, S., & Sarhyal, A. (2021). Ayurveda management of Major Depressive Disorder: A case study. *Journal of Ayurveda and Integrative Medicine*, *12*(2), 378–383. doi:10.1016/j.jaim.2021.03.012 PMID:34024690

Uebaba, K., Xu, F., Ogawa, H., Tatsuse, T., Wang, B., Hisajima, T., & Venkatraman, S. (2008). Psychoneuroimmunologic effects of Ayurvedic Oil-Dripping Treatment. *Journal of Alternative and Complementary Medicine (New York, N.Y.)*, *14*(10), 1189–1198. doi:10.1089/acm.2008.0273 PMID:19123874

Verma, K., Deepeshwar, S., & Srivastava, A. (n.d.). Comparative impact of yoga and ayurveda practice in insomnia: A randomized controlled trial. *PubMed*, *12*, 160. doi:10.4103/jehp.jehp_1489_22 PMID:37404923

World Health Organization. (2022). *Ageing and health*. WHO. https://www.who.int/news-room/fact-sheets/detail/ageing-and-health

Yadav, D. (2014a). *Ashtangahridaya: Vol. Sutra Sthana. Ch.13, Ver. 1-12*. Chaukhamba Surbharati Prakashan.

Yadav, D. (2014b). *Ashtangahridaya: Vol. Sutrasthana, Chapter 1, Ver. 6,20*. [Sanskrit]. Chaukhambha Subharati Prakashan.

Compilation of References

Aakash. (2021). *Introduction to the Indian Psychology concept.* Mantracare. https://mantracare.org/therapy/therapy-types/indian-psychology

Acharya, P. S. S. (2003). *Eternity of Sound and the Science of Mantras.* Shri Vedmata Gayatri Trust-Uttarakhand.

Adams, G. A., & Webster, J. R. (2021, November 18). Relating supervisor interpersonal emotion management- and task-oriented leadership to adaptive performance: A moderated-mediation model incorporating trust and gender. *Equality, Diversity and Inclusion: An International Journal.* https://www.emerald.com/insight/content/doi/10.1108/EDI-07-2021-0174/full/html

Adams, G., Kurtiş, T., Ordóñez, L. G., Molina, L. E., & Oropeza, I. D. (2018). Decolonizing Knowledge in Hegemonic Psychological Science. In N. N. Wane & K. L. Todd (Eds.), *Decolonial Pedagogy: Examining Sites of Resistance, Resurgence, and Renewal* (pp. 35–53). Springer International Publishing. doi:10.1007/978-3-030-01539-8_3

Adey, P., Csapó, B., Demetriou, A., Hautamäki, J., & Shayer, M. (2007). Can we be intel-ligent about intelligence? Why education needs the concept of plastic general ability. *Educational Research Review, 2*(2), 75–97. doi:10.1016/j.edurev.2007.05.001

Adgadanand, S. (2010). *Maharishi Patanjali's - Yog-Darshan: Yoga Sūtras of Patañjali.* Shree Paramhans Swami Adgadanandji Ashram Trust.

Aditya, A. (2020). Counselling in an Ancient Hindu text: A case for CBT in the Sri MadSrimad Bhagavad Gita Focusing on Arjuna's Distress. The European Journal of Social &Behavioural Sciences, *XXVIII*, 2301–2218.

Agarwal, A., & Agarwal, A. (2013). Impact of mantra chanting on stress coping. *Indian Journal of Positive Psychology, 4*(1), 96.

Agarwal, A., Malini, S., Bairy, L. K., & Rao, M. S. (2002). EFFECT OF TINOSPORA CORDIFOLIA ON LEARNING AND MEMORY IN NORMAL AND MEMORY DEFICIT RATS. *Indian Journal of Pharmacology, 34*(5), 339–349. https://www.researchgate.net/profile/Laxminarayana_Bairy/publication/228366221_Effect_of_Tinospora_cardifolia_on_learning_and_memory_in_normal_and_memory_deficit_rats/links/00463514b28a457b90000000.pdf

Agarwalla, S., Seshadri, B., & Krishnan, V. R. (2015). Impact of Gunas and Karma Yoga on Transformational Leadership. *Journal of Human Values, 21*(1), 11–22. doi:10.1177/0971685815569590

Agrawal, J., & Cornelissen, R. M. (2020). *Yoga and positive mental health.* OSF.

Agrawal, J. (2021). Sattva enhancement therapy: An illustrative report. *Indian Journal of Clinical Psychology, 48*(2), 3–6.

Ahir, Y. (2005). *Clinico-experimental study of Kushmandadi Ghrita in Generalized Anxiety Disorder(DSM-IV) w.s.r.to Chittodvega.* IPGT and RA, Gujarat Ayurveda University, Jamnaga.

Ahmad, A., Khan, M. U., Kumar, B. D., Kumar, G. S., Rodriguez, S. P., & Patel, I. (2015). Beliefs, attitudes and selfuse of Ayurveda, Yoga and Naturopathy, Unani, Siddha, and Homeopathy medicines among senior pharmacy students: An exploratory insight from Andhra Pradesh, India. *Pharmacognosy Research, 7*(4). PMID:26692742

Ahmed, I. (2020, February 17). How To Achieve Mindfulness In Islam. *The Siasat Daily*. https://www.siasat.com/how-achieve-mindfulness-islam-1828249/

Aich, T. K. (2013). Buddha philosophy and Western psychology. *Indian Journal of Psychiatry, 55*(6), 165. doi:10.4103/0019-5545.105517 PMID:23858249

Aishe. (2021). Rise in Number of Foreign Students Studying in India, BTech Most opted Course. *News18*. https://www.news18.com/news/education-career/rise-in-number-of-foreign-students-studying-in-india-rises-btech-most-opted-course-3863621.html

Akhgarjand, C., Asoudeh, F., Bagheri, A., Kalantar, Z., Vahabi, Z., Shab-Bidar, S., Rezvani, H., & Djafarian, K. (2022). Does Ashwagandha supplementation have a beneficial effect on the management of anxiety and stress? A systematic review and meta-analysis of randomized controlled trials. *Phytotherapy Research, 36*(11), 4115–4124. doi:10.1002/ptr.7598 PMID:36017529

Akthar, S. E. (2005). *Freud along the Ganges psychoanalytical reflections on the people and culture of India*. Rave Media.

Al-Farabi, A. N. (1995). *Tahsil Al-Sa'ada* [Attainment of Happiness]. Ja'far Al Yasin.

All About Sikhs. (2017, February 12). The Sikh Perspective Of Meditation. *Gateway to Sikhism*. https://www.allaboutsikhs.com/scriptures/guru-granth-sahib/the-sikh-perspective-of-meditation/

Allen, M. N., & Jensen, L. (1990). Hermeneutical inquiry meaning and scope. *Western Journal of Nursing Research, 12*(2), 241–253. doi:10.1177/019394599001200209 PMID:2321377

American Psychiatric Association. (2013). *Diagnostic and Statistical Manual of Mental Disorders* (5th ed.). American Psychiatric Association Publishing., DSM-5.

Anālayo, B. (2022). Eightfold Path in Early Buddhism. Springer eBooks. doi:10.1007/978-3-030-90465-4_38-1

Anand, T., Naika, M., Phani, K. G., & Khanum, F. (2010). Antioxidant and DNA Damage Preventive Properties of Centella asiatica (L) Urb. *Pharmacognosy Journal, 2*(17), 53–58. doi:10.1016/S0975-3575(10)80010-0

Andrade, C. (2008). The National Institute of Open Schooling. *Indian Journal of Psychiatry, 50*(3), 227–228. doi:10.4103/0019-5545.43618 PMID:19742229

Andrews, C. F. (1938). An open-air school. *Visva-Bharati News. Bulletin*, 1930.

Antić, A. (2021). Transcultural Psychiatry: Cultural Difference, Universalism and Social Psychiatry in the Age of Decolonisation. *Culture, Medicine and Psychiatry, 45*(3), 359–384. doi:10.100711013-021-09719-4 PMID:33905076

Anuradha, M. V., & Kumar, Y. L. N. (2015). Trigunas in organizations: Moving toward an east-west synthesis. *International Journal of Cross Cultural Management, 15*(2), 195–214. doi:10.1177/1470595815594636

Apolinário-Hagen, J., Drüge, M., & Fritsche, L. (2020). Cognitive behavioural therapy, mindfulness-based cognitive therapy and acceptance commitment therapy for anxiety disorders: integrating traditional with digital treatment approaches. *Anxiety Disorders: Rethinking and Understanding Recent Discoveries*, (pp. 291-329). Springer. https://link.springer.com/chapter/10.1007/978-981-32-9705-0_17

Apte, V. S. (Ed.). (1975). The practical Sanskrit – English dictionary. (4 th Ed.). Delhi: Motilal Banarsidass.

Arrowsmith, J., & Parker, J. (2013). The meaning of 'employee engagement' for the values and roles of the HRM function. *International Journal of Human Resource Management, 24*(14), 2692–2712. doi:10.1080/09585192.2013.763842

Ashmos, D. P., & Duchon, D. (2000). Spirituality at Work: A Conceptualization and Measure. *Journal of Management Inquiry, 9*(2), 134–145. doi:10.1177/105649260092008

Atwal, S. (2010). *Indian psychology: The connection between mind, body, and the universe*. Pepperdine University.

Avasthi, A., Kate, N., & Grover, S. (2013). Indianization of psychiatry utilizing Indian mental concepts. *Indian Journal of Psychiatry, 55*(6, Suppl 2), S136–S144. doi:10.4103/0019-5545.105508 PMID:23858244

Ayurvedic Pharmacoepia of India. (2016). Dept. of AYUSH, Ministry of Health and Family Welfare, Govt. of India.

Ayyathan, D. M., Chandrasekaran, R., & Kalaivani, T. (2015). Neuroprotective effect of Tagara, an Ayurvedic drug against methyl mercury induced oxidative stress using rat brain mitochondrial fractions. *BMC Complementary and Alternative Medicine, 15*(1), 268. doi:10.118612906-015-0793-2 PMID:26264039

Baer, R. A., Smith, G. T., Hopkins, J., Krietemeyer, J., & Toney, L. (2006). Using self-report assessment methods to explore facets of mindfulness. *Assessment, 13*(1), 27–45. doi:10.1177/1073191105283504 PMID:16443717

Bajaj, B., Gupta, R., & Sengupta, S. (2018, October 19). Emotional Stability and Self-Esteem as Mediators Between Mindfulness and Happiness. *Journal of Happiness Studies*. Advance online publication. doi:10.100710902-018-0046-4

Bajpai, P., Yadav, R., & Tripathi, M. (2019). Srimad Bhagavad Gita: A path leading to Consciousness andSelf Realization. *Journal of Emerging Technologies and Innovative Research, 6*(3), 351–356.

Bala, S. (2005). Gandhian conception of education – It's relevance in present times. *Indian Journal of Poultry Science, 66*(3), 531–548.

Balasubramaniam, M., Telles, S., & Doraiswamy, P. M. (2013a). Yoga on Our Minds: A Systematic Review of Yoga for Neuropsychiatric Disorders. *Frontiers in Psychiatry, 3*. https://www.frontiersin.org/articles/10.3389/fpsyt.2012.00117

Baldo, J. V., Schendel, K., Lewis, S. J., Herron, T. J., Dempsey, D. G., Muir, J. J., Curran, B., Paulraj, S., Chok, J. M., & Cole, M. (2021). Mindfulness-Based Stress Reduction Intervention in Chronic Stroke: A Randomized, Controlled Pilot Study. *Mindfulness, 12*(12), 2908–2919. doi:10.100712671-021-01751-0

Balkrishna, V., Sanghvi, L. D., Rana, K., Doongaji, D. R., & Vahia, N. S. (1977). The comparison of psychophysiological therapy with drug therapy. *Indian Journal of Psychiatry, 19*, 87–89.

Balodhi, J. P. (Ed.). (1984). *Relationship of Ithihasa and Puranas to Vedas: Our Vedic Heritage* (pp. 64–68). Chinmayanada Mission.

Balodi, G., & Raina, D. (2014). A comparative study of emotional maturity and values in Bhagavad Gita readers and non-readers. *Indian Journal of Positive Psychology, 5*(4), 415.

Banerjee, N., Das, A., & Ghosh, M. S. (2021). National Educational Policy (2020): A critical analysis. *Towards Excellence*, 13(3).

Bangalore, N. G. (2012). Yoga therapy for Schizophrenia. *International Journal of Yoga, 5*(2), 85–91. doi:10.4103/0973-6131.98212 PMID:22869990

Bansal, C., Upadhyay, A., & Shukla, U. (2020). Efficacy of Brimhana Nasya and Ashwagandha (Withania somnifera (L.) Dunal) root powder in primary insomnia in elderly male: A randomized open-label clinical study. *Ayu, 41*(3), 159. doi:10.4103/ayu.AYU_177_19 PMID:35370376

Baron, R. A., Mueller, B. A., & Wolfe, M. T. (2016). Self-efficacy and entrepreneurs' adoption of unattainable goals: The restraining effects of self-control. *Journal of Business Venturing*, *31*(1), 55–71. doi:10.1016/j.jbusvent.2015.08.002

Basler, A. J. (2011). Pilot Study Investigating the Effects of Ayurvedic *Abhyanga* Massage on Subjective Stress Experience. *Journal of Alternative and Complementary Medicine (New York, N.Y.)*, *17*(5), 435–440. doi:10.1089/acm.2010.0281 PMID:21568717

Bates, T. C., Enkhbat, T., Gray, E., Lee, J., & Zakharin, M. (2023, July 14). How to get things done: Tight linkage of conscientiousness with twelve mechanisms of goal setting theory. *Personality and Individual Differences*. Science Direct. https://www.sciencedirect.com/science/article/pii/S0191886923002544

Baykal, E. (2022). The Relationship Between Spiritual Well-Being and Life Satisfaction During COVID-19. In Handbook of Research on Interdisciplinary Perspectives on the Threats and Impacts of Pandemics (pp. 425-443). IGI Global.

Baykal, E. (2019a). Person Organization Fit: Spiritual Way to Boost Performance. *Asya Studies*, *3*(9), 31–43. doi:10.31455/asya.597151

Baykal, E. (2019b). Effect of Workplace Spirituality on Work Engagement Mediator Effect of Altruistic Love. *PressAcademia Procedia*, *9*(1), 61–64. doi:10.17261/Pressacademia.2019.1066

Baykal, E. (2019c). Creating Organizational Commitment Through Spiritual Leadership: Mediating Effect Of Meaning At Work. *Business & Management Studies: An International Journal*, *7*(2), 837–855. doi:10.15295/bmij.v7i2.1113

Baykal, E. (2021). Understanding Religion As a Phenomenon in Workplace Sprituality: A Durkheimian Approach. *Spiritual Psychology and Counseling*, *6*(2), 27–41. doi:10.37898pc.2021.6.2.134

Beehner, C. G., & Blackwell, M. J. (2016). The impact of workplace spirituality on food service worker turnover intention. *Journal of Management, Spirituality & Religion*, *13*(4), 304–323. doi:10.1080/14766086.2016.1172251

Behere, P. B., Das, A., Yadav, R., & Behere, A. P. (2013). Ayurvedic concepts related to psychotherapy. *Indian Journal of Psychiatry*, *55*(6), 310. doi:10.4103/0019-5545.105556 PMID:23858273

Behere, R. V., Arasappa, R., Jagannathan, A., Varambally, S., Venkatasubramanian, G., Thirthalli, J., Subbakrishna, D. K., Nagendra, H. R., & Gangadhar, B. N. (2011). Effect of yoga therapy on facial emotion recognition deficits, symptoms and functioning in patients with schizophrenia. *Acta Psychiatrica Scandinavica*, *123*(2), 147–153. doi:10.1111/j.1600-0447.2010.01605.x PMID:20846271

Benfey, T. (Ed.). (1982). Sanskrit English dictionary. New Delhi: Milan.

Bhajanananda, S. (2006). *Selfless work: Its basis, methods, and fulfillment. Belur Math.* Ramakrishna Mission Vivekananda University Press.

Bhargava, R., Kumar, N., & Gupta, A. (2017). Indian perspective on psychotherapy: Cultural issues. *Journal of Contemporary Psychotherapy*, *47*(2), 95–103. doi:10.100710879-016-9348-1

Bhargav, H., George, S., & Varambally, S. (2022). Yoga and mental health: What every psychiatrist needs to know. *BJPsych Advances*, *29*(1), 1–12. doi:10.1192/bja.2022.22

Bhargav, H., Jasti, N., More, P., Kumar, V., Chikkanna, U., Kumar, R. K., & Varambally, S. (2021). Correlation of prakriti diagnosis using AyuSoft prakriti diagnostic tool with clinician rating in patients with psychiatric disorders. *Journal of Ayurveda and Integrative Medicine*, *12*(2), 365–368. doi:10.1016/j.jaim.2021.01.012 PMID:33750638

Bhat, R. (2013). Effect of Madhookasaradi Nasya in the Management of Positive Symptoms of Schizophrenia. *Int. J. Ayu. Alt. Med, 1.*

Bhat, S. G. S., Arasappa, R., Jagannathan, A., & Varambally, S. (2021). Yoga therapy for Obsessive Compulsive Disorder (OCD): A case series from India. *Asian Journal of Psychiatry*, *62*, 102739. doi:10.1016/j.ajp.2021.102739

Bhatia, S. C., Madabushi, J., Kolli, V., Bhatia, S. K., & Madaan, V. (2013). The Bhagavad Gita and contemporary psychotherapies. *Indian Journal of Psychiatry*, *55*(6, Suppl 2), S315–S321. doi:10.4103/0019-5545.105557 PMID:23858274

Bhatnagar, M., Sisodia, S. S., & Bhatnagar, R. (2005). Antiulcer and Antioxidant Activity of Asparagus racemosus WILLD and Withania somnifera DUNAL in Rats. *Annals of the New York Academy of Sciences*, *1056*(1), 261–278. doi:10.1196/annals.1352.027 PMID:16387694

Bhattacharjee, A., & Singh, S. (2021). Zoroastrian Ethics in Business. *IIMS Journal of Management Science, 3si*, 133–143. doi:10.5958/0976-173X.2021.00010.5

Bhattacharya, H. (1975). Yoga Psychology, Nature of Mind and Its Activities. *Indian Psychology*.. The Ramakrishna Mission Institute of Culture.

Bhavanani, A. (2012). OBSTACLES ON THE PATH OF YOGA. *Yoga Life*, *43*, 3–9.

Bhawuk, D. P., & Bhawuk, D. P. (2011). Indian concept of self. *Spirituality and Indian Psychology: Lessons from the Bhagavad-Gita*, (pp. 65-91). Springer.

Bhawuk, D. (2011). *Spirituality and Indian psychology: lessons from the Bhagavad-Gita*. Springer Science & Business Media. doi:10.1007/978-1-4419-8110-3

Bhawuk, D. P. (2010). Methodology for building psychological models from scriptures: Contributions of Indian psychology to indigenous and universal psychologies. *Psychology and Developing Societies*, *22*(1), 49–93. doi:10.1177/097133360902200103

Bhovi, P., Hegde, R., K., S., & D'Souza, V. (2020). A Clinical Study To Evaluate The Efficacy Of Nasya With Sarshapataila In Vishada (Depression). *International Ayurvedic Medical Journal*.

Bhugra, D. (1992). Psychiatry in ancient Indian texts: A review. *History of Psychiatry*, *3*(10), 167–186. doi:10.1177/0957154X9200301002 PMID:11623029

Bicer, C. (2022, January 1). *Avoiding halo effect in employee selection: Implementing effective techniques in hiring*. Fiscaoeconomia. https://www.ceeol.com/search/article-detail?id=1046177

Biswas, S. K., & Debnath, M. (2017). *Yoga and Ayurveda: Concomitant preventive therapeutics for some important lifestyle disorders*.

Bodhi, B. (2011). What does mindfulness really mean? A canonical perspective. *Contemporary Buddhism*, *12*(1), 19–39. doi:10.1080/14639947.2011.564813

Boffetta, P., & Collatuzzo, G. (2022). Application of P4 (Predictive, Preventive, Personalized, Participatory) approach to Occupational Medicine. *PubMed*, *113*(1), e2022009. doi:10.23749/mdl.v113i1.12622 PMID:35226650

Bond, M. H., Leung, K., Au, A., Tong, K. K., De Carrasquel, S. R., Murakami, F., Yamaguchi, S., Bierbrauer, G., Singelis, T. M., Broer, M., Boen, F., Lambert, S. M., Ferreira, M. C., Noels, K. A., van Bavel, J., Safdar, S., Zhang, J., Chen, L., Solcova, I., & Lewis, J. R. (2004). Culture-level dimensions of social axioms and their correlates across 41 cultures. *Journal of Cross-Cultural Psychology*, *35*(5), 548–570. doi:10.1177/0022022104268388

Bose, G. (1931). A new technique of psychoanalysis. *The International Journal of Psycho-Analysis*, *12*, 387–388.

Braun, V., & Clarke, V. (2006). Using thematic analysis in psychology. *Qualitative Research in Psychology*, *3*(2), 77–101. doi:10.1191/1478088706qp063oa

Bredesen, D. E., & Rao, R. V. (2017). Ayurvedic profiling of Alzheimer's disease. *PubMed, 23*(3), 46–50. https://pubmed.ncbi.nlm.nih.gov/28236613

Bremner, J. D., Moazzami, K., Wittbrodt, M. T., Nye, J. A., Lima, B. B., Gillespie, C. F., Rapaport, M. H., Pearce, B. D., Shah, A. J., & Vaccarino, V. (2020). Diet, Stress and Mental Health. *Nutrients, 12*(8), 2428. doi:10.3390/nu12082428 PMID:32823562

Brems, C., Colgan, D., Freeman, H., Freitas, J., Justice, L., Shean, M., & Sulenes, K. (2016). Elements of yogic practice: Perceptions of students in healthcare programs. *International Journal of Yoga, 9*(2), 121. doi:10.4103/0973-6131.183710 PMID:27512319

Brenes, G. A., Sohl, S., Wells, R. E., Befus, D., Campos, C. L., & Danhauer, S. C. (2019). The Effects of Yoga on Patients with Mild Cognitive Impairment and Dementia: A Scoping Review. *The American Journal of Geriatric Psychiatry, 27*(2), 188–197. doi:10.1016/j.jagp.2018.10.013 PMID:30413292

Bridges, L. & Sharma, M. (2017). The Efficacy of Yoga as a Form of Treatment for Depression. *Journal of Evidence-Based Complementary & Alternative Medicine*. doi:10.1177/2156587217715927

Britton, A. (2018). Applied Yogic Wisdom: Ancient Science, Contemporary Recovery [Doctoral dissertation, Loyola Marymount University].

Broderick, J., Vancampfort, D., Mockler, D., Bennett, K., Waugh, A., McDonough, C., Cramer, H., & Walshe, M. (2018). Yoga for schizophrenia. *Cochrane Database of Systematic Reviews, 2018*(12), CD013213. doi:10.1002/14651858.CD013213

Brooks ; Scarano. (1989). Transcendental Meditation in the treatment of post-vietnam adjustment. *Journal of Counseling and Development, 64*, 212–215.

Brown, J. L. C., Eubanks, C., & Keating, A. (2017). Yoga, quality of life, anxiety, and trauma in low-income adults with mental illness: A mixed-methods study. *Social Work in Mental Health, 15*(3), 308–330. doi:10.1080/15332985.2016.1220441

Brown, K. W., & Ryan, R. M. (2003, April). The benefits of being present: Mindfulness and its role in psychological well-being. *Journal of Personality and Social Psychology, 84*(4), 822–848. doi:10.1037/0022-3514.84.4.822 PMID:12703651

Burnette, J. (2000). *Assessment of culturally and linguistically diverse students for special education eligibility* (Report No. EDO-EC-00–13). Arlington, VA: ERIC Clearinghouse on Disabilities and Gifted Education. (ERIC Document Reproduction Service No. ED449637)

Cabral, P., Meyer, H. B., & Ames, D. (2011). *Effectiveness of yoga therapy as a complementary treatment for major psychiatric disorders: A meta-analysis*. Prim Care Companion CNS Disorder.

Capon, H. O., Shea, M., & McIver, S. (2019). Yoga and mental health: A synthesis of qualitative findings. *Complementary Therapies in Clinical Practice, 37*, 122–132. doi:10.1016/j.ctcp.2019.101063 PMID:31587992

Carmody, J., Baer, R. A., & Lykins, LB, E., & Olendzki, N. (. (2009). An empirical study of the mechanisms of mindfulness in a mindfulness-based stress reduction program. *Journal of Clinical Psychology, 65*(6), 613–626. doi:10.1002/jclp.20579 PMID:19267330

Carrithers, M., & Humphrey, C. (1991). *The assembly of listeners: Jains in society*. Cambridge University Press. doi:10.1017/CBO9780511896637

Casebeer, A. J. (1952). *"Philosophy, Religion and Theology". Concepts of self-realization (a comparison of the concept of self-realization in the "Bhagavadgita" with that concept in the Pauline Epistles)* [Thesis, University of Southern California]. ProQuest LLC. doi:10.25549/usctheses-c40-1215

Caulfield, J. (2023). *How to Do Thematic Analysis | Step-by-Step Guide & Examples*. Scribbr. https://www.scribbr.com/methodology/thematic-analysis/

Centre for Yoga Studies. (2023, May 14). *Sāṃkhya Kārikā verse 2*. Centre for Yoga Studies. https://yogastudies.org/samkhya/samkhya-verse-2/

Chacko, D., & Vidhukumar, K. (2020). The Prevalence of Specific Learning Disorder among School-going Children in Ernakulam District, Kerala, India: Ernakulam Learning Disorder (ELD) Study. *Indian Journal of Psychological Medicine*, *42*(3), 250–255. doi:10.4103/IJPSYM.IJPSYM_199_19 PMID:32612329

Chadda, R.K. & Rajhans, P. (2021). Learnings from Ancient India: Relevance to Contemporary Psychiatry. *Perspective/Viewpoint, 3*(150-153)

Chadda, R. K., & Deb, K. S. (2013). Indian family systems, collectivistic society and psychotherapy. *Indian Journal of Psychiatry*, *55*(6, Suppl 2), S299–S309. doi:10.4103/0019-5545.105555 PMID:23858272

Chamorro-Premuzic, T., & Lovric, D. (2022, June 20). How to move from strategy to execution. *Harvard Business Review*. https://hbr.org/2022/06/how-to-move-from-strategy-to-execution

Chandna, S., Sharma, P. K., & Vasudevan, M. (2022). The Mindful Self: Exploring Mindfulness in Relation with Self-esteem and Self-efficacy in Indian Population. *Psychological Studies*, *67*(2), 261–272. doi:10.100712646-021-00636-5 PMID:35125522

Charak Samhita. (n.d.). SBP Nirnay Sagar.

Charak Samhita: Vol. Sutrasthana. (1998). Chaukhamba Bharti Academy. [Hindi]

Charaka Samhita. (1998a). Chaukhamba Bharti Academy.

Charaka Samhita: Vol. Sutrasthana. (1998b). Chaukhambha Bharati Academy. [Hindi]

Charan, C. (2020). *Bhagavad Gita: 365 Reflections for Daily Mindfulness*. Wikas Printing & Carriers Pvt. Ltd.

Chatterjee, B., & Pancholi, J. (2011). Prakriti -based medicine: A step towards personalized medicine. *Ayu*, *32*(2), 141. doi:10.4103/0974-8520.92539 PMID:22408293

Chaudhary, N., Misra, G., Bansal, P., Valsiner, J., & Singh, T. (2022). Making Sense of Culture for the Psychological Sciences. *Review of General Psychology*, *26*(4), 399–415. doi:10.1177/10892680211066473

Chaudhry, N., Bhandari, R. B., & Gaur, V. (2023). Yoga perspective on personal excellence and well-being. *Journal of Ayurveda and Integrative Medicine*, *14*(3), 100717. doi:10.1016/j.jaim.2023.100717 PMID:37224682

Chaudhuri, H. (1953). The Integralism of Sri Aurobindo. *Philosophy East & West*, *3*(2), 131–136. doi:10.2307/1397259

Chavan, S. (2013). Approach towards life style modification plan as per ayurveda and modern technique for prevention of geriatrics. *Int Res J Pharm*.

Chawla, V., & Guda, S. (2010). Individual spirituality at work and its relationship with job satisfaction, propensity to leavand job commitment: An exploratory study among sales professionals. *Journal of Human Values*, *16*(2), 157–167. doi:10.1177/097168581001600203

Chen, C. Y., & Li, C. I. (2013). Assessing the spiritual leadership effectiveness: The contribution of follower's self-concept and preliminary tests for moderation of culture and managerial position. *The Leadership Quarterly*, *24*(1), 240–255. doi:10.1016/j.leaqua.2012.11.004

Cheung, S. Y., Huang, E. G., Chang, S., & Wei, L. (2020, July). Does being mindful make people more creative at work? The role of creative process engagement and perceived leader humility. *Organizational Behavior and Human Decision Processes*, *159*, 39–48. doi:10.1016/j.obhdp.2019.12.003

ChhakoV. (2021, May 28). Wikipedia. Retrieved from https://en.wikipedia.org/wiki/Vand_Chhako

Chinmayananda, S. (1982). *ATMABODHA*. Central Chinmaya Mission Trust.

Chinmayananda, S. (2021, September 8). *Bhagavad Gita chapter 3 - verse 17 - 3.17 Yas tvatma-ratir*. Shlokam. https://shlokam.org/bhagavad-gita/3-17/

Chong, S., Kim, Y. J., Lee, H. W., Johnson, R. E., & Lin, S.-H. (2020, July). Mind your own break! The interactive effect of workday respite activities and mindfulness on employee outcomes via affective linkages. *Organizational Behavior and Human Decision Processes*, *159*, 64–77. doi:10.1016/j.obhdp.2019.11.001

Choudhary, K., Maitreya, Kumar, K., & Richa. (2021). Meditative Therapies in Clinical Psychology. *Indian Journal of Clinical Psychology*, *48*(1).

Chowdhary, S., & Gopinath, J. K. (2013). Clinical hypnosis and Patanjali yoga sutras. *Indian Journal of Psychiatry*, *55*(6, Suppl 2), S157–S164. doi:10.4103/0019-5545.105516 PMID:23858248

Chully, A. A., Jose, J., & M, L. (2022, August 4). *Authentic leadership in a pandemic world: An exploratory study in the Indian context*. Journal of Management Development. https://www.emerald.com/insight/content/doi/10.1108/JMD-10-2021-0281/full/html?casa_token=6U6Idw9AS5AAAAAA%3ALfnipb5fIGa2lJ-UYJa-PxqFVC4dcIc6du1qyuVPF_iBiwfek3C-u-lo8j1yOurLeLSKhF_852PKW7NIWRaTkRDrNo-pVwcQBn2OmvkxP3g-CgkSfyI

C-IAYT Portfolio Review—International Association of Yoga Therapists IAYT. (n.d.). IAYT. https://www.iayt.org/page/PRE_Eligibility

Cillessen, L., Compen, F., & Speckens, A. E. M. (2020). Mindfulness-Based interventions. In Springer eBooks (pp. 1396–1399). Springer. doi:10.1007/978-3-030-39903-0_101983

Clay, R. A. (2002). *A renaissance for humanistic psychology*. APA. Https://Www.Apa.Org. https://www.apa.org/monitor/sep02/renaissance

Clothey, F. W. (2007). *Religion in India: A historical introduction*. Routledge. doi:10.4324/9780203967836

Cohen, E. (2015). The hold and release practice: A new way into meditation and mindfulness. *Transpersonal Psychology Review*, *17*(1), 9–19. https://eprints.leedsbeckett.ac.uk/id/eprint/3470/. doi:10.53841/bpstran.2015.17.1.9

Colagiuri, B., Schenk, L. A., Kessler, M. D., Dorsey, S. G., & Colloca, L. (2015). The placebo effect: From concepts to genes. *Neuroscience*, *307*, 171–190. doi:10.1016/j.neuroscience.2015.08.017 PMID:26272535

Conboy, L. A., Noggle, J. J., Frey, J. L., Kudesia, R. S., & Khalsa, S. B. S. (2013). Qualitative evaluation of a high school yoga program: Feasibility and perceived benefits. *Explore (New York, N.Y.)*, *9*(3), 171–180. doi:10.1016/j.explore.2013.02.001 PMID:23643372

Contrada, R., & Baum, A. (Eds.). (2010). *The handbook of stress science: Biology, psychology, and health*. Springer Publishing Company.

Conze, E. (2012). *Buddhism: Its essence and development*. Courier Corporation.

Coo, C., & Salanova, M. (2017, May 31). Mindfulness Can Make You Happy-and-Productive: A Mindfulness Controlled Trial and Its Effects on Happiness, Work Engagement and Performance. *Journal of Happiness Studies*, *19*(6), 1691–1711. doi:10.100710902-017-9892-8

Cornelissen, M. (2011). *Foundations of Indian Psychology Volume 2: Practical Applications*. Pearson Education India.

Cornelissen, M. (2013). *Foundations and applications of Indian psychology* (G. Misra, Ed.; 2nd ed.). Pearson.

Corsini, R. J. (2002). *The dictionary of psychology*. Brunner-Routledge.

D'cruz, M., & Andrade, C. (2022). Potential clinical applications of Ashwagandha (*Withania somnifera*) in medicine and neuropsychiatry. *Expert Review of Clinical Pharmacology, 15*(9), 1067–1080. doi:10.1080/17512433.2022.2121699 PMID:36062480

D'Souza, J., & Gurin, M. (2016). The universal significance of Maslow's concept of self-actualization. *The Humanistic Psychologist, 44*(2), 210–214. doi:10.1037/hum0000027

Daaleman, T. P., Cobb, A. K., & Frey, B. B. (2001). Spirituality and well-being: An exploratory study of the patient perspective. *Social Science & Medicine, 53*(11), 1503–1511. doi:10.1016/S0277-9536(00)00439-1 PMID:11710425

Dalal, A. K. (2011). A journey back to the roots: Psychology in India. In *Foundations of Indian Psychology* (p. 39). https://www.ipi.org.in/texts/ajit/dalal-joureny-to-the-roots.pdf

Dalal, A. K. (2006). Social interventions to moderate discriminatory attitudes: The case of the physically challenged in India. *Psychology Health and Medicine, 11*(3), 374–382. doi:10.1080/13548500600595392 PMID:17130074

Dalal, A. K., & Misra, G. (2010). The Core and Context of Indian Psychology. *Psychology and Developing Societies, 22*(1), 121–155. doi:10.1177/097133360902200105

Dalal, R. (2010). *Hinduism: An Alphabetical Guide*. Penguin Books.

Danielly, Y., & Silverthorne, C. (2017). Psychological Benefits of Yoga for Female Inmates. *International Journal of Yoga Therapy, 27*(1), 9–14. doi:10.17761/1531-2054-27.1.9 PMID:29131730

Daniels, R. J., Trebilcock, M. J., & Carson, L. D. (2011). The Legacy of Empire: The Common Law Inheritance and Commitments to Legality in Former British Colonies. *The American Journal of Comparative Law, 59*(1), 111–178. doi:10.5131/AJCL.2010.0015

Das, Ajay, & Kuyini, Ahmed Bawa & Desai. (2013). Inclusive Education in India: Are the Teachers Prepared? *International Journal of Special Education*, 28.

Dasgupta, S. D. (2015). (Un) Holy Connections? Understanding Woman Abuse in Hinduism. In *Religion and Men's Violence Against Women* (pp. 371–382). Springer New York. doi:10.1007/978-1-4939-2266-6_23

Dasgupta, S. N. (1975). *A history of Indian philosophy* (Indian ed., Vol. 1–5). Motilal Banarsidass. (Original work published 1922)

Debroy, B., & Debroy, D. (2006). *The Holy Vedas: Rig Veda, Yajur Veda Sama Veda and Atharva Veda* (13th ed.). BR Publishing Corporation.

Deshmukh, D. S. K. (2021). Effect of Pragya Yoga and Pranakarshan Pranayama (Popounded by Acharya Sriram Sharma) on aggression level of Juvenile delinquents. International Journal of Yogic, *Human Movement and Sports Sciences, 6*(2), 81–84.

Deshpande, S., Nagendra, H. R., & Raghuram, N. (2008). A randomized control trial of the effect of Yoga on Gunas (personality) and Health in normal healthy volunteers. *International Journal of Yoga, 1*(1), 2–10. doi:10.4103/0973-6131.36785 PMID:21829278

Devi, U. K., & Swarup, A. (2000). Evaluation of Clinical Efficacy of Menotab in Alleviating Symptoms of Menopausal Syndrome: Phase III Open Clinical Trial. *The Antiseptic*, *98*. https://www.himalayawellness.com/pdf_files/menosan001.pdf

Dhar, B. K., & Stasi, A. Döpping, J. O., Gazi, M. A. I., Shaturaev, J., & Sarkar, S. M. (2022, July 14). *Mediating role of strategic flexibility between leadership styles on strategic execution: A study on bangladeshi private enterprises - global journal of flexible systems management*. Springer. https://link.springer.com/article/10.1007/s40171-022-00310-3

Dhillon, M. (2023). Weaving Together the Ancient and the Contemporary: Intersections of the Bhagavad Gita with Modern Psychology. *Pastoral Psychology*, *72*(4), 1–13. doi:10.100711089-023-01070-2 PMID:37359496

Dhiman, S. (2019). Karma Yoga: The Path of Enlightened Action. In: Bhagavad Gītā and Leadership. Palgrave Studies in Workplace Spirituality and Fulfillment. Palgrave Macmillan, Cham. doi:10.1007/978-3-319-67573-2_5

Dhingra, D., Parle, M., & Sk, K. (2004). Memory enhancing activity of Glycyrrhiza glabra in mice. *Journal of Ethnopharmacology*, *91*(2–3), 361–365. doi:10.1016/j.jep.2004.01.016 PMID:15120462

Dhingra, D., & Sharma, A. (2006). Antidepressant-like activity of Glycyrrhiza glabra L. in mouse models of immobility tests. *Progress in Neuro-Psychopharmacology & Biological Psychiatry*, *30*(3), 449–454. doi:10.1016/j.pnpbp.2005.11.019 PMID:16443316

Diggory, J. C., & Mehta, M. L. (1959). Jaina Psychology: A Psychological Analysis of the Jaina Doctrine of Karma. *Journal of the American Oriental Society*, *79*(2), 136–138. doi:10.2307/595861

Dillbeck, M. C. (1991). The Bhagavad-Gita: A case study. *Modern Science and Vedic Science*, *4*, 96–134.

Dindo, L., Van Liew, J. R., & Arch, J. J. (2017). Acceptance and commitment therapy: A transdiagnostic behavioural intervention for mental health and medical conditions. *Neurotherapeutics; the Journal of the American Society for Experimental NeuroTherapeutics*, *14*(3), 546–553. https://link.springer.com/article/10.1007/s13311-017-0521-3. doi:10.100713311-017-0521-3 PMID:28271287

Dobkin, P. L., Irving, J. A., & Amar, S. (2012). For Whom May Participation in a Mindfulness-Based Stress Reduction Program be Contraindicated? *Mindfulness*, *3*(1), 44–50. doi:10.100712671-011-0079-9

Doria, S., de Vuono, A., Sanlorenzo, R., Irtelli, F., & Mencacci, C. (2015). Anti-anxiety efficacy of Sudarshan Kriya Yoga in general anxiety disorder: A multicomponent, yoga based, breath intervention program for patients suffering from generalized anxiety disorder with or without comorbidities. *Journal of Affective Disorders*, *184*, 310–317. doi:10.1016/j.jad.2015.06.011 PMID:26142611

Douglass, B. G., & Moustakas, C. (1985). Heuristic inquiry: The internal search to know. *Journal of Humanistic Psychology*, *25*(3), 39–55. doi:10.1177/0022167885253004

Dreeben, S. J., Mamberg, M. H., & Salmon, P. (2013). The MBSR body scan in clinical practice. *Mindfulness*, *4*(4), 394–401. https://link.springer.com/article/10.1007/s12671-013-0212-z. doi:10.100712671-013-0212-z

Dubey, S., Tripathi, J. N., Gupta, S., & Reddy, K. R. C. (2010). A comparative clinical trial on the role of Panchakarma therapy and Unmada Gajankusha Rasa in the cases of major depressive disorder vis-à-vis kaphaja Unmada. *Ayu*, *31*(2), 205. doi:10.4103/0974-8520.72396 PMID:22131711

Duckworth, A. (2016). *Grit: The power of passion and perseverance* (Vol. 234). Scribner.

Durai, S. (2023). Truth-based leadership: Lessons from thirukural. In A. K. Maheshwari (Ed.), Consciousness-Based Leadership and Management, Volume 1: Vedic and Other Philosophical Approaches to Oneness and Flourishing (pp. 319–338). Springer International Publishing. doi:10.1007/978-3-031-06234-6_14

Dwivedi, Y. K., Kshetri, N., Hughes, L., Slade, E. L., Jeyaraj, A., Kar, A. K., Baabdullah, A. M., Koohang, A., Raghavan, V., Ahuja, M., Albanna, H., Albashrawi, M. A., Al-Busaidi, A. S., Balakrishnan, J., Barlette, Y., Basu, S., Bose, I., Brooks, L., Buhalis, D., & Wright, R. (2023). "So what if ChatGPT wrote it?" Multidisciplinary perspectives on opportunities, challenges and implications of generative conversational AI for research, practice and policy. *International Journal of Information Management*, *71*, 102642. doi:10.1016/j.ijinfomgt.2023.102642

Eby, L. T., Allen, T. D., Conley, K. M., Williamson, R. L., Henderson, T. G., & Mancini, V. S. (2019, June). Mindfulness-based training interventions for employees: A qualitative review of the literature. *Human Resource Management Review*, *29*(2), 156–178. doi:10.1016/j.hrmr.2017.03.004

Education World. (2013, September 7). Chapter 68: Mode of execution. *Thirukkural in English*. https://thirukkural133.wordpress.com/2013/09/07/chapter-68-mode-of-execution/

Eerde, W. V. (2003). Procrastination at work and time management training. *The Journal of Psychology*, *137*(5), 421–434. doi:10.1080/00223980309600625 PMID:14629073

Ehri, L. C., Nunes, S. R., Willows, D. M., Schuster, B. V., Yaghoub-Zadeh, Z., & Shanahan, T. (2001). Phonemic awareness instruction helps children learn to read: Evidence from the National Reading Panel's meta-analysis. *Reading Research Quarterly*, *36*(3), 250–287. doi:10.1598/RRQ.36.3.2

Emmons, R. (2000b). Spirituality and intelligence: Problems and prospects. *The International Journal for the Psychology of Religion*, *10*(1), 57–64. doi:10.1207/S15327582IJPR1001_6

Emmons, R. A. (1999). *The psychology of ultimate concerns*. Guilford Press.

Emmons, R. A. (2000a). Is spirituality an intelligence? Motivation, cognition, and the psychology of ultimate concern. *The International Journal for the Psychology of Religion*, *10*(1), 3–26. doi:10.1207/S15327582IJPR1001_2

Everett, F., Proctor, N., & Cartmell, B. (1983). Providing psychological services to american indian children and families. *Professional Psychology, Research and Practice*, *14*(5), 588–603. doi:10.1037/0735-7028.14.5.588

Fallot, R. D. (2001). Spirituality and religion in psychiatric rehabilitation and recovery from mental illness. *International Review of Psychiatry (Abingdon, England)*, *13*(2), 110–116. doi:10.1080/09540260120037344

Farb, N. A. (2014). From retreat centre to clinic to boardroom? Perils and promises of the modern mindfulness movement. *Religions*, *5*(4), 1062–1086. doi:10.3390/rel5041062

Finegan, J. E. (2000). The impact of person and organizational values on organizational commitment. *Journal of Occupational and Organizational Psychology*, *73*(2), 149–169. doi:10.1348/096317900166958

Forjan, D. N., Tuckey, M. R., & Li, Y. (2020, January 20). Problem solving and affect as mechanisms linking daily mindfulness to task performance and job satisfaction. *Stress and Health*, *36*(3), 338–349. doi:10.1002mi.2931 PMID:31957967

Frank, P., & Marken, M. (2021). Developments in Qualitative Mindfulness Practice Research: A Pilot Scoping Review. *Mindfulness*, *13*(1), 17–36. doi:10.100712671-021-01748-9

Fredrickson, B. L. (2001). The role of positive emotions in positive psychology: The broaden-and-build theory of positive emotions. *The American Psychologist*, *56*(3), 218–226. doi:10.1037/0003-066X.56.3.218 PMID:11315248

Fredrickson, B. L. (2013). Positive emotions broaden and build. In Vol. 47, pp. 1–53). Advances in experimental social psychology. Academic Press.

Freud, S. (2015). Beyond the pleasure principle. *Psychoanalysis and History*, *17*(2), 151–204. https://www.euppublishing.com/doi/full/10.3366/pah.2015.0169. doi:10.3366/pah.2015.0169

Fry, L. W., & Matherly, L. L. (2006). *Spiritual leadership and organizational performance: An exploratory study.* In Annual Meeting of the Academy of Management, Atlanta-Georgia. http://www. tarleton. edu/~ fry/sltorgperf. pdf

Fry, L. W. (2003). Toward a theory of spiritual leadership. *The Leadership Quarterly, 14*(6), 693–727. doi:10.1016/j.leaqua.2003.09.001

Fry, L. W., & Cohen, M. P. (2009). Spiritual leadership as a paradigm for organizational transformation and recovery from extended work hours cultures. *Journal of Business Ethics, 84*(S2), 265–278. doi:10.100710551-008-9695-2

Fry, L. W., & Slocum, J. W. Jr. (2008). Maximizing the triple bottom line through spiritual leadership. *Organizational Dynamics, 37*(1), 86–96. doi:10.1016/j.orgdyn.2007.11.004

Fry, L., & Kriger, M. (2009). Towards a theory of Being-centered Leadership: Multiple Levels of Being as Context for Effective Leadership. *Human Relations, 62*(11), 1667–1696. doi:10.1177/0018726709346380

Fry, L., & Nisiewicz, M. (2013). *Maximizing the Triple Bottom Line through Spiritual Leadership.* Stanford University Press.

Fullan, M. (2015). The new meaning of educational change. Teachers college press.

Gabriel, M. G., Curtiss, J., Hofmann, S. G., & Khalsa, S. B. S. (2018). Kundalini Yoga for Generalized Anxiety Disorder: An Exploration of Treatment Efficacy and Possible Mechanisms. *International Journal of Yoga Therapy, 28*(1), 97–105. doi:10.17761/2018-00003 PMID:29698081

Gagné, M., & Deci, E. L. (2005). *Self-determination theory and work motivation.* Wiley Online Library. https://onlinelibrary.wiley.com/doi/abs/10.1002/job.322

Gallegos, A. M., Crean, H. F., Pigeon, W. R., & Heffner, K. L. (2017). Meditation and yoga for posttraumatic stress disorder: A meta-analytic review of randomized controlled trials. *Clinical Psychology Review, 58,* 115–124. doi:10.1016/j.cpr.2017.10.004 PMID:29100863

Gambhirananda, S. (1965). *Brahma sutra bhasva.* Calcutta, India: Sun lithographing Co.

Gangadhar, B., & Varambally, S. (2011). Yoga as Therapy in Psychiatric Disorders: Past, Present, and Future. *Biofeedback, 39*(2), 60–63. doi:10.5298/1081-5937-39.2.03

Garg, N., & Saini, D. (2023). Workplace spirituality to cultivate innovative work behaviour: The moderating role of perceived working conditions. *The International Journal of Sociology and Social Policy.* doi:10.1108/IJSSP-03-2023-0050

Garland, E. L., Farb, N. A., Goldin, P. R., & Fredrickson, B. L. (2015, November 24). Mindfulness Broadens Awareness and Builds Eudaimonic Meaning: A Process Model of Mindful Positive Emotion Regulation. *Psychological Inquiry, 26,* 293–314. doi:10.1080/1047840X.2015.1064294 PMID:27087765

Garland, E., Gaylord, S., & Park, J. (2009). The role of mindfulness in positive reappraisal. *Explore (New York, N.Y.), 5*(1), 37–44. doi:10.1016/j.explore.2008.10.001 PMID:19114262

Gavin, D. (1996). *Flood, An introduction to Hinduism.* Cambridge University Press.

Gayathri, N., & Meenakshi, K. (2012). Emotional intelligence through the Bhagavad-Gita. *International Journal of Research Studies in Psychology, 1*(2), 73–80. doi:10.5861/ijrsp.2012.v1i2.83

George, A. J., John, R., & Rajkumar, E. (2021d). Mindfulness-based positive psychology interventions: A systematic review. *BMC Psychology, 9*(1), 116. doi:10.118640359-021-00618-2 PMID:34362457

Gergen, K. J., Gulerce, A., Lock, A., & Misra, G. (1996). Psychological science in cultural context. *The American Psychologist, 51*(5), 496–503. doi:10.1037/0003-066X.51.5.496

Gerhard, W. A. (1964). Heimann," Facets of Indian Thought"(Book Review). *The Journal of Asian Studies, 24*(1), 182. doi:10.2307/2050470

Ghodke-Puranik, Y., Joshi, K., & Patwardhan, B. (2011). Traditional Medicine to Modern Pharmacogenomics: Ayurveda*Prakriti*Type and CYP2C19 Gene Polymorphism Associated with the Metabolic Variability. *Evidence-Based Complementary and Alternative Medicine, 1–5*, 1–5. doi:10.1093/ecam/nep206

Ghosh, A., & Deb, A. (2016). Positive Psychology Progress in India: Accomplishments and Pathways Ahead. *Psychological Studies, 61*(3), 113–125. doi:10.100712646-016-0367-5

Giacalone, R., & Jurkiewicz, C. (2003). Toward a science of workplace spirituality. In R. Giacalone, & C. Jurkiewicz (Eds.), Handbook of workplace spirituality and organizational performance (pp. 3–28). Armonk, NY7 Sharpe.

Gold, E., Smith, A. M. S., Hopper, I., Herne, D., Tansey, G., & Hulland, C. (2009). Mindfulness-Based Stress Reduction (MBSR) for primary school teachers. *Journal of Child and Family Studies, 19*(2), 184–189. doi:10.100710826-009-9344-0

Goldin, P. R., & Gross, J. J. (2010). Effects of mindfulness-based stress reduction (MBSR) on emotion regulation in social anxiety disorder. *Emotion (Washington, D.C.), 10*(1), 83–91. doi:10.1037/a0018441 PMID:20141305

Gómez-Pinilla, F. (2008). Brain foods: The effects of nutrients on brain function. *Nature Reviews. Neuroscience, 9*(7), 568–578. doi:10.1038/nrn2421 PMID:18568016

Gone, J., & Alcántara, C. (2007). Identifying effective mental health interventions for american indians and alaska natives: A review of the literature. *Cultural Diversity & Ethnic Minority Psychology, 13*(4), 356–363. doi:10.1037/1099-9809.13.4.356 PMID:17967104

GopalA.SharmaA.SubramanyamM. (2020). Dynamics of psychological responses to covid-19 in india: a longitudinal study. doi:10.1101/2020.06.12.20129791

Gopalacharya, C. S. (Ed.). (1967). *Shabdārthakausthubha* [Sanskrit- Kannada Dictionary]. Vol. 1–6). Bangalore Press.

Gordon, J. S. (1982). Holistic medicine: advances and shortcomings. *PubMed, 136*(6), 546–551. https://pubmed.ncbi.nlm.nih.gov/7113200

Goswamee, G., & Saikia, R. (2017). A study on the educational philosophy of Rabindranath Tagore and its influence on elementary education with special reference to Assam. *The Clarion- International Multidisciplinary Journal, 6*, 71-74.

Gothe, N. P., Hayes, J. S., Temali, C., & Damoiseaux, J. S. (2018). Differences in Brain Structure and Function Among Yoga Practitioners and Controls. *Frontiers in Integrative Neuroscience, 12*, 26. doi:10.3389/fnint.2018.00026 PMID:29988397

Gothe, N. P., Khan, I., Hayes, J. S., Erlenbach, E., & Damoiseaux, J. S. (2019). Yoga Effects on Brain Health: A Systematic Review of the Current Literature. *Brain Plasticity, 5*(1), 105–122. doi:10.3233/BPL-190084 PMID:31970064

Gould-Williams, J. S., Mostafa, A. M. S., & Bottomley, P. (2015). Public service motivation and employee outcomes in the Egyptian public sector: Testing the mediating effect of person-organization fit. *Journal of Public Administration: Research and Theory, 25*(2), 597–622. doi:10.1093/jopart/mut053

Goyal, M. (2018). *Rasayana* in perspective of the present scenario. *Ayu, 39*(2), 63. doi:10.4103/ayu.AYU_300_18 PMID:30783358

Grace, S. (2020, June 16). *65 Bible Verses That Show Mindfulness Was God's Idea*. Calming Grace. https://www.calming-grace.com/bible-verses-about-mindfulness/

Grassini, S. (2023). Shaping the Future of Education: Exploring the Potential and Consequences of AI and ChatGPT in Educational Settings. *Education Sciences*, *13*(7), 7. doi:10.3390/educsci13070692

Gupta, P. (2015). Pharmacogenetics, Pharmacogenomics and Ayurgenomics for Personalized Medicine: a Paradigm Shift. *Indian J. Pharm. Sci.*, *77*(2). doi:10.4103/0250-474X.156543

Gupta, A. (2015). pedagogy of third space: A multidimensional early childhood curriculum. *Policy Futures in Education*, *13*(2), 260–272. doi:10.1177/1478210315579540

Gupta, N., Khera, S., Vempati, R. P., Sharma, R., & Bijlani, R. L. (n.d.). Effect Of Yoga Based Lifestyle Intervention On State And Trait Anxiety. *Indian Journal of Physiology and Pharmacology*. PMID:16850902

Gupta, S. K. (2019). Meditation, Yoga and Health. *Think India Journal*, *23*(3), 188–191.

Gurchiek, K. (3 C.E.). *Prayer and Meditation Rooms Can Increase Inclusion*. SHRM; SHRM. https://www.shrm.org/resourcesandtools/hr-topics/behavioral-competencies/global-and-cultural-effectiveness/pages/prayer-meditation-rooms-can-increase-inclusion.aspx

Gutek, G. (2004). *The Montessori Method: The Origins of an Educational Innovation: Including an Abridged and Annotated Edition of Maria Montessori's The Montessori Method*. Rowman & Littlefield Publishers, Inc.

Güven, C. (2023, January 27). *Promoting religious diversity in the workplace - Ruul*. Ruul I Worktech Solutions for Modern and Global Work. https://ruul.io/blog/promoting-religious-diversity-in-the-workplace#:~:text=The%20importance%20of%20religious%20diversity%20in%20the%20workplace,-More%20than%2085&text=A%20diverse%20workforce%20is%20essential,come%20up%20with%20versatile%20solutions

Hafenbrack, A. C., Cameron, L. D., Spreitzer, G. M., Zhang, C., Noval, L. J., & Shaffakat, S. (2020, July). Helping People by Being in the Present: Mindfulness Increases Prosocial Behavior. *Organizational Behavior and Human Decision Processes*, *159*, 21–38. doi:10.1016/j.obhdp.2019.08.005

Haneef, S. (1979, January 1). What Everyone Should Know about Islam and Muslims. (pp. 4-25).

Hanh, T. N. (1991). *Old path, white clouds: walking in the footsteps of the Buddha*. Parallax Press.

Harnack, A. (2006). *What is Christianity?* Book Tree.

Harne, B. P., & Hiwale, A. S. (2018). EEG spectral analysis on OM mantra meditation: A pilot study. *Applied Psychophysiology and Biofeedback*, *43*(2), 123–129. doi:10.100710484-018-9391-7 PMID:29752573

Hausknecht, J. P., & Trevor, C. O. (2011). Collective turnover at the group, unit, and organizational levels: Evidence, issues, and implications. *Journal of Management*, *37*(1), 352–388. doi:10.1177/0149206310383910

Heylighen, F. (1992). A cognitive-systemic reconstruction of maslow's theory of self-actualization. *Behavioral Science*, *37*(1), 39–58. doi:10.1002/bs.3830370105

Hobfoll, S. E. (2001, December 21). The Influence of Culture, Community, and the Nested-Self in the Stress Process: Advancing Conservation of Resources Theory. *Applied Psychology*, *50*(3), 337–421. doi:10.1111/1464-0597.00062

Hodge, D. R. (2004). Spirituality and people with mental illness: Developing spiritual competency in assessment and intervention. *Families in Society*, *85*(1), 36–44. doi:10.1606/1044-3894.257

Hooi, L. W., & Chan, A. J. (2022, September 20). Innovative culture and rewards-recognition matter in linking Transformational leadership to workplace digitalisation? *Leadership & Organization Development Journal.* https://www.emerald.com/insight/content/doi/10.1108/LODJ-07-2021-0349/full/html?casa_token=E5olx2zLS6QAAAAA%3Av9IS4q9Efyr8WvZO4_CAUC0Pkz0J9rXD3QmpfIkgTrDIJFVNdrwhn3HUwvHbc1dP1tcRpMAIfuTm4bGECkJgJ9LF-bYy7CwmpgR7-Op7q3cjduz0XA40

Hoshmand, L. T. (2007). Cultural–Ecological Perspectives on the Understanding and Assessment of Trauma. In J. P. Wilson & C. S. Tang (Eds.), Cross-Cultural Assessment of Psychological Trauma and PTSD (pp. 31–50). Springer US. doi:10.1007/978-0-387-70990-1_2

Howarth, A., Smith, J. G., Perkins-Porras, L., & Ussher, M. (2019). Effects of Brief Mindfulness-Based Interventions on Health-Related Outcomes: A Systematic Review. *Mindfulness, 10*(10), 1957–1968. doi:10.100712671-019-01163-1

Huang, Z., Chavda, V. P., Bezbaruah, R., Uversky, V. N., Sucharitha, P., Patel, A., & Chen, Z. (2022a). An Ayurgenomics Approach: Prakriti-Based Drug Discovery and Development for Personalized care. *Frontiers in Pharmacology, 13*, 866827. doi:10.3389/fphar.2022.866827 PMID:35431922

Hudson, R. (2014). The question of theoretical foundations for the spirituality at work movement. *Journal of Management, Spirituality & Religion, 11*(1), 27–44. doi:10.1080/14766086.2013.801031

Hung, S. H., & Wa, J. Y. S. (2021). Dharma therapy: A Buddhist counselling approach to acknowledging and enhancing perspectives, attitudes and values. *International Perspectives in Values-based Mental Health Practice: Case Studies and Commentaries*, 305-311.

Huppes, N. (2011). *Teaching Indian Psychology—Challenges and Prospects An application-oriented paper.* Indian Psychology Institute. https://www.ipi.org.in/texts/neeltje/nh-teaching-indian-psychology.php

Huxter, M. (2015). *Mindfulness and the Buddha's noble eightfold path.* Buddhist Foundations of Mindfulness. https://link.springer.com/chapter/10.1007/978-3-319-18591-0_3

Hwang, K.-K. (2004). *The Epistemological Goal of Indigenous Psychology: The Perspective of Constructive Realism* [National Taiwan University]. https://scholarworks.gvsu.edu/iaccp_papers?utm_source=scholarworks.gvsu.edu%2Fiaccp_papers%2F265&utm_medium=PDF&utm_campaign=PDFCoverPages

Hwang, K. K., & Chang, J. (2009). Self-cultivation: Culturally sensitive psychotherapies in Confucian societies. *The Counseling Psychologist, 37*(7), 1010–1032. doi:10.1177/0011000009339976

Hwong, A. R., Wang, M., Khan, H., Chagwedera, D. N., Grzenda, A., Doty, B., Benton, T., Alpert, J., Clarke, D., & Compton, W. M. (2022). Climate change and mental health research methods, gaps, and priorities: A scoping review. *The Lancet. Planetary Health, 6*(3), e281–e291. doi:10.1016/S2542-5196(22)00012-2 PMID:35278392

India's most respected special schools 2022-2023. (2022, October). Education World. https://www.educationworld.in/indias-most-respected-special-needs-schools-2022-2023/

Iqbal, N., Singh, A., & Aleem, S. (2015). Effect of dynamic meditation on mental health. *Journal of Religion and Health, 55*(1), 241–254. doi:10.100710943-015-0082-x PMID:26179581

Isaeva, N. V. (1993). *Shankara and Indian Philosophy.* SUNY Press.

Ivtzan, I., & Papantoniou, A. (2014). Yoga meets positive psychology: Examining the integration of hedonic (gratitude) and eudaimonic (meaning) wellbeing in relation to the extent of yoga practice. *Journal of Bodywork and Movement Therapies, 18*(2), 183–189. doi:10.1016/j.jbmt.2013.11.005 PMID:24725784

Iyer, M. (2009). *Faith & philosophy of Zoroastrianism* (Vol. 7). Gyan Publishing House.

Iyer, S. (2022). Mindfulness-based Interventions: Can They Improve Self-care and Psychological Well-being? [Google Scholar]. *Indian Journal of Critical Care Medicine : Peer-Reviewed, Official Publication of Indian Society of Critical Care Medicine, 26*(4), 407–408. doi:10.5005/jp-journals-10071-24194 PMID:35656051

Jabin, N., Wohra, S., & Das, A. (2022). Education in India and the Post- Colonial Perspective. *Analysis*, 487–498.

Jackson, J. J., Wood, D., Bogg, T., Walton, K. E., Harms, P. D., & Roberts, B. W. (2010, August 1). What do conscientious people do? development and validation of the behavioral indicators of conscientiousness (BIC). *Journal of research in personality.* https://www.ncbi.nlm.nih.gov/pmc/articles/PMC3028204/

Jagadeesan, T., R, A., R, K., Jain, T., Allu, A. R., Selvi G, T., Maveeran, M., & Kuppusamy, M. (2022). Effect of Bhramari Pranayama intervention on stress, anxiety, depression and sleep quality among COVID 19 patients in home isolation. *Journal of Ayurveda and Integrative Medicine, 13*(3), 100596. doi:10.1016/j.jaim.2022.100596 PMID:35693195

Jain, P. (2021, May 25). Living with Mindfulness — Parveen Jain. Parveen Jain. Retrieved from https://www.parveenjain.com/blog/living-with-mindfulness

Jaini, P. (2000). *Collected papers on Jaina studies.* Motilal Banarsidass.

Jainism Says. (2020). Jainism: Know It, Understand It & Internalize It. *Jainism Says.* https://jainism-says.blogspot.com/2020/05/yoga-and-meditation-in-jainism.html

Jaiswal, Y. S., & Williams, L. L. (2016). A glimpse of Ayurveda – The forgotten history and principles of Indian traditional medicine. *Journal of Traditional and Complementary Medicine, 7*(1), 50–53. doi:10.1016/j.jtcme.2016.02.002 PMID:28053888

Janetius, S. T. (2011). *Indigenous therapeutic counselling in the Indian context.* Research gate.

Janssen, M., Heerkens, Y., Kuijer, W., Van Der Heijden, B., & Engels, J. (2018). Effects of Mindfulness-Based Stress Reduction on employees' mental health: A systematic review. *PLoS One, 13*(1), e0191332. doi:10.1371/journal.pone.0191332 PMID:29364935

JapoN. (2023, September 27). Wikipedia. Retrieved from https://en.wikipedia.org/wiki/Naam_Japo#:~:text=In%20Sikhism%2C%20N%C4%81m%20Jap%C5%8D%20

Jas (2022, May 7). Conquer your mind and Conquer the world - ReflectandRespond. ReflectandRespond. https://reflectandrespond.com/guru-nanak-conquer-your-mind-conquer-the-world/

Jayaram, V. (2019). The Samkhya Yoga of the Bhagavadgita, An Analysis. *Hindu Website.* https://www.hinduwebsite.com/samkhya.asp

Jensen, C. G., Vangkilde, S., Frokjaer, V., & Hasselbalch, S. G. (2012). Mindfulness training affects attention—Or is it attentional effort? *Journal of Experimental Psychology. General, 141*(1), 106–123. doi:10.1037/a0024931 PMID:21910559

Jeste, D., & Vahia, I. (2008). Comparison of the conceptualization of wisdom in ancient Indian literature with modern views: Focus on the Bhagavad Gita. *Psychiatry, 71*(3), 197–209. doi:10.1521/psyc.2008.71.3.197 PMID:18834271

Jha, A. P., Stanley, E. A., Kiyonaga, A., Wong, L., & Gelfand, L. (2010). Examining the protective effects of mindfulness training on working memory capacity and affective experience. *Emotion (Washington, D.C.), 10*(1), 54–64. doi:10.1037/a0018438 PMID:20141302

Jiménez-Gómez, L., Bernabé, J. R. Y., Crego, A., Ventola, A. R. M., & Gómez-Martínez, M. Á. (2022). Effectiveness of the Mindfulness-Based Stress Reduction (MBSR) vs. the Mindful Self-Compassion (MSC) Programs in Clinical and Health Psychologist Trainees. *Mindfulness, 13*(3), 584–599. doi:10.100712671-021-01814-2

Jin, M. H., McDonald, B., & Park, J. (2018). Person–organization fit and turnover intention: Exploring the mediating role of employee followership and job satisfaction through conservation of resources theory. *Review of Public Personnel Administration, 38*(2), 167–192. doi:10.1177/0734371X16658334

Jm, G., Brar, J. S., Rai, A., & Knr, C. (2019). Effects of a standardized extract of Withania somnifera (Ashwagandha) on depression and anxiety symptoms in persons with schizophrenia participating in a randomized, placebo-controlled clinical trial. *PubMed, 31*(2), 123–129. https://pubmed.ncbi.nlm.nih.gov/31046033

Junglas, I., Johnson, N., Steel, D., Abraham, D., & Loughlin, P. (2007). Identity formation, learning styles and trust in virtual worlds. *The Data Base for Advances in Information Systems, 38*(4), 90–96. doi:10.1145/1314234.1314251

Juntunen, C., Barraclough, D., Broneck, C., Seibel, G., Winrow, S., & Morin, P. (2001). American indian perspectives on the career journey. *Journal of Counseling Psychology, 48*(3), 274–285. doi:10.1037/0022-0167.48.3.274

Juyal, R. C., Negi, S., Wakhode, P., Bhat, S., Bhat, B., & Thelma, B. (2012). Potential of Ayurgenomics Approach in Complex Trait Research: Leads from a Pilot Study on Rheumatoid Arthritis. *PLoS One, 7*(9), e45752. doi:10.1371/journal.pone.0045752 PMID:23049851

Kalra, V. (2020). *Psychotherapy Model for the Training Counsellors in India*. National Louis University. https://digitalcommons.nl.edu/cgi/viewcontent.cgi? article= 1443&context=diss

Kamradt, J. M. (2017). Integrating yoga into psychotherapy: The ethics of moving from the mind to the mat. *Complementary Therapies in Clinical Practice, 27*, 27–30. doi:10.1016/j.ctcp.2017.01.003 PMID:28438276

Kapur, M., John, A., Rozario, J., & Oommen, A. (1991) NIMHANS Index for Specific Learning Disabilities. Department of Clinical Psychology, NIMHANS Publication, Bangalore.

Karkada, G., Shenoy, K., Halahalli, H. N., & Karanth, K. S. (2012). Nardostachys jatamansi extract prevents chronic restraint stress-induced learning and memory deficits in a radial arm maze task. *Journal of Natural Science, Biology, and Medicine, 3*(2), 125. doi:10.4103/0976-9668.101879 PMID:23225973

KaroK. (2022, August 17). Wikipedia. Retrieved from https://en.wikipedia.org/wiki/Kirat_Karo

Kaur, P., & Sinha, A. K. (1992). Dimensions of guna in organizational setting. *Vikalpa, 17*(3), 27–32. doi:10.1177/0256090919920303

Kay, A. A., & Skarlicki, D. P. (2020, July). Cultivating a conflict-positive workplace: How mindfulness facilitates constructive conflict management. *Organizational Behavior and Human Decision Processes, 159*, 8–20. doi:10.1016/j.obhdp.2020.02.005

Keir, S. T. (2010). Effect of massage therapy on stress levels and quality of life in brain tumor patients—Observations from a pilot study. *Supportive Care in Cancer, 19*(5), 711–715. doi:10.100700520-010-1032-5 PMID:21046417

Keng, S., Tong, E. M. W., Yan, E. T. L., Ebstein, R. P., & Lai, P. (2021). Effects of mindfulness-based stress reduction on affect dynamics: A randomized controlled trial. *Mindfulness, 12*(6), 1490–1501. doi:10.100712671-021-01617-5

Keown, D. (2022). Origins of Buddhist ethics. Encyclopedia of Religious Ethics, (pp. 602–610). Wiley. doi:10.1002/9781118499528.ch71

Keshavan, M. S. (2020). Building resilience in the COVID-19 era: Three paths in the Bhagavad Gita. *Indian Journal of Psychiatry, 62*(5), 459–461. doi:10.4103/psychiatry.IndianJPsychiatry_829_20 PMID:33678824

Khalsa, S. (2017). A perspective on yoga research: Past to present. *Yoga Mimamsa., 49*(1), 1–2. doi:10.4103/ym.ym_10_17

Khanna, D., & Peterson, A. (2023). *State-led education reform in Delhi, India, A case study of the Happiness Curriculum.* Brookings Institution. https://policycommons.net/artifacts/4139426/state-led-education-reform-in-delhi-india-a-case-study-of-the-happiness-curriculum/4948375/

Khemka, S. S., Ramarao, N. H., & Hankey, A. (2011). Effect of integral yoga on psychological and health variables and their correlations. *International Journal of Yoga*, *4*(2), 93–99. doi:10.4103/0973-6131.85492 PMID:22022128

Kilamarva, K. (1994). Clinical evaluation of Smrtisagararasa in cases of residual schizophrenia. *J Research Ayurveda Siddha, 15.*

Kilpatrick, L. A., Suyenobu, B. Y., Smith, S. R., Bueller, J. A., Goodman, T., Creswell, J. D., Tillisch, K., Mayer, E. A., & Naliboff, B. D. (2011). Impact of mindfulness-based stress reduction training on intrinsic brain connectivity. *NeuroImage*, *56*(1), 290–298. doi:10.1016/j.neuroimage.2011.02.034 PMID:21334442

Kim, U., Yang, G., & Hwang, K. K. (Eds.). (2006). *Indigenous and cultural psychology: Understanding people in context.* Springer. doi:10.1007/0-387-28662-4

King, D. B. (2008). Brighter paths to wellbeing: An integrative model of human intelligence and health. Trent University Centre for Health Studies Showcase 2008, pp. 12–13. King, D. B. (2010). Personal meaning production as a component of spiritual intelligence. *International Journal of Existential Psychology & Psychotherapy*, *3*(1), 1–5.

Kirk, M. L., Boon, B., & DiTuro, D. (2005). *Hatha Yoga Illustrated.* Human Kinetics.

Kirk, S. A., & Kirk, W. D. (1971). *Psycholinguistic learning disabilities: Diagnosis and remediation.* University of Illinois Press.

Kirmayer, L. J. (2015). Mindfulness in cultural context. *Transcultural Psychiatry*, *4*(4), 447–469. doi:10.1177/1363461515598949 PMID:26264787

Kishore, R. K., Ashok, A. H., Udupa, K., Thirthalli, J., Lavekar, G. S., Gangadhar, B. N., Raju, T., & Sathyaprabha, T. (2014). Evaluation of the influence of ayurvedic formulation (Ayushman-15) on psychopathology, heart rate variability and stress hormonal level in major depression (Vishada). *Asian Journal of Psychiatry*, *12*, 100–107. doi:10.1016/j.ajp.2014.07.002 PMID:25219946

Koleci, V., & Koleci, R. (2022). *(PDF) objectives of Modern Management Psychology.* Research Gate. https://www.researchgate.net/publication/364642679_Objectives_of_modern_management_psychology

Komito, D. R., Rinchen, G. S., & Dorjee, T. (1987). *Nagarjuna's Seventy Stanzas.* Snow Lion.

Kongkeaw, C., Dilokthornsakul, P., Thanarangsarit, P., Limpeanchob, N., & Scholfield, C. N. (2014). Meta-analysis of randomized controlled trials on cognitive effects of Bacopa monnieri extract. *Journal of Ethnopharmacology*, *151*(1), 528–535. doi:10.1016/j.jep.2013.11.008 PMID:24252493

Koo, B., Park, K., Ha, J., Park, J. H., Lim, J., & Lee, D. (2003). Inhibitory Effects of the Fragrance Inhalation of Essential Oil from Acorus gramineus on Central Nervous System. *Biological & Pharmaceutical Bulletin*, *26*(7), 978–982. doi:10.1248/bpb.26.978 PMID:12843622

Kornfielf, J. (2011). *Teachings of the Buddha.* Shambala Publications.

Kraines, M. A., Peterson, S. K., Tremont, G., Beard, C., Brewer, J. A., & Uebelacker, L. A. (2022). Mindfulness-based stress reduction and cognitive therapy for depression: A systematic review of cognitive outcomes. *Mindfulness*, *13*(5), 1126–1135. doi:10.100712671-022-01841-7 PMID:36059888

Kreyenbroek, P. G. (2013). *Living Zoroastrianism: urban Parsis speak about their religion.* Routledge. doi:10.4324/9780203037133

Krishnan, H. A. (2021). Mindfulness as a strategy for sustainable competitive advantage. *Business Horizons, 64*(5), 697–709. doi:10.1016/j.bushor.2021.02.023

Krishnan, R. (2022). The bhagavad gita as the epitome of indian psychology vis-à-vis modern psychology. *Mind & Society, 11*(01), 62–66. doi:10.56011/mind-mri-111-20228

Krishnan, V. R., & Mulla, Z. R. (2022). Karma-yoga: philosophy of moral development and work motivation. In *Indigenous Indian Management: Conceptualization, Practical Applications and Pedagogical Initiatives* (pp. 127–156). Springer International Publishing. doi:10.1007/978-3-030-87906-8_5

Kristof-Brown, A. L., Zimmerman, R. D., & Johnson, E. C. (2005). Consequences of individuals' fit at work: A meta-analysis of person-job, person-organization, person-group, and person-supervisor fit. *Personnel Psychology, 58*(2), 281–342. doi:10.1111/j.1744-6570.2005.00672.x

Kudesia, R. S. (2019). Mindfulness as Metacognitive Practice. *Academy of Management Review, 44*(2), 405–423. doi:10.5465/amr.2015.0333

Kulamarva, K., Shivakumar, V., Chikkanna, U., Ramakrishna, K. K., Bhargav, H., & Varambally, S. (2023, May). Role of Ayurveda in the management of psychotic disorders: A systematic review of clinical evidence. *Journal of Ayurveda and Integrative Medicine, 14*(3), 100720. doi:10.1016/j.jaim.2023.100720 PMID:37290315

Kulkarni, R. (1995). Synergetic effect of Vallarai and Brahmi on learning ability of albino mice and school children. *International Seminar on Recent Trends in Pharmaceutical Sciences.*

Kulkarni, R., Girish, K., & Kumar, A. (2012a). Nootropic herbs (Medhya Rasayana) in Ayurveda: An update. *Pharmacognosy Reviews, 6*(12), 147. doi:10.4103/0973-7847.99949 PMID:23055641

Kumar, M. (2023). *Indian Psychology in the New Millennium.* Tutorials Point. https://www.tutorialspoint.com/indian-psychology-in-the-new-millennium

Kumar, M. (2023). *Indian Psychology: Implications and Applications.* Tutorials Point. https://www.tutorialspoint.com/indian-psychology-implications-and-applications

Kumar, M. (2023). *Psychotherapy and Indian thought.* Tutorials Point. https://www. tutorialspoint.com/ psychotherapy-and-indian-thought.

Kumar, S. K. (2008). Indian thought and tradition: A psycho-historical perspective. Handbook of Indian psychology, (pp. 19-52). Cambridge Press.

Kumar, A., & Sk, K. (2006). Protective effect of BR-16A, a polyherbal preparation against social isolation stress: Possible GABAergic mechanism. *Phytotherapy Research, 20*(7), 538–541. doi:10.1002/ptr.1873 PMID:16691632

Kumar, D., & Singh, D. (2022). India's New Education Policy (NEP) 2020 Creating Children with Disability. *International Journal of Advanced Research in Science. Tongxin Jishu,* •••, 70–74.

Kumar, K., Prakash, A., & Singh, K. (2020). How National Education Policy 2020 can be a lodestar to transform future generation in India. *Journal of Public Affairs, 21*(3), e2500. Advance online publication. doi:10.1002/pa.2500

Kumar, R. S., Britto, J., Ilavarasu, J., & Rajesh, S. K. (2022). Study of Emotion Regulation Based on Yogic Personality Using Implicit, Explicit, and Eye Tracking Techniques. *International Journal of Yoga, 15*(2), 122–129. doi:10.4103/ijoy.ijoy_36_22 PMID:36329772

Kumar, S., & Nathani, N. (2014). Preventative and therapeutic measures of Ayurveda for mental health care. *Pharma Science Monitor*, *5*(1), 176–183.

Kumar, V. (2006). Potential medicinal plants for CNS disorders: An overview. *Phytotherapy Research*, *20*(12), 1023–1035. doi:10.1002/ptr.1970 PMID:16909441

Kuppuswamy, B. (1977). *Dharma and Society*. Macmillan.

Kwok, J. Y. Y., Kwan, J. C. Y., Auyeung, M., Mok, V. C. T., & Chan, H. Y. L. (2017). The effects of yoga versus stretching and resistance training exercises on psychological distress for people with mild-to-moderate Parkinson's disease: Study protocol for a randomized controlled trial. *Trials*, *18*(1), 1–13. https://trialsjournal.biomedcentral.com/articles/10.1186/s13063-017-2223-x. doi:10.118613063-017-2223-x PMID:28049491

Lai, X., Liang, H., & Zhao, Y. (2002). A survey of the studies on chemical constituents and pharmacological activities of Acorus plants. *PubMed*, *27*(3), 161–165, 198. https://pubmed.ncbi.nlm.nih.gov/12807142

Lal, S. (1984). Rabindranāth Tagore's Ideals of Aesthetic Education. *Journal of Aesthetic Education*, *18*(2), 31–39. doi:10.2307/3332497

Lauver, K. J., & Kristof-Brown, A. (2001). Distinguishing between employees' perceptions of person–job and person–organization fit. *Journal of Vocational Behavior*, *59*(3), 454–470. doi:10.1006/jvbe.2001.1807

Lawler, V. V. & Lyman Porter, E. (2005). Expectancy theories. In Organizational Behavior 1. Routledge.

Lazaridou, A., & Pentaris, P. (2016). Mindfulness and spirituality: Therapeutic perspectives. *Person-Centered and Experiential Psychotherapies*, *15*(3), 235–244. doi:10.1080/14779757.2016.1180634

Lazarus, R., & Folkman, S. (1984). *Stress, appraisal, and coping*. Springer.

Lee, J., Kim, K. H., Webster, C., & Henning, M. A. (2021). The evolution of mindfulness from 1916 to 2019. *Mindfulness*, *12*(8), 1849–1859. doi:10.100712671-021-01603-x

Lee, T. R., Chen, S. Y., Wang, S. H., & Dadura, A. (2010). The relationship between spiritual management and determinants of turnover intention. *European Business Review*, *22*(1), 102–116. doi:10.1108/09555341011009034

Lengacher, C. A., Gruss, L. F., Kip, K. E., Reich, R. R., Chauca, K. G., Moscoso, M. S., Joshi, A., Tinsley, S., Shani, B., Cousin, L., Khan, C. P., Goodman, M., & Park, J. Y. (2021). Mindfulness-based stress reduction for breast cancer survivors: Evaluating mediators of psychological and physical outcomes in a large randomized controlled trial. *Journal of Behavioral Medicine*, *44*(5), 591–604. doi:10.100710865-021-00214-0 PMID:33963420

Lim, S. J. (2007). Effects of fractions of Benincasa hispida on antioxidant status in Streptozotocin induced Diabetic rats. *Korean J Nutr, 40*.

Linley, P. A., & Joseph, S. (Eds.). (2004). *Positive Psychology in Practice*. Wiley. doi:10.1002/9780470939338

Liu, S., Xin, H., Shen, L., Hi, J., & Liu, J. (2020, January 21). The Influence of Individual and Team Mindfulness on Work Engagement. *Frontiers in Psychology*, *10*, 2928. doi:10.3389/fpsyg.2019.02928 PMID:32038356

Li, Y., Wu, L., Chang, C., Wang, L., Guo, C., Zhao, X., Zhao, T., Wang, X., Liu, A., & Zhang, Y. (2020). Serum Metabolic Profiling Reveals the Antidepressive Effects of the Total Iridoids of Valeriana jatamansi Jones on Chronic Unpredictable Mild Stress Mice. *Frontiers in Pharmacology*, *11*, 338. doi:10.3389/fphar.2020.00338 PMID:32265710

Locke, E. A., & Latham, G. P. (2006). New directions in goal-setting theory. *Current Directions in Psychological Science*, *15*(5), 265–268. doi:10.1111/j.1467-8721.2006.00449.x

Lolla, A. (2018). Mantras help the general psychological well-being of college students: A pilot study. *Journal of Religion and Health, 57*(1), 110–119. doi:10.100710943-017-0371-7 PMID:28271341

Lv, J., Sun, Z., Li, H., & Hou, Y. (2023, June 26). *The role of negative perfectionism and the relationship between critical thinking and the halo effect: Insights from Corporate Managers in human resources*. MDPI. https://www.mdpi.com/2076-328X/13/7/533

Lynch, J., Prihodova, L., Dunne, P. J., O'Leary, C., Breen, R., Carroll, Á., Walsh, C., McMahon, G., & White, B. (2018). Mantra meditation programme for emergency department staff: A qualitative study. *BMJ Open, 8*(9), e020685. doi:10.1136/bmjopen-2017-020685 PMID:30249626

Lyubomirsky, S., & Layous, K. (2013). How do simple positive activities increase well-being? *Current Directions in Psychological Science, 22*(1), 57–62. doi:10.1177/0963721412469809

Macdonell, A. A. (Ed.). (1924). *A Practical Sanskrit Dictionary*. Oxford University Press.

MacPherson, S. A., Grabovac, A. D., Collins, E. J., Heath, T., Rockman, P., & Winston, D. (2022). Transprofessional competencies across clinical, organizational, and educational professions: The case of mindfulness-based teaching and learning (MBTL). *Professional Development in Education*, 1–17. doi:10.1080/19415257.2022.2143863

Madahavananda, S. (1982). *Vivekacudamani*. The Indian Press.

Maehle, G. (2011). *Ashtanga Yoga: Practice and Philosophy*. New World Library.

Mahakul, B. K. (2020). Mahatma Gandhi's vision on education: its relevance in the 21st century. *International Journal of Creative Research Thoughts (IJCRT), 8*(2,).

Maharishi Mahesh Yogi. (1963). *The science of being and the art of living: Transcendental meditation*. Signet.

Maharishi Mahesh Yogi. (1967). *On the Bhagavad-Gita: A translation and commentary*. Penguin/Arkana.

Malviya, S. (2021, September 12). Influence of western culture on Indian society. *The Times of India*. https://timesofindia.indiatimes.com/readersblog/know-your-rights/influence-of-western-culture-on-indian-society-37332/

Manickam, L. (2008). Research on Indian Concepts of psychology: Major Challenges and Perspectives for future action. In *Handbook of Indian Psychology* (pp. 492–505). https://www.researchgate.net/publication/312056622_Research_on_Indian_Concepts_of_psychology_Major_Challenges_and_Perspectives_for_future_action

Manickam, L. S. S., & Sahya. (2004). The concept in Indian philosophical psychology and its contemporary relevance. In: Joshi K. & Cornelissen M. (eds.), *Yoga and Indian approaches to psychology*. New-Delhi: Centre for the Study of Civilizations.

Marballi., G.K (2013). *Journey Through The Srimad Bhagavad Gita - A Modern Commentary With Word-To-Word Sanskrit-English Translation*. Lulu.

Marques, J. (2022). Treading the noble eightfold path: A leadership development strategy in a VUCA world. In Developing Leaders for Real: Proven Approaches That Deliver Impact (pp. 163–173). Emerald Publishing. doi:10.1108/978-1-80071-364-220221024

Marrie, R. A., Walld, R., Bolton, J. M., Sareen, J., Walker, J. R., Patten, S. B., Singer, A., Lix, L. M., Hitchon, C., El-Gabalawy, R., Katz, A., Fisk, J. D., & Bernstein, Ç. N. (2017a). Increased incidence of psychiatric disorders in immune-mediated inflammatory disease. *Journal of Psychosomatic Research, 101*, 17–23. doi:10.1016/j.jpsychores.2017.07.015 PMID:28867419

Marutham, P., Balodhi, J. P., & Mishra, H. (1998). Sattva, Rajas, Tamas (SRT) Inventory. *Nimhans Journal*, 15–19.

Mason, R., & De la Torre, M. (2000). Heritage conservation and values in globalizing societies. In *World culture report 2000: Cultural Diversity, Conflict and Pluralism*. UNESCO PUBLISHING, UNESCO Digital Library. https://unesdoc.unesco.org/ark:/48223/pf0000121094

Matasci, D., Jerónimo, M. B., & Dores, H. G. (Eds.). (2020). *Education and Development in Colonial and Postcolonial Africa: Policies, Paradigms, and Entanglements* (pp. 1890s–1980s). Springer International Publishing., doi:10.1007/978-3-030-27801-4

Mathew, V. G. (2001). *A Short History of Indian Psychology*. Psychology4All. https://www.psychology4all.com/HistoryI.htm

Mathias, K., Kermode, M., Goicolea, I., Seefeldt, L., Shidhaye, R., & San Sebastian, M. (2018). Social Distance and Community Attitudes Towards People with Psycho-Social Disabilities in Uttarakhand, India. *Community Mental Health Journal*, *54*(3), 343–353. doi:10.100710597-017-0211-y PMID:29143156

Mazumdar, D. A. (2021). Importance of Jain values in shaping. *Business Ethics (Oxford, England).*

McCarty, T. L., Borgoiakova, T., Gilmore, P., Lomawaima, K. T., & Romero, M. E. (2005). Indigenous Epistemologies and Education—Self-Determination, Anthropology, and Human Rights. *Anthropology & Education Quarterly*, *36*(1), 1–7. doi:10.1525/aeq.2005.36.1.001

McQuaid, E. L., & Spirito, A. (2012). Integrating Research Into Clinical Internship Training Bridging the Science/Practice Gap in Pediatric Psychology. *Journal of Pediatric Psychology*, *37*(2), 149–157. doi:10.1093/jpepsy/jsr114 PMID:22286345

Mehta, K., Mehta, S., Chalana, H., Singh, H., & Thaman, R. G. (2020). Effectiveness of Rajyoga meditation as an adjunct to first-line treatment in patients with obsessive compulsive disorder. *Indian Journal of Psychiatry*, *62*(6), 684–689. doi:10.4103/psychiatry.IndianJPsychiatry_401_19 PMID:33896974

Mekong Cultural Hub. (n.d.). *Anmol Vellani*. Mekong Cultural Hub. https://www.mekongculturalhub.org/people/anmol/

Memon, M. A., Salleh, R., Nordin, S. M., Cheah, J. H., Ting, H., & Chuah, F. (2018). Person-organisation fit and turnover intention: The mediating role of work engagement. *Journal of Management Development*, *37*(3), 285–298. doi:10.1108/JMD-07-2017-0232

Menon,S.(2005). What is Indian psychology: Transcendence in and while thinking. *The Journal of Transpersonal Psychology, 37*(2), 83-98.

Menon, S. (2005). What is Indian psychology: Transcendence in and while thinking. *Journal of Transpersonal Psychology*, *37*, 2.

Meuller. (2021). *Aspects of Purusha (Consciousness) and Prakriti(Nature)*. LinkedIn. .https://www.linkedin.com/pulse/aspects-purusha-consciousness-prakritinature-erica-mueller

Miller, J. (2003). Daoism and nature. *Nature across cultures: Views of nature and the environment in non-western cultures*, (pp. 393–409). Springer. https://link.springer.com/chapter/10.1007/978-94-017-0149-5_20

Miller, R. (n.d.). *Yoga Therapy: Definition, Perspective and Principles*. International Association of Yoga Therapists (IAYT). https://www.iayt.org/page/YogaTherapyDefinitio

Miller, C. J., McNear, J., & Metz, M. J. (2013). A comparison of traditional and engaging lecture methods in a large, professional-level course. *Advances in Physiology Education*, *37*(4), 347–355. doi:10.1152/advan.00050.2013 PMID:24292912

Milliman, J., Czaplewski, A. J., & Ferguson, J. (2003). Workplace spirituality and employee work attitudes: An exploratory empirical assessment. *Journal of Organizational Change Management*, *16*(4), 426–447. doi:10.1108/09534810310484172

Mills, P. J., Peterson, C. T., Wilson, K., Pung, M. A., Patel, S. V., Weiss, L., Kshirsagar, S. G., Tanzi, R. E., & Chopra, D. (2019). Relationships among classifications of ayurvedic medicine diagnostics for imbalances and western measures of psychological states: An exploratory study. *Journal of Ayurveda and Integrative Medicine*, *10*(3), 198–202. doi:10.1016/j.jaim.2018.02.001 PMID:30385015

Miranda, A., & Gutter, P. (2002). Diversity research literature in school psychology: 1990-1999. *Psychology in the Schools*, *39*(5), 597–604. doi:10.1002/pits.10051

Miranda, E. (2002). Planning and executing time-bound projects. *Computer*, *35*(3), 73–79. doi:10.1109/2.989933

Mishra, Sreetama. (2014). Some Reflections on Pedagogy: In the Light of Paulo Freire and Rabindranath Tagore. *Indian Journal of Applied Research*, *4*(1).

Mishra, A. K., & Padalia, D. (2021). Re-envisioning Psychology: A Critical History of Psychology in India. In G. Misra, N. Sanyal, & S. De (Eds.), *Psychology in Modern India: Historical, Methodological, and Future Perspectives* (pp. 163–201). Springer. doi:10.1007/978-981-16-4705-5_10

Mishra, A. S., Sk, R., Hs, V., Nagarathna, R., Anand, A., Bhutani, H., Sivapuram, M. S., Singh, A., & Nagendra, H. R. (2020). Knowledge, Attitude, and Practice of Yoga in Rural and Urban India, KAPY 2017: A Nationwide Cluster Sample Survey. *Medicines (Basel, Switzerland)*, *7*(2), 8. doi:10.3390/medicines7020008 PMID:32033426

Mishra, L. C., Singh, B. B., & Dagenais, S. (2001). Ayurveda: A historical perspective and principles of the traditional healthcare system in India. *Alternative Therapies in Health and Medicine*, *7*(2), 36–43. PMID:11253415

Mishra, R. C. (1994). Individualist-collectivist orientations across generations. In U. Kim, H. C. Triandis, C. Kagitcibasi, S. Choi, & G. Yoon (Eds.), *Individualism and collectivism: Theory, method, and practice* (pp. 225–238). SAGE Publications.

Mishra, R. C. (2013). Moksha and the Hindu worldview. *Psychology and Developing Societies*, *25*(1), 21–42. doi:10.1177/0971333613477318

Monier Williams, M. (1964). *A Sanskrit – English Dictionary* (Rev. ed.). Motilal Banarsidass.

Moniz, R. J. (2010). 1 - History of managerial thought: A brief overview. In R. J. Moniz (Ed.), *Practical and Effective Management of Libraries* (pp. 1–18). Chandos Publishing. doi:10.1016/B978-1-84334-578-7.50001-3

Monro, R. (1997). Yoga therapy. *Journal of Bodywork and Movement Therapies*, *1*(4), 215–218. doi:10.1016/S1360-8592(97)80047-2

Montiel-Castro, A. J., González-Cervantes, R. M., Bravo-Ruiseco, G., & Pacheco-López, G. (2013). The microbiota-gut-brain axis: Neurobehavioral correlates, health and sociality. *Frontiers in Integrative Neuroscience*, *7*. doi:10.3389/fnint.2013.00070 PMID:24109440

Mooventhan, A., & Nivethitha, L. (2017). Evidence based effects of yoga in neurological disorders. *Journal of Clinical Neuroscience*, *43*, 61–67. doi:10.1016/j.jocn.2017.05.012 PMID:28599839

Morgan, A. K., & Stevens, J. D. (2010). Does *Bacopa monnieri* Improve Memory Performance in Older Persons? Results of a Randomized, Placebo-Controlled, Double-Blind Trial. *Journal of Alternative and Complementary Medicine (New York, N.Y.)*, *16*(7), 753–759. doi:10.1089/acm.2009.0342 PMID:20590480

Moynihan, D. P., & Pandey, S. K. (2007). The ties that bind: Social networks, person-organization value fit, and turnover intention. *Journal of Public Administration: Research and Theory*, *18*(2), 205–227. doi:10.1093/jopart/mum013

Mukherjee, M. (2019, January 1). *Culturally Responsive Teaching Learning in Indian Multicultural Context: Review of Contemporary Policy & Practice*. 25th International Multi-disciplinary Conference On Arts, Social Science, Management and Technology. Research Gate.

Mukherjee, M. (2015). Indian education at the crossroads of postcoloniality, globalization and the 21st century Knowledge Economy (Part 1). *Policy Futures in Education, 13*(2), 165–170. doi:10.1177/1478210314568180

Mukherjee, P. K., Venkatesan, K., Mal, M., & Houghton, P. J. (2007). *In vitro* Acetylcholinesterase Inhibitory Activity of the Essential Oil from *Acorus calamus* and its Main Constituents. *Planta Medica, 73*(3), 283–285. doi:10.1055-2007-967114 PMID:17286241

Mukundananda, S. (n.d.). Bhagavad Gita, The Song of God – Swami Mukundananda (Chapter 14, Verse 20). *Holy Bhagavad Gita*. https://www.holy-bhagavad-gita.org/chapter/14/verse/20

Mulla, Z. R., & Krishnan, V. R. (2006). Karma Yoga: A conceptualization and validation of the Indian philosophy of work. *Journal of Indian Psychology, 24*(1/2), 26–43.

Mulla, Z. R., & Krishnan, V. R. (2008). Karma-Yoga, the Indian work ideal, and its relationship with empathy. *Psychology and Developing Societies, 20*(1), 27–49. doi:10.1177/097133360702000102

Mulla, Z. R., & Krishnan, V. R. (2014). Karma-yoga: The Indian model of moral development. *Journal of Business Ethics, 123*(2), 339–351. doi:10.100710551-013-1842-8

Müller, F. M. (1879). *Taittiriya Upanishad. The sacred books of the East* (Vol. 15). Oxford University Press. https://holybooks-lichtenbergpress.netdna-ssl.com/wp-content/uploads/15.SacredBooksEast.VarOrSch.v15.Muller.Hindu_.Mull_.Upanishads.p2.KathMundTait.Mait_.Oxf_.1884.pdf

Murthy, P. K., & Kumar, S. K. (2007). The concept of Triguna: A critical analysis and synthesis. *Psychological Studies, 52*(2), 103–113.

Murthy, S. (2010). From local to global contributions of Indian psychiatry to international psychiatry. [PUBMED]. *Indian Journal of Psychiatry, 52*(7), 30–37. doi:10.4103/0019-5545.69202 PMID:21836699

Myers, J. E., & Williard, K. (2003). Integrating spirituality into counselor preparation: A developmental, wellness approach. *Counseling and Values, 47*(2), 142–155. doi:10.1002/j.2161-007X.2003.tb00231.x

Nagendra, H. R. (2013). Integrated yoga therapy for mental illness. *Indian Journal of Psychiatry, 55*(7, Suppl 3), S337. doi:10.4103/0019-5545.116299 PMID:24049195

Nahavandi, A., & Krishnan, H. A. (2017). Indo-European Leadership (IEL): A Non-Western Leadership Perspective. *Global and Culturally Diverse Leaders and Leadership (Building Leadership Bridges*, (PP. 105-123). Emerald. doi:10.1108/S2058-880120170000003006

Nandram, S., & Bindlish, P. (2017). *Managing VUCA through integrative self-management.* Springer. https://link.springer.com/book/10.1007%2F978-3-319-52231-9

Narayan J. (1997). *Grade Level Assessment Device for Children with Learning Problems in Schools (GLAD)*. Secunderabad: National Institute for the Mentally Handicapped (NIMH).

Narayanan, Y. (2010). Sustainable consumption as a means to self-realization: A Hindu perspective on when enough is enough. *Sustainable Development (Bradford), 18*(5), 252–259. doi:10.1002d.476

Narcıkara, E. (2017). *Spiritüel liderlik davranışının algılanan performans üzerine etkisi.* Yayınlanmış Doktora Tezi, Yıldız Teknik Üniversitesi.

Narcıkara, E. B. (2018). Spiritüelite (Ruhsallık) ve iş ortamında anlam arayışı. *Alanya Akademik Bakış*, *2*(1), 11–25. doi:10.29023/alanyaakademik.337789

Narcıkara, E. B., & Zehir, C. (2016). Effect of Organizational Support in the Relationship between Spiritual Leadership and Performance. *International Journal of Humanities and Social Science*, *6*(12), 29–42.

National Education Policy. (2020) *NEP Final*. NEP. https://www.education.gov.in/sites/upload_files/mhrd/files/NEP_Final_English_0.pdf

NCERT. (2022). *National Curriculum Framework for Foundational Stage, 2022*. Government of India.

Nedungottil, C., Agrawal, J., Sharma, M. P., & Murthy, P. (2021). *Men with and without alcohol dependence: A comparative study of Triguna*. Anasakti, Personality and Subjective Well-being.

Neki, J. S. (1973). Guru-Chela relationship: The possibility of therapeutic paradigm. *The American Journal of Orthopsychiatry*, *43*(5), 755–766. doi:10.1111/j.1939-0025.1973.tb00847.x PMID:4742816

Neki, J. S. (1977). Psychotherapy in India. *Indian Journal of Psychiatry*, *19*, 1–10.

Neumark-Sztainer, D. (2014). Yoga and eating disorders: Is there a place for yoga in the prevention and treatment of eating disorders and disordered eating behaviours? *Advances in Eating Disorders (Abingdon, England)*, *2*(2), 136–145. doi:10.1080/21662630.2013.862369 PMID:24955291

Newberg, A. & Waldman, M. (2012). *Words can Change your Brain*. A Plume Book.

Ninivaggi, F. (2010). *A comprehensive guide to traditional Indian medicine for the west-anatomy* (Vol. 3). Rowman & Littlefield Publishers.

Noggle, J. J., Steiner, N. J., Minami, T., & Khalsa, S. B. S. (2012). Benefits of yoga for psychosocial well-being in a US high school curriculum: A preliminary randomized controlled trial. *Journal of Developmental and Behavioral Pediatrics*, *33*(3), 193–201. doi:10.1097/DBP.0b013e31824afdc4 PMID:22343481

Nowicki, E. A., & Sandieson, R. (2002). A meta-analysis of school-age children's attitudes towards persons with physical or intellectual disabilities. *International Journal of Disability Development and Education*, *49*(3), 243–265. doi:10.1080/1034912022000007270

O'Connell, K. M. (2010) Tagore and Education: Creativity, Mutuality and Survival. *Asiatic: IIUM Journal of English Language and Literature*, *4*(1), 65–76. https://journals.iium.edu.my/asiatic/index.php/ajell/article/view/518

O'Keefe, V. M., Cwik, M. F., Haroz, E. E., & Barlow, A. (2021). Increasing Culturally Responsive Care and Mental Health Equity With Indigenous Community Mental Health Workers. *Psychological Services*, *18*(1), 84–92. doi:10.1037er0000358 PMID:31045405

Obeyesekere, G. (1970). Ayurveda and mental illness. *Comparative Studies in Society and History*, *12*(3), 292–296. doi:10.1017/S0010417500005867 PMID:11614363

Olkin, R., & Pledger, C. (2003). Can disability studies and psychology join hands? *The American Psychologist*, *58*(4), 296–304. doi:10.1037/0003-066X.58.4.296 PMID:12866396

Ong, J. C., & Smith, C. E. (2017). Using mindfulness for the treatment of insomnia. *Current Sleep Medicine Reports*, *3*, 57–65. https://link.springer.com/article/10.1007/s40675-017-0068-1

Osborne, A. (1970). *Ramana Maharshi and the path of self-knowledge*. Rider & Co.

Osho International. (2015). *Being Free in an Unfree Society: Different Approaches of Western Psychology and the Eastern Concept of Meditation*. The Concept of No-Mind. https://pragyata.com/the-concept-of-no-mind/

Osho. (2005). *Jeevan kya hai (What is life?)*. New Delhi: Hind Pocket Books.

Ouchi, Y., Kanno, T., Okada, H., Yoshikawa, E., Shinke, T., Nagasawa, S., Minoda, K., & Doi, H. (2006). Changes in cerebral blood flow under the prone condition with and without massage. *Neuroscience Letters*, *407*(2), 131–135. doi:10.1016/j.neulet.2006.08.037 PMID:16973270

Padesky, C. A. (1993a). *Socratic Questioning: Changing minds or guiding discovery?* Keynote address to European Congress of Behavioural and Cognitive Therapies, London.

Panara, K., Nariya, M., & Nishteswar, K. (2020). Central nervous system depressant activity of Jatamansi (Nardostachys jatamansi DC.) rhizome. *Ayu*, *41*(4), 250. doi:10.4103/ayu.AYU_251_20 PMID:35813358

Panda, S. N. (2017). The bhagavad gitā and health management of psychotherapy. *Odisha journal of social science, 106.*

Pandey, A., Gupta, V., & Gupta, R. K. (2019). Spirituality and innovative behaviour in teams: Examining the mediating role of team learning. *IIMB Management Review*, *31*(2), 116–126. doi:10.1016/j.iimb.2019.03.013

Pandurangi, A., Keshavan, M., Ganapathy, V., & Gangadhar, B. (2017). Yoga: Past and present. *The American Journal of Psychiatry*, *174*(1), 16–17. doi:10.1176/appi.ajp.2016.16080853 PMID:28040996

Panesar, D. S. (2017). Meditation (Sikhism). In Encyclopedia of Scientific Dating Methods (pp. 238–241). Springer Netherlands. doi:10.1007/978-94-024-0846-1_498

Paranjpe, A. C. (2002). Indigenous Psychology in the Post- Colonial Context: An Historical Perspective. *Psychology and Developing Societies*, *14*(1), 27–43. doi:10.1177/097133360201400103

Paranjpe, A. C. (2011). Indian Psychology and the International Context. *Psychology and Developing Societies*, *23*(1), 1–26. doi:10.1177/097133361002300101

Pardasani, R., Sharma, R. R., & Bindlish, P. (2014). Facilitating workplace spirituality: Lessons from Indian spiritual traditions. *Journal of Management Development*, *33*(8/9), 847–859. doi:10.1108/JMD-07-2013-0096

Park, C. L., Finkelstein-Fox, L., Sacco, S. J., Braun, T. D., & Lazar, S.C. L. (2021). How does yoga reduce stress? A clinical trial testing psychological mechanisms. *Stress and Health*, *37*(1), 116–126. doi:10.1002mi.2977 PMID:32797683

Parott (2017, November 21) How to be a Mindful Muslim: An Exercise in Islamic Meditation | Yaqeen Institute for Islamic Research. Retrieved from Yaqeen Institute for Islamic Research. https://yaqeeninstitute.org/read/paper/how-to-be-a-mindful-muslim-an-exercise-in-islamic-meditation

Patañjali. (1978). *The Yoga Sutras of Patanjali*. Patanjali. http://ci.nii.ac.jp/ncid/BA24616006

Patel, B. (n.d.). Pulin K Garg. *Archives*. https://archives.iima.ac.in/faculty/Pulin-K-Garg.html

Paterson, J. (2000). Workers of south India their attitudes and their education. *Asia Pacific Disability Rehabilitation Journal*, *10*(1), 1–16.

Patil, M. & Patwardhan, B. (1997). Antistress activity of Tinospora cordifolia (Willd) Meirs. *Indian Drugs, 34.* https://api.semanticscholar.org/Corpus

Paul, D. P. (2015, December 5). *Bhagvad Gita's Guide to Mindfulness*. Atlantadunia. https://www.atlantadunia.com/dunia/Features/F242.htm#:~:text=It's%20succinctly%20stated%20in%20Bhagvad,and%20his%20enemy%20as%20well

Peddireddy, V. (2016). Quality of life, psychological interventions and treatment outcome in tuberculosis patients: The indian scenario. *Frontiers in Psychology*, *7*. doi:10.3389/fpsyg.2016.01664 PMID:27833578

Pedersen, P. (2003). Culturally biased assumptions in counseling psychology. *The Counseling Psychologist*, *31*(4), 396–403. doi:10.1177/0011000003031004002

Peltokorpi, V., Allen, D. G., & Froese, F. (2015). Organizational embeddedness, turnover intentions, and voluntary turnover: The moderating effects of employee demographic characteristics and value orientations. *Journal of Organizational Behavior*, *36*(2), 292–312. doi:10.1002/job.1981

Penberthy, J. K., König, A., Gioia, C. J., Rodríguez, V. M., Starr, J., Meese, W., Worthington-Stoneman, D., Kersting, K., & Natanya, E. (2013). Mindfulness-based relapse prevention: History, mechanisms of action, and effects. *Mindfulness*, *6*(2), 151–158. doi:10.100712671-013-0239-1

Petryszak, N. G. (1981). Tabula rasa–its origins and implications. *Journal of the History of the Behavioral Sciences*, *17*(1), 15–27. doi:10.1002/1520-6696(198101)17:1<15::AID-JHBS2300170104>3.0.CO;2-3 PMID:11608578

Phiri, P., Sajid, S., & Delanerolle, G. (2023). Decolonising the psychology curriculum: A perspective. *Frontiers in Psychology*, *14*, 1193241. https://www.frontiersin.org/articles/10.3389/fpsyg.2023.1193241. doi:10.3389/fpsyg.2023.1193241 PMID:37388662

Pickar, D. (2008). Countertransference bias in the child custody evaluator. *Journal of Child Custody*, *4*(3), 45–67. doi:10.1300/J190v04n03_04

Piparaiya, R. K. (2003). *Ten Upanishads of Four Vedas*. Motilal Banarsidass Publishing House. https://www.mlbd.in/products/ten-upanishads-of-four-vedas-ram-k-piparaiya-9788178221595-8178221594

Podsakoff, N. P., LePine, J. A., & LePine, M. A. (2007). Differential challenge stressor-hindrance stressor relationships with job attitudes, turnover intentions, turnover, and withdrawal behavior: A meta-analysis. *The Journal of Applied Psychology*, *92*(2), 438–454. doi:10.1037/0021-9010.92.2.438 PMID:17371090

Pollock, S. (2006). *The Language of the Gods in the World of Men: Sanskrit, Culture, and Power in Premodern India*. University of California Press. doi:10.1525/9780520932029

Pomfrey, P. L. (2002). *The return of the self: Transcendence and transformation. A case study of the Bhagavad-Gita in the light of Vedic psychology* [Doctoral dissertation, The Wright Institute].

Prabhu, H. R., & Bhat, P. S. (2013). Mind and consciousness in yoga — Vedanta: A comparative analysis with western psychological concepts. *Indian Journal of Psychiatry*, *55*(6, Suppl S2), 182–186. doi:10.4103/0019-5545.105524 PMID:23858252

Prabhu, J., Prabhu, K., Chaudhuri, A., Rao, M. R. K., Selvi, V., Balaji, T., & Dinakar, S. (2020). Neuro-protective effect of Ayurveda formulation, Saraswatharishtam, on scopolamine induced memory impairment in animal model. *Pharmacognosy Journal*, *12*(1), 6–13. doi:10.5530/pj.2020.12.2

Prasher, B., Negi, S., Aggarwal, S., Mandal, A. K., Sethi, T., Deshmukh, S., Purohit, S. G., Sengupta, S., Khanna, S., Mohammad, F., Garg, G., Brahmachari, S. K., & Mukerji, M. (2008a). Whole genome expression and biochemical correlates of extreme constitutional types defined in Ayurveda. *Journal of Translational Medicine*, *6*(1), 48. doi:10.1186/1479-5876-6-48 PMID:18782426

Prince, P. S. M., & Menon, V. P. (2001). Antioxidant action ofTinospora cordifolia root extract in alloxan diabetic rats. *Phytotherapy Research*, *15*(3), 213–218. doi:10.1002/ptr.707 PMID:11351355

Puni, A., Agyemang, C. B., & Asamoah, E. S. (2016). Leadership styles, employee turnover intentions and counterproductive work behaviours. *International Journal of Innovative Research and Development, 5*(1), 1–7.

Purvya, M. C., & Meena, M. (2011). A review on role of prakriti in aging. *Ayu, 32*(1), 20. doi:10.4103/0974-8520.85719 PMID:22131753

Pyles, L. (2018). *Healing justice: Holistic self-care for change makers.* Oxford University Press., https://global.oup.com/academic/product/healing-justice-9780190663087

Qaradawi, Y. (2010). *Islam: an introduction.* The Other Press.

Qiu, J., Shen, B., Zhao, M., Wang, Z., Xie, B., & Xu, Y. (2020). A nationwide survey of psychological distress among chinese people in the covid-19 epidemic: Implications and policy recommendations. *General Psychiatry, 33*(2), e100213. doi:10.1136/gpsych-2020-100213 PMID:32215365

Querstret, D., Morison, L., Dickinson, S., Cropley, M., & John, M. (2020). Mindfulness-based stress reduction and cognitive therapy for psychological health and well-being in nonclinical samples: A systematic review and meta-analysis. *International Journal of Stress Management, 27*(4), 394–411. doi:10.1037tr0000165

Quranic. (2022, November 29). *Mindfulness in Islam - Quranic Arabic For Busy People.* Quranic Arabic For Busy People. https://www.getquranic.com/mindfulness-in-islam/

Radhakrishnan, S. (1948). *Indian Philosophy* (Vol. I). George Allen and Unwin Ltd.

Raghav, S., Singh, H., Dalal, P. K., Srivastava, J. S., & Asthana, O. P. (2006). Randomized controlled trial of standardized Bacopa monniera extract in age-associated memory impairment. *Indian Journal of Psychiatry, 48*(4), 238. doi:10.4103/0019-5545.31555 PMID:20703343

Raghuwanshi, A. (2011). A Review: History of Revival of Yoga in the 20th Century and Establishment of Yoga as a Science in the 21st Century. *International Scientific Yoga Journal: Sense, 1*(1).

Raja, B., Dharma, & K, Selvi. (2011). Causes of Problems in Learning English as A Second Language as Perceived by Higher Secondary Students. *i-manager's Journal on English Language Teaching, 1*, 40-45. . doi:10.26634/jelt.1.4.1604

Rajan, S., Shamkuwar, M. K., & Tanwar, A. K. (2021). Impact of Shirodhara on biological markers of stress: A case study. *Journal of Ayurveda and Integrative Medicine, 12*(1), 178–181. doi:10.1016/j.jaim.2021.01.008 PMID:33637424

Rakhshani, A., Maharana, S., Raghuram, N., Nagendra, H. R., & Venkatram, P. (2010). Effects of integrated yoga on quality of life and interpersonal relationship of pregnant women. *Quality of Life Research: An International Journal of Quality of Life Aspects of Treatment, Care and Rehabilitation, 19*(10), 1447–1455. doi:10.100711136-010-9709-2 PMID:20632115

Ramaa, S. (2000). Two decades of research on learning disabilities in India. *Dyslexia (Chichester, England), 6*(4), 268–283. doi:10.1002/1099-0909(200010/12)6:4<268::AID-DYS177>3.0.CO;2-A PMID:11129452

Ramanathan, M. (2007). Neuroprotective evaluation of standardized extracts of Centella asiatica in monosodium glutamate treated rats. *Indian J Exp Biol., 45.*

Ramaprasad, D. (2013). Emotions: An Indian perspective. *Indian Journal of Psychiatry, 55*(6, Suppl 2), S153. doi:10.4103/0019-5545.105514 PMID:23858247

Ramirez, L., & Hammack, P. (2014). Surviving colonization and the quest for healing: Narrative and resilience among california indian tribal leaders. *Transcultural Psychiatry, 51*(1), 112–133. doi:10.1177/1363461513520096 PMID:24459128

Rani C (2017). A Study of Educational Vision of Aurobindo Ghosh. *International Journal of Indian Psychology*, *5*(1). doi:10.25215/0501.125

Rani, A. (2016). Sri Aurobindo Ghosh's Philosophy of Education. *International Education and Research Journal*, 157–157.

Rani, J. N. (2007). Impact of yoga training on triguna and self-ideal disparity. Psychological Studies. *Natl Acad Psychol India.*, *52*, 174–177.

Rao, K. R. (2008). Introducing Indian Psychology. In K. R. Rao, A. Paranjpe, & A. K. Dalal (Eds.), Handbook of Indian Psychology (pp. 7–18). essay, Foundation Books.

Rao, K. G. M., Rao, S., & Rao, S. (2006). Centella asiatica (L.) Leaf Extract Treatment During the Growth Spurt Period Enhances Hippocampal CA3 Neuronal Dendritic Arborization in Rats. *Evidence-Based Complementary and Alternative Medicine*, *3*(3), 349–357. doi:10.1093/ecam/nel024 PMID:16951719

Rao, K. R., & Paranjpe, A. C. (2016). *Psychology in the Indian tradition*. Springer India. doi:10.1007/978-81-322-2440-2

Rao, K. R., Paranjpe, A. C., & Dalal, A. K. (2008). *Handbook of Indian Psychology*. Foundation Books. doi:10.1017/UPO9788175968448

Rao, P. S. (2010). *Organizational behaviour*. Himalaya Publishing House.

Rao, P. V. K., & Harigopal, K. (1979). The three gunas and ESP: An exploratory investigation. *Journal of Indian Psychology*, *2*(1), 63–68.

Rao, R. V. (2018). Ayurveda and the science of aging. *Journal of Ayurveda and Integrative Medicine*, *9*(3), 225–232. doi:10.1016/j.jaim.2017.10.002 PMID:29276113

Rao, S. K. R. (1979). *Consciousness in Advaita*. IBH Prakashana for Sri Abhinava Vidyatheerta Swamigal Scientific Research Academy.

Rastogi, R., Saxena, M., Maheshwari, M., Garg, P., Gupta, M., Shrivastava, R., & Gupta, H. (2020). Yajna and mantra science bringing health and comfort to the Indo-Asian public: a healthcare 4.0 approach and computational study. *Machine Learning with Health Care Perspective: Machine Learning and Healthcare*, 357-390.

Ravindra, P. N., & Babu, P. (2021). A Correlation Study between Tri-Guna and Emotional Style: A Theoretical Approach toward Developing a Working Model to Integrate Tri-Guna with Affective Neuroscience and Well-Being. *International Journal of Yoga*, *14*(3), 213–221. doi:10.4103/ijoy.ijoy_52_21 PMID:35017863

Ravishankar, B., & Shukla, V. J. (2007). Indian systems of medicine: A brief profile. *African Journal of Traditional, Complementary, and Alternative Medicines*, *4*(3), 319–337. doi:10.4314/ajtcam.v4i3.31226 PMID:20161896

Reat, N. R. (1990). *The origins of Indian psychology*. Jain Publishing Company.

Reb, J., Allen, T., & Vogus, T. J. (2020, July). Mindfulness arrives at work: Deepening our understanding of mindfulness in organizations. *Organizational Behavior and Human Decision Processes*, *159*, 1–7. doi:10.1016/j.obhdp.2020.04.001

Rego, A., & Cunha, M. P. (2008). Workplace spirituality and organizational commitment: An empirical study. *Journal of Organizational Change Management*, *21*(1), 53–75. doi:10.1108/09534810810847039

Reina, C. S., & Kudesia, R. S. (2020, July). Wherever you go, there you become: How mindfulness arises in everyday situations. *Organizational Behavior and Human Decision Processes*, *159*, 78–96. doi:10.1016/j.obhdp.2019.11.008

Reinhardt, K. M., Noggle Taylor, J. J., Johnston, J., Zameer, A., Cheema, S., & Khalsa, S. B. S. (2018). Kripalu Yoga for Military Veterans With PTSD: A Randomized Trial. *Journal of Clinical Psychology*, *74*(1), 93–108. doi:10.1002/jclp.22483 PMID:28524358

Rieber, R. W., & Robinson, D. K. (Eds.). (2001). *Wilhelm Wundt in history: The making of a scientific psychology*. Springer Science & Business Media. doi:10.1007/978-1-4615-0665-2

Ross, A., Bevans, M., Friedmann, E., Williams, L., & Thomas, S. (2014). "I Am a Nice Person When I Do Yoga!!!" A Qualitative Analysis of How Yoga Affects Relationships. *Journal of Holistic Nursing*, *32*(2), 67–77. doi:10.1177/0898010113508466 PMID:24166108

Rotti, H., Guruprasad, K. P., Nayak, J., Kabekkodu, S. P., Kukreja, H., Mallya, S., Nayak, J. N., Bhradwaj, R. C., Gangadharan, G. G., Prasanna, B. V., Raval, R., Kamath, A., Gopinath, P. M., Kondaiah, P., & Satyamoorthy, K. (2014). Immunophenotyping of normal individuals classified on the basis of human dosha prakriti. *Journal of Ayurveda and Integrative Medicine*, *5*(1), 43. doi:10.4103/0975-9476.128857 PMID:24812475

Rotti, H., Raval, R., Anchan, S., Bellampalli, R., Bhale, S., Bharadwaj, R., Bhat, B. K., Dedge, A. P., Dhumal, V. R., Gangadharan, G. G., Girijakumari, T. K., Gopinath, P. M., Govindaraj, P., Halder, S., Joshi, K., Kabekkodu, S. P., Kamath, A., Kondaiah, P., Kukreja, H., & Valiathan, M. V. S. (2014). Determinants of Prakriti, the Human Constitution Types of Indian Traditional Medicine and its Correlation with Contemporary Science. *Journal of Ayurveda and Integrative Medicine*, *5*(3), 166. doi:10.4103/0975-9476.140478 PMID:25336848

Roy, A. G. (2021) Reflection of Tagore's educational thought on his dream school Patha Bhavana, Santiniketan. *International Journal of creative research thoughts-IJCRT*.

Roy, G., & Kumar, R. (2023). Construction of Asakti Model from Shrimad Bhagavad Gita: An Understanding of Attachment from Indian Ethos. *Psychological Studies*, 1–11. doi:10.100712646-023-00750-6

Rudraprasad Sengupta. (2012). Wikipedia. https://en.wikipedia.org/wiki/Rudraprasad_Sengupta

Ryan, R. M., Huta, V., & Deci, E. L. (2008). Living well: A self-determination theory perspective on eudaimonia. *Journal of Happiness Studies*, *9*(1), 139–170. doi:10.100710902-006-9023-4

Sachin, K. S. & Pranati, C.R., (2020). Reiki: Old Indian therapy as new methodology. International Journal of creative research thoughts, 8, 694- 703.

Sadler, J. Z. (1992). Clinical problem solving and the biopsychosocial model. *The American Journal of Psychiatry*, *149*(10), 1315–1323. doi:10.1176/ajp.149.10.1315 PMID:1530068

Sahoo, M. K., Biswas, H., & Padhy, S. K. (2015). Psychological Co-morbidity in Children with Specific Learning Disorders. *Journal of Family Medicine and Primary Care*, *4*(1), 21–25. doi:10.4103/2249-4863.152243 PMID:25810984

Saini, D. (2020). Does Mindfulness & Happiness Predict Job Satisfaction among Indian Employees? *Indian Journal of Industrial Relations*, *56*(1).

Sakthivel, A., Kalyan, P., Bhattacharjee, R., & Ramkumar, A. (2023). Novel Chakra Sadhana Yoga-Based Treatment Approach For Posttraumatic Stress Disorder (Ptsd) And Dissociative Identity Disorder (Did)-A Case Study. *Proceedings of the International Conference on Public Health*. ACM. 10.17501/24246735.2022.7201

Salagame, K. K. K. (2011). Indian Psychology. In *The Encyclopedia of Cross-Cultural Psychology* (pp. 695–698). John Wiley & Sons, Ltd. doi:10.1002/9781118339893.wbeccp283

Salmon, P., & Loo, J. L. (2023). Mindfulness-based cognitive therapy. In Springer eBooks (pp. 1–19). doi:10.1007/978-3-030-42825-9_75-1

Samal, J. (2014). Indian public health standards for Ayurveda, Yoga and Naturopathy, Unani, Siddha and Homoeopathy facilities: An assessment. [Google Scholar]. *International Journal of Medicine and Public Health, 4*(4), 331. doi:10.4103/2230-8598.144058

Samarakoon, S., Chandola, H., & Ravishankar, B. (2011). Effect of dietary, social, and lifestyle determinants of accelerated aging and its common clinical presentation: A survey study. *Ayu, 32*(3), 315. doi:10.4103/0974-8520.93906 PMID:22529643

Sandberg, J., & Tsoukas, H. (2011, April 1). Grasping the Logic of Practice: Theorizing Through Practical Rationality. *Academy of Management Review, 36*(2), 338–360. doi:10.5465/amr.2009.0183

Santos, J. L., Bashaw, M. A., Mattcham, W., Cutcliffe, J. R., & Vedana, K. G. G. (2018). The Biopsychosocial Approach: Towards Holistic, Person-Centred Psychiatric/Mental Health Nursing Practice. In *Principles of specialty nursing* (pp. 89–101). Springer International Publishing. https://doi.org/8 doi:10.1007/978-3-319-31772-4_

Saripudin, W., & Rosari, R. (2019). Does Spiritual Leadership Model Enhance Work Engagement? Empirical Evidence From an Islamic Hospital in Yogyakarta. *Journal of Leadership in Organizations, 1*(2). Advance online publication. doi:10.22146/jlo.45520

Sathiyaseelan, A., Balasundaram, S., & Zirkler, M. (2022). Indian Perspectives of Mindful Leadership. In *International Research Conference on Mindfulness 2022* (IRCM 2022).

Sathiyaseelan, A., Balasundaram, S., & Zirkler, M. (2022). Indian perspectives on mindful leadership. In *Proceedings of the International Research Conference on Mindfulness 2022 (IRCM 2022).* Research Gate. https://www.researchgate.net/profile/Sathiyaseelan-Balasundaram/publication/359199972_Indian_Perspectives_on_Mindful_Leadership/links/622da88797401151d216376b/Indian-Perspectives-on-Mindful-Leadership.pdf

Sathyanarayanan, G., Vengadavaradan, A., & Bharadwaj, B. (2019). Role of Yoga and Mindfulness in Severe Mental Illnesses: A Narrative Review. *International Journal of Yoga, 12*(1), 3–28. doi:10.4103/ijoy.IJOY_65_17 PMID:30692780

Sayegh, P., Vivian, D., Heller, M., Kirk, S., & Kelly, K. (2023). Racial, cultural, and social injustice in psychological assessment: A brief review, call to action, and resources to help reduce inequities and harm. *Training and Education in Professional Psychology, 17*(4), 366–374. Advance online publication. doi:10.1037/tep0000451

Schaap, J. (2012). Toward strategy implementation success: An empirical study of the role of senior-level leaders in the nevada gaming industry. *UNLV Gaming Research & Review Journal, 10*(2). https://digitalscholarship.unlv.edu/grrj/vol10/iss2/2

Schaffer, J., & Rodolfa, E. (2020). Reflecting on reflective practice. *Clinical Psychology : a Publication of the Division of Clinical Psychology of the American Psychological Association, 27*(4). Advance online publication. doi:10.1111/cpsp.12361

Schmid, A. A., Sternke, E., L, A., DO, Conner, N., Starnino, V. R., & Davis, L. W. (2021). The eight limbs of yoga can be maintained in a veteran friendly yoga program. *International Journal of Yoga, 14*(2), 127.. doi:10.4103/ijoy.IJOY_106_20

Schneider, B. (1987). The people make the place. *Personnel Psychology, 40*(3), 437–453. doi:10.1111/j.1744-6570.1987.tb00609.x

Schultz, P. D., & Schultz, E. (2011). A History of Modern Psychology (10th ed.). Cengage Learning.

Sebastian, K. A., & Mathew, G. V. (2002). Three gunas and PSI experience; a study of PSI experience in relation to inertia, activation, and stability. *Journal of Indian Psychology, 20*(2), 44–48.

Sedlmeier, P., & Srinivas, K. (2016). How Do Theories of Cognition and Consciousness in Ancient Indian Thought Systems Relate to Current Western Theorizing and Research? *Frontiers in Psychology*, *7*, 343. doi:10.3389/fpsyg.2016.00343 PMID:27014150

Seligman, M. E. (2002). Positive psychology, positive prevention, and positive therapy. Handbook of positive psychology, 2(2002), 3-12.

Seminar on research in Ayurveda and Sidha. (1995). CCRAS.

Shah, A. M. (2005). The foundations of successful strategy implementation: Overcoming obstacles. *Global Business Review*, *6*(2), 293–302. doi:10.1177/097215090500600208

Shahbaz, W., & Parker, J. (2021, June 26). Workplace mindfulness: An integrative review of antecedents, mediators, and moderators. *Human Resource Management Review*. doi:10.1016/j.hrmr.2021.100849

Shamasundar, C. (2008). Relevance of ancient Indian wisdom to modern mental health a few examples. [PUBMED]. *Indian Journal of Psychiatry*, *50*(2), 138–143. doi:10.4103/0019-5545.42404 PMID:19742213

Shannahoff-Khalsa, D., Fernandes, R. Y., Pereira, C. A. D. B., March, J. S., Leckman, J. F., Golshan, S., Vieira, M. S. R., Polanczyk, G. V., Miguel, E. C., & Shavitt, R. G. (2019). Kundalini yoga meditation versus the relaxation response meditation for treating adults with obsessive-compulsive disorder: A randomized clinical trial. *Frontiers in Psychiatry*, *10*, 793. doi:10.3389/fpsyt.2019.00793 PMID:31780963

Sharma, N., & Soni, D. (2022). *Effect of Gayatri Mantra on Health: A Narrative Review*. OSF.

Sharma, P. (2005). *Database on Medicinal plants used in Ayurveda and Sidha* (Vol. 1). CCRAS, Dept. of AYUSH, Ministry of Health and Family Welfare, Govt. of India.

Sharma, S. (1998). Life force as a unique Divine greatness (2nd ed.). Akhand Jyoti Institution, Mathura.

Sharma, A., Sabharwal, P., & Dada, R. (2021). Herbal medicine—An introduction to its history. In *Herbal Medicine in Andrology* (pp. 1–8). Academic Press. doi:10.1016/B978-0-12-815565-3.00001-1

Sharma, A., & Singh, R. (2014). Combating educational stress in adolescents: The miraculous role of chanting mantras. *Indian Journal of Psychological Science*, *5*(1), 25–37.

Sharma, G., Gujral, J. S., Agarwal, A., Jat, M., Mohanty, S., & Pandey, R. M. (2022). Exploring knowledge, attitude and practice regarding yoga among patients attending cardiology and neurology clinics in a tertiary care hospital in northern India. *The National Medical Journal of India*, *34*(4), 201–205. doi:10.25259/NMJI_11_20 PMID:35112541

Sharma, M. (2021). *Indian Psychology-Exploring the Historical Roots*. Emerging Trends and Future Implications., doi:10.25215/0902.168

Sharma, N. (2014). Cognitive behaviour therapy in perspective of the Bhagwat Gita. *International Journal of Humanities and Social Science Invention*, *3*(1), 2319–7722.

Sharma, R. (1999). Self-concept and job satisfaction in sattva rajas and tamas personalities. *Journal of Indian Psychology*, *17*(2), 9–17.

Sharma, S. (2006). Psychiatry, colonialism and Indian civilization: A historical appraisal. *Indian Journal of Psychiatry*, *48*(2), 109–112. doi:10.4103/0019-5545.31600 PMID:20703396

Sharma, V. K., Das, S., Mondal, S., & Goswami, U., & Gandhi, A. (n.d.). Effect of sahaj yoga on depressive disorders. *Indian Journal of Physiology and Pharmacology*. PMID:16579401

Shearer, A. (1982). *(Trans.). Effortless being. The yoga sutras of Patanjali.* Wildwood House Limited.

Sheep, M. L. (2004). Nailing Down Gossamer: A Valid Measure Of The Person-Organization Fit Of Workplace Sprituality. In Academy of Management Proceedings, Briarcliff Manor, Academy of Management. doi:10.5465/ambpp.2004.13862520

Sheikh, A. A., Inam, A., Rubab, A., Najam, U., Rana, N. A., & Awan, H. M. (2019). The Spiritual Role of a Leader in Sustaining Work Engagement: A Teacher-Perceived Paradigm. *SAGE Open, 9*(3), 2158244019863567. doi:10.1177/2158244019863567

Shetty, K. T., Subbakrishna, D. K., & Meti, B. L., & Raju, T. R. (1998). Therapeutic Efficacy of Sudarshan Kriya Yoga (SKK) in Dysthymic Disorder. *Nimhans Journal*, 21–28.

Shilpa, S., & Murthy, C. V. (2011). Understanding personality from Ayurvedic perspective for psychological assessment: A case. *Ayu, 32*(1), 12. doi:10.4103/0974-8520.85716 PMID:22131752

Shirazi, B. A. K. (2011). Integral education: Founding vision and principles. *Integral Review, 7*(1), 4–10.

Shroff, F. M., & Asgarpour, M. (2017). *Yoga and Mental Health: A Review. Journal of Physiotherapy &amp.* Physical Rehabilitation. doi:10.4172/2573-0312.1000132

Shroff, F. M., Asgarpour, M., & Fm, S. (2017). Yoga and mental health: A review. *Physiother Rehabil, 2*(132), 2573–0312.

Shukla, P. K., Khanna, V. K., Ali, M. M., Maurya, R., Khan, M. Y., & Srimal, R. C. (2006). Neuroprotective effect of Acorus calamus against middle cerebral artery occlusion–induced ischaemia in rat. *Human and Experimental Toxicology, 25*(4), 187–194. doi:10.1191/0960327106ht613oa PMID:16696294

Shukla, R. (2013). Indian perspective of spiritual well-being. *Indian Journal of Positive Psychology, 4*(1), 114–116.

Shukla, S. (2020). Spirituality in Ayurveda. *Spirituality in Clinical Practice, 7*(2), 103–113. doi:10.1037cp0000181

Silva, R. & Padakannaya, P. (2007). An Analysis of Early Literacy Skills among Indian Children at Lower Kindergarten. *Indian Journal of Applied Linguistics, 33*(2) p129-140

Silva, Reena & Padakannaya, P. (2009). Spelling homophonic words in Kannada and English: A cross-linguistic study. *Journal of Psychosomatic Research, 4*, 183–191.

Silver, L. B. (1986). Learning disabilities. The primary care role in multidisciplinary management. *Postgraduate Medicine, 79*(8), 285–296. doi:10.1080/00325481.1986.11699438 PMID:3714591

Singh, N., & Krishnan, V. R. (2005a). *Toward a Better Understanding of Transformational Leadership: Differentiating between Altruism and Self-sacrifi ce.* Proceedings of the Australian and New Zealand Academy of Management Conference, Canberra.

Singh, A. D. (2017). Yoga for Mental Health: Opportunities and Challenges. MOJ Yoga &amp. *Physical Therapy, 2*(1). Advance online publication. doi:10.15406/mojypt.2017.02.00009

Singhal, M., & Chatterjee, L. (2006). A person–organization fit-based approach for spirituality at work: Development of a conceptual framework. *Journal of Human Values, 12*(2), 161–178. doi:10.1177/097168580601200205

Singha, R., & Kanna, S. Y. (2022). Women's empowerment, mindfulness, and role of women in eradicating alcohol and drug addiction from Indian society. *Journal of International Women's Studies, 24*(7), 7. https://vc.bridgew.edu/jiws/vol24/iss7/7/

Singh, C., & Reddy, T. O. (2018). Yoga origin, history and development in India. [IJMEES]. *Indian Journal of Movement Education and Exercise Sciences, 8*(1), 9–12.

Singh, K., Raina, M., & Oman, D. (2023). Positive Psychology and Hinduism. In E. B. Davis, E. L. Worthington Jr, & S. A. Schnitker (Eds.), *Handbook of Positive Psychology, Religion, and Spirituality*. Springer. doi:10.1007/978-3-031-10274-5_13

Singh, K., Raina, M., & Sahni, P. (2017). The concept and measure of Sukha–Dukha: An Indian perspective on well-being. *Journal of Spirituality in Mental Health*, *19*(2), 116–132. doi:10.1080/19349637.2016.1231604

Singh, K., & Smith, A. (2007). *Sikhism*. QED.

Singh, R. P., Narsimhamurthy, K., & Singh, G. (2008). Neuronutrient impact of Ayurvedic Rasayana therapy in brain aging. *Biogerontology*, *9*(6), 369–374. doi:10.100710522-008-9185-z PMID:18931935

Singh, R., Banerjee, S., Kumar, P., Raveesha, K. A., & Rao, A. (2006). Tinospora cordifolia induces enzymes of carcinogen/drug metabolism and antioxidant system, and inhibits lipid peroxidation in mice. *Phytomedicine*, *13*(1–2), 74–84. doi:10.1016/j.phymed.2004.02.013 PMID:16360936

Singh, R., & Oberhummer, I. (1980). Behavior therapy within a setting of karma yoga. *Journal of Behavior Therapy and Experimental Psychiatry*, *11*(2), 135–141. doi:10.1016/0005-7916(80)90012-9

Sinha, D., & Tripathi, R. (1994). Individualism in a collectivist culture: A case of coexistence of dichotomies. In U. Kim, H. C. Triandis, C. Kacitçibabi, S. C. Choi & G. Yoon (Eds.), Individualism and Collectivism: Theory, Method and Applications (pp. 123-136). Thousand Oaks, CA: Sage.

Sinha, C., & Fox Lee, S. (2017). Note on "History of psychology in India: Problems and prospects.". *History of Psychology*, *20*(1), 126–128. doi:10.1037/h0101578 PMID:28150967

Sinha, P., Hussain, T., Boora, N. K., Rao, G. N., Varghese, M., Gururaj, G., & Benegal, V. (2021). Prevalence of Common mental disorders in older adults: Results from the National Mental Health Survey of India. *Asian Journal of Psychiatry*, *55*, 102463. doi:10.1016/j.ajp.2020.102463 PMID:33212298

Siperstein, G. N. Sugumaran, K., Bardon, J., Norins & Parker, R. C. (2004). *Attitudes of the Public in India towards People with Intellectual Disabilities*. University of Massachusetts Boston. https://media.specialolympics.org/soi/files/healthy- athletes/ResearchStudies/India_FullReport.pdf

Sipe, W. E., & Eisendrath, S. J. (2012). Mindfulness-based cognitive therapy: Theory and practice. *Canadian Journal of Psychiatry*, *57*(2), 63–69. https://journals.sagepub.com/doi/pdf/10.1177/070674371205700202. doi:10.1177/070674371205700202 PMID:22340145

Sitamma, M., Sridevi., & Rao, P. V. K. (1995). Three gunas and cognitive characteristics: A study of field dependence independence and perceptual acuity. *Journal of Indian Psychology*, *13*(2), 13–20.

Sivachandrakumar., A. (2019, January). Classic Poem (Puram - 206) – A Management view. *International Journal of Emerging Technologies and Innovative Research*, *.6*(1), 42-46. https://www.jetir.org/papers/JETIRT006007.pdf

Sivananda Radha, S. (2005). *Mantras: Words of Power*. Timeless Books.

Sivananda, S. (1986). *Mind: Its Mysteries and Control*.

Sivananda, S. S. (1999). *Guru Tattva – The Divine Life Society* (6th ed.). The Divine Life Society. https://www.dlshq.org/download/guru-tattva/

Sivananda, S. (1974). *Mind: Its Mysteries and Control*. Divine Life Society.

Skoog, I. (2011). Psychiatric disorders in the elderly. *Canadian Journal of Psychiatry*, *56*(7), 387–397. doi:10.1177/070674371105600702 PMID:21835102

Slade, M. (2010). Mental illness and well-being: The central importance of positive psychology and recovery approaches. *BMC Health Services Research, 10*(1), 1–14. doi:10.1186/1472-6963-10-26 PMID:20102609

Smith, K. G., Locke, E. A., & Barry, D. (1990). Goal setting, planning, and organizational performance: An experimental simulation. *Organizational Behavior and Human Decision Processes, 46*(1), 118–134. doi:10.1016/0749-5978(90)90025-5

Sondhi, S., & Sakti, S. (2021). Power of Words in India's Linguistic Tradition. *Kalakalpa IGNCA Journal for Arts, 6*(1). https://ssrn.com/abstract=3874909

Sood, M., Singh, S., & Chadda, R. (2017). Relevance of traditional Indian medical concepts in psychosomatic medicine. [India]. *Annals of the National Academy of Medical Sciences (India), 53*(3), 148–155. doi:10.1055-0040-1712757

Sotillos, S. B. (2022, December 20). *Book review – Perennial psychology of the Bhagavad Gita*. Academia. https://www.academia.edu/45645129/Book_Review_Perennial_Psychology_of_the_Bhagavad_Gita

Soumya, R. R., & Sathiyaseelan, A. (2021). Mindfulness: An emotional aid to the glass ceiling experiences. *Cogent Psychology, 8*(1), 1907911. doi:10.1080/23311908.2021.1907911

Srivastava, K. (2012). Concept of personality: Indian perspective. *Industrial Psychiatry Journal, 21*(2), 89.

Srivastava, K. (2010). Human nature: Indian perspective revisited. [Google Scholar]. *Industrial Psychiatry Journal, 19*(2), 77–81. doi:10.4103/0972-6748.90335 PMID:22174527

Srivastava, S., Patel, A., Tiwari, S. K., & Gupta, K. (2019). Effectiveness of Pranic Healing on Mental Health. *Journal of Psychosomatic Research, 14*(1), 163–168.

Starnino, V. R. (2016). When trauma, spirituality, and mental illness intersect: A qualitative case study. *Psychological Trauma: Theory, Research, Practice, and Policy, 8*(3), 375–383. doi:10.1037/tra0000105 PMID:26783761

Stead, T. (2017). *Mindfulness and Christian Spirituality*. Presbyterian Publishing Corp.

Stone, M. (2009). *Yoga for a World Out of Balance: Teachings on Ethics and Social Action*. Shambhala Publications.

Streeter, C. C., Jensen, J., Perlmutter, R. M., Cabral, H., Shu, G., Terhune, D. B., & Ciraulo, D. A. (2007). Yoga Asana Sessions Increase Brain GABA Levels: A Pilot Study. *Journal of Alternative and Complementary Medicine (New York, N.Y.), 13*(4), 419–426. doi:10.1089/acm.2007.6338 PMID:17532734

Subrahmanyam, S., & Porkodi, K. (1980). Neurohumoral correlates of Transcendental Meditation. *Journal of Biomedicine (Sydney, NSW), 1*, 73–88.

Subudhi, C. (2014). Culture and mental illness. *Social Work Practice in Mental Health: Cross-Cultural Perspectives, 141*, 132–140.

Sudha, R. (2020). Gayathri Mantra and Social Skills Training for Social Anxiety, Stress, Self Concept, and Well Being among School Students with Learning Difficulties. *International Journal of Psychosocial Rehabilitation, 24*(3), 1983–2004. doi:10.37200/IJPR/V24I3/PR200946

Sun, S., Nardi, W., Loucks, E. B., & Operario, D. (2021). Mindfulness-based interventions for sexual and gender minorities: A systematic review and evidence evaluation. *Mindfulness, 12*(10), 2439–2459. https://link.springer.com/article/10.1007/s12671-021-01710-9. doi:10.100712671-021-01710-9

Suntharesan, V. (2012). Role of Mother Tongue in Teaching English as a Second Language to Tamil Students (Special Reference to Undergraduates of the University of Jaffna, Sri Lanka). *Language in India, 12*(12).

Suresh, N. C., & Srilakshmidevi, N. B., & Suresh, V. (. (2020). Yogic Diet, Trigunas and Mental Health: Implications for Research. *Indian Journal of Health Studies, 02*(02), 64–73. doi:10.56490/IJHS.2020.2204

Suthren Hirst, J. G. (2005). *Śaṃkara's Advaita Vedānta: A Way of Teaching*. Routledge. doi:10.4324/9780203001929

Sutras Ch 4 PH Notes. (n.d.). Sanskrit Documents. https://sanskritdocuments.org/sites/athayoga/sutra_ch4phn.html

Swami Krishnananda. (2023). *The Teachings of the Bhagavadgita*. Swami Krishnananda. https://www.swami-krishnananda.org/bhagavad/bhagavad_pub.html

Swami Vireshananda. (2023) *How Each Chapter of the Bhagavadgita is a Yoga?* Swami Krishnananda. https://advaita-ashrama.org/how-each-chapter-of-the-bhagavadgita-is-a-yoga/

Szwajkowski, E. (2000). Simplifying the principles of stakeholder management: The three most important principles. *Business & Society, 39*(4), 379–396. doi:10.1177/000765030003900403

Tagore, R. (1931). *My Educational Mission*. The Modern Review.

Tajfel, H. (1981). *Human groups and social categories*. Cambridge University Press.

Tajfel, H. (1982). *Social identity and intergroup relations*. Cambridge University Press.

Talukder, M. M. H. (2016). On "Self-realization" – the Ultimate Norm Of Arne Naess's Ecosophy T. *Symposion (Los Angeles, Calif.), 2*(3), 219–235. doi:10.5840ymposion20163217

Tan, M. Y. L., McConnell, B. L., & Barlas, J. (2022). Application of dialectical behaviour therapy in treating common psychiatric disorders: Study protocol for a scoping review. *BMJ Open, 12*(9), e058565. doi:10.1136/bmjopen-2021-058565 PMID:36167385

Tatta, J., Willgens, A. M., & Palombaro, K. M. (2022). Mindfulness and acceptance–based interventions in physical therapist practice: The time is now. *Physical Therapy, 102*(3), pzab293. doi:10.1093/ptj/pzab293 PMID:35079796

Taylor, E. (1999). *Shadow culture: Psychology and spirituality in America*. Counterpoint. [Google Scholar]

Tett, R. P., & Burnett, D. D. (2003). A personality trait-based interactionist model of job performance. *The Journal of Applied Psychology, 88*(3), 500–517. doi:10.1037/0021-9010.88.3.500 PMID:12814298

Thapar, A. (2002). *The Penguin History of Early India: From the Origins to AD 1300*. Penguin Books.

The Dhammapada. Verses and Stories. (n.d.). Retrieved from https://www.tipitaka.net/tipitaka/dhp/

Therapuetic Approaches. (2021). *National Council of Educational Research and Training*. NCERT. https://ncert.nic.in

Thoma, M. V., Rohleder, N., & Rohner, S. L. (2021). Clinical Ecopsychology: The Mental Health Impacts and Underlying Pathways of the Climate and Environmental Crisis. *Frontiers in Psychiatry, 12*, 675936. doi:10.3389/fpsyt.2021.675936 PMID:34093283

Thomas, R. (2001). *Folk psychologies across cultures*. Sage Publications, Inc. doi:10.4135/9781452233901

Thomas, S., & Rao, S. L. (2016). Effect of Gayatri mantra meditation on naive subjects: An EEG and fMRI pilot study. *International Journal of Indian Psychology, 3*(7), 14–18.

Thoroughgood, C. N., Sawyer, K. B., & Webster, J. R. (2020, July). Finding calm in the storm: A daily investigation of how trait mindfulness buffers against paranoid cognition and emotional exhaustion following perceived discrimination at work. *Organizational Behavior and Human Decision Processes, 159*, 49–63. doi:10.1016/j.obhdp.2019.02.004

Tikhe, S. G., Nagendra, H. R., & Tripathi, N. (2012). Ancient science of yogic life for academic excellence in university students. *Ancient Science of Life*, *31*(3), 80–83. doi:10.4103/0257-7941.103179 PMID:23284211

Timbers, V. L., & Hollenberger, J. C. (2022). Christian Mindfulness and Mental Health: Coping through Sacred Traditions and Embodied Awareness. *Religions*, *1*(1), 62. doi:10.3390/rel13010062

Tiwari, P., & Patel, R. (2013). Estimation of total phenolics and flavonoids and antioxidant potential of ashwagandharishta prepared by traditional and modern methods. *Asian Journal of Pharmaceutical Analysis*, *3*(4), 147–152. https://www.indianjournals.com/ijor.aspx?target=ijor:ajpa&volume=3&issue=4&article=009&type=pdf

Tiwari, S. K., & Pandey, N. M. (2012). Status and requirements of geriatric mental health services in India: An evidence-based commentary. *Indian Journal of Psychiatry*, *54*(1), 8. doi:10.4103/0019-5545.94639 PMID:22556431

Toolika, E., Bhat, N. P., & Shetty, S. K. (2015). A comparative clinical study on the effect of Tagara (Valeriana wallichii DC.) and Jatamansi (Nardostachys jatamansi DC.) in the management of Anidra (primary insomnia). *Ayu*, *36*(1), 46. doi:10.4103/0974-8520.169008 PMID:26730138

Torres, S. (2019). *Beyond Colonizing Epistemicides: Toward a Decolonizing Framework for Indigenous Education.* [Thesis, LMU]. https://digitalcommons.lmu.edu/etd/895

Townley, G., Brown, M., & Sylvestre, J. (2018). Community Psychology and Community Mental Health: A Call for Reengagement. *American Journal of Community Psychology*, *61*(1–2), 3–9. doi:10.1002/ajcp.12225 PMID:29315707

Trammel, R. (2018). Effectiveness of an MP3 Christian mindfulness intervention on mindfulness and perceived stress. *Mental Health, Religion &amp. Mental Health, Religion & Culture*, *5*(5), 500–514. doi:10.1080/13674676.2018.1505837

Travis, F. T., & Wallace, R. K. (1977). Autonomic patterns during respiratory suspensions: Proposed markers of transcendental consciousness. *Psychophysiology*, *34*(1), 39–46. doi:10.1111/j.1469-8986.1997.tb02414.x PMID:9009807

Tripathi, J., & Singh, R. (1994). Concept of deha prakriti vis-à-vis human constitution in ayurveda. *PubMed.* https://pubmed.ncbi.nlm.nih.gov/22556666

TrustsT.AboutS. D. T. (2023, July 18), Retrieved from https://www.tatatrusts.org/about-tatatrusts/about-sir-dorabji-tata

Tsoukas, H. (1994). Refining Common Sense: Types of Knowledge in Management Studies. *Journal of Management Studies*, *31*(6), 761–780. doi:10.1111/j.1467-6486.1994.tb00638.x

Tsui, K. T., Lee, J. C. K., Zhang, Z., & Wong, P. H. (2019). The Relationship Between Teachers' Perceived Spiritual Leadership and Organziational Commitment: A Multilevel Analysis in the Hong Kong Context. *Asian Journal of Social Sciences & Humanities*, *8*, 3.

Tubaki, B. R., Chandake, S., & Sarhyal, A. (2021). Ayurveda management of Major Depressive Disorder: A case study. *Journal of Ayurveda and Integrative Medicine*, *12*(2), 378–383. doi:10.1016/j.jaim.2021.03.012 PMID:34024690

Udupa, K. N., & Prasad, R. (1985). Stress and its management by yoga. In *Motilal Banarsidass eBooks*. https://ci.nii.ac.jp/ncid/BA47667811

Uebaba, K., Xu, F., Ogawa, H., Tatsuse, T., Wang, B., Hisajima, T., & Venkatraman, S. (2008). Psychoneuroimmunologic effects of Ayurvedic Oil-Dripping Treatment. *Journal of Alternative and Complementary Medicine (New York, N.Y.)*, *14*(10), 1189–1198. doi:10.1089/acm.2008.0273 PMID:19123874

Uma, K., Lakshmi, Y. S., & Parameshwaran, E. G. (1971). Construction of a personality inventory based on the doctrine of three gunas. *Research Bulletin (International Commission for the Northwest Atlantic Fisheries)*, *6*, 49–58.

UNESCO. (2020). *Towards inclusion in education: status, trends and challenges: the UNESCO Salamanca Statement 25 years on*. UNESCO.

UNICEF. (2017). Improving Education Participation. Policy and Practice Pointers for Enrolling All Children and Adolescents in School and Preventing Dropout. UNICEF.

Upadhyay, N. (2023, April 4). *Managing Neurological Disorders with Mindfulness Meditation: A Jainism Philosophy Perspective*. LinkedIn.

Vadivale, A. M., & Sathiyaseelan, A. (2019). Mindfulness-based relapse prevention–A meta-analysis. *Cogent Psychology*, *6*(1), 1567090. doi:10.1080/23311908.2019.1567090

Vadivale, A. M., & Sathiyaseelan, A. (2022). Need for mindfulness-based relapse prevention strategies for postpartum smoking relapse prevention. *Indian Journal of Public Health*, *66*(3), 334–336. https://journals.lww.com/IJPH/Fulltext/2022/66030/Need_for_Mindfulness_based_Relapse_Prevention.20.aspx. doi:10.4103/ijph.ijph_1494_21 PMID:36149116

Vahia, N. S., Jeste, D. V., Kapoor, S. N., Ardhapurkar, I., & Nath, R. S. (1973). Further experience with the therapy based upon concepts of Patanjali in the treatment of psychiatric disorders. *Indian Journal of Psychiatry*, *15*, 32–37.

Vahia, N., Vinekar, S., & Doongaji, D. (1966). Some ancient Indian concepts in the treatment of psychiatric disorders. *The British Journal of Psychiatry*, *112*(492), 1089–1096. doi:10.1192/bjp.112.492.1089 PMID:5971528

Vancampfort, D., Vansteelandt, K., Scheewe, T., Probst, M., Knapen, J., De Herdt, A., & De Hert, M. (2012). Yoga in schizophrenia: A systematic review of randomized controlled trials. *Acta Psychiatrica Scandinavica*, *126*(1), 12–20. doi:10.1111/j.1600-0447.2012.01865.x PMID:22486714

Varambally, S., & Gangadhar, B. (2012). Yoga: A spiritual practice with therapeutic value in psychiatry. *Asian Journal of Psychiatry*, *5*(2), 186–189. doi:10.1016/j.ajp.2012.05.003 PMID:22813667

Varma, V. K. (1982). Present state of psychotherapy in India. *Indian Journal of Psychiatry*, *24*, 209–226. PMID:21965915

Verma, G. (2021). The Effect of Swadhyay on the Mental Health Using Statistical Approach. *IOSR Journal of Humanities and Social Science*, *26*(3). doi: 2603051921 doi:10.9790/0837-

Verma, K., Deepeshwar, S., & Srivastava, A. (n.d.). Comparative impact of yoga and ayurveda practice in insomnia: A randomized controlled trial. *PubMed*, *12*, 160. doi:10.4103/jehp.jehp_1489_22 PMID:37404923

Verma, R. (2009). *Faith & philosophy of hinduism* (Vol. 1). Gyan Publishing House.

Vijayabanu, C., Therasa, C., & Daisy, S. A. (2019). Impression Management Tactics as a psychological booster for the communication of IT employees–SMART PLS Approach. *Revista de Psicología*, *37*(2), 683–707. doi:10.18800/psico.201902.012

Vivekananda, S. (2009). *Karma-Yoga: The Yoga of action*. Advaita Ashrama.

Von Glasenapp, H. (1999). *Jainism: An Indian religion of salvation, 14*.

Walker, L. H., & Colosimo, K. (2011, January). Mindfulness, self-compassion, and happiness in non-meditators: A theoretical and empirical examination. *Personality and Individual Differences*, *50*(2), 222–227. doi:10.1016/j.paid.2010.09.033

Walsh, R., & Roche, L. (1979). Precipitation of acute psychotic episodes by intensive meditation in individuals with a history of schizophrenia. *The American Journal of Psychiatry*, *136*(8), 1085–1086. doi:10.1176/ajp.136.8.1085 PMID:380368

Webster, M. (2011). Introduction to acceptance and commitment therapy. *Advances in Psychiatric Treatment, 17*(4), 309–316. doi:10.1192/apt.bp.107.005256

Weinstein, N., Brown, K. W., & Ryan, R. M. (2009, June). A multi-method examination of the effects of mindfulness on stress attribution, coping, and emotional well-being. *Journal of Research in Personality, 43*(3), 374–385. doi:10.1016/j.jrp.2008.12.008

Weiss, H. M., & Cropanzano, R. (1996). Affective events theory: A theoretical discussion of the structure, causes and consequences of affective experiences at work. *Research in Organizational Behavior, 18*, 1–7.

West, J., Liang, B., & Spinazzola, J. (2017). Trauma Sensitive Yoga as a complementary treatment for posttraumatic stress disorder: A Qualitative Descriptive analysis. *International Journal of Stress Management, 24*(2), 173–195. doi:10.1037tr0000040 PMID:28458503

Whitfield, T., Barnhofer, T., Acabchuk, R. L., Cohen, A., Lee, M., Schlosser, M., Arenaza-Urquijo, E. M., Böttcher, A., Britton, W. B., Coll-Padrós, N., Collette, F., Chételat, G., Dautricourt, S., Demnitz-King, H., Dumais, T., Klimecki, O., Meiberth, D., Moulinet, I., Müller, T., & Marchant, N. L. (2021). The Effect of mindfulness-based programs on Cognitive Function in Adults: A systematic review and meta-analysis. *Neuropsychology Review, 32*(3), 677–702. doi:10.100711065-021-09519-y PMID:34350544

Wig, N. (1989). Indian concepts of mental health and their impact on care of the mentally ill. *International Journal of Mental Health, 18*(3), 71–80. doi:10.1080/00207411.1989.11449136

Wig, N. (2004). Hanuman complex and its resolution: An illustration of psychotherapy from Indian mythology. *Indian Journal of Psychiatry, 46*, 25–28. PMID:21206772

Wikipedia. (2015). *Na. Muthuswamy*. Wikipedia. https://en.wikipedia.org/wiki/Na._Muthuswamy

Wikipedia. (2017). *T. K. V. Desikachar*. Wikipedia. https://en.wikipedia.org/wiki/T._K._V._Desikachar

Williams, J. M. G., & Kuyken, W. (2012). Mindfulness-based cognitive therapy: A promising new approach to preventing depressive relapse. *The British Journal of Psychiatry, 200*(5), 359–360. doi:10.1192/bjp.bp.111.104745 PMID:22550328

Wilson, J. P. (2007). The Lens of Culture: Theoretical and Conceptual Perspectives in the Assessment of Psychological Trausma and PTSD. In J. P. Wilson & C. S. Tang (Eds.), Cross-Cultural Assessment of Psychological Trauma and PTSD (pp. 3–30). Springer US. doi:10.1007/978-0-387-70990-1_1

Wolf, D. B. (1998). The Vedic Personality Inventory: A study of gunas. *Journal of Indian Psychology, 16*(1), 26–43.

Wolpe, J. (1973). *The Practice of Behavior Therapy*. Pergamon Press.

Wood, J. J. (2006). Effect of anxiety reduction on children's school performance and social adjustment. *Developmental Psychology, 42*(2), 345–349. doi:10.1037/0012-1649.42.2.345 PMID:16569172

Woods, S. L., & Rockman, P. (2021). *Mindfulness-based stress reduction: Protocol, practice, and teaching skills*. New Harbinger Publications. https://www.newharbinger.com/9781684035601/mindfulness-based-stress-reduction

Woodyard, C. D. (2011). Exploring the therapeutic effects of yoga and its ability to increase quality of life. *International Journal of Yoga, 4*(2), 49. doi:10.4103/0973-6131.85485 PMID:22022122

World Health Organization. (1993). *The ICD-10 classification of mental and behavioural disorders: Diagnostic criteria for research*. WHO.

World Health Organization. (2022). *Ageing and health*. WHO. https://www.who.int/news-room/fact-sheets/detail/ageing-and-health

Xiang, W., Chen, X., & Zhang, F. (2019). The Diffusion of Green Technology Innovation Based on Cloud Platform for Energy Saving. *Ekoloji Dergisi*, (107), 1641–1650.

Xu, W., Itagi, R. K., & Thaiyar, M. S. (2021). Impact of yama and niyama on psychospiritual factors in young adults: A randomized controlled trial. *International Journal of Yoga - Philosophy Psychology and Parapsychology, 9*(1), 32. doi:10.4103/ijoyppp.ijoyppp_17_20

Xu, R. (2020). Analysis of the concept of self between Brahmanism and Buddhism. *In 5th International Conference on Contemporary Education, Social Sciences and Humanities-Philosophy of Being Human as the Core of Interdisciplinary Research (ICCESSH 2020)* (pp. 103–106). Atlantis Press. 10.2991/assehr.k.200901.021

Yadav, D. (2014a). *Ashtangahridaya: Vol. Sutra Sthana. Ch.13, Ver. 1-12*. Chaukhamba Surbharati Prakashan.

Yadav, D. (2014b). *Ashtangahridaya: Vol. Sutrasthana, Chapter 1, Ver. 6,20*. [Sanskrit]. Chaukhambha Subharati Prakashan.

Yusof, J. M., Zulkiffli, S. N. A., & Muda, M. S. (2016). The Influence Of Spiritual Leadership On Intention To Leave Of The Employees. *International Journal of Applied Business and Economic Research, 14*(9), 113–9124.

Zaki, S. (2022). Relevance of Sri Aurobindo's philosophy of education to national education policy 2020. *International Journal of Health Sciences, 6*(S3), 9601–9608. doi:10.53730/ijhs.v6nS3.8288

Zenger, J., & Folkman, J. (2016, May 23). 4 ways to be more effective at execution. *Harvard Business Review*. https://hbr.org/2016/05/4-ways-to-be-more-effective-at-execution

Zhang, D., Lee, K., Mák, E., Ho, C. Y., & Wong, S. Y. S. (2021). Mindfulness-based interventions: An overall review. *British Medical Bulletin, 138*(1), 41–57. doi:10.1093/bmb/ldab005 PMID:33884400

Zohar, D., & Marshall, I. (2000). *SQ: Spiritual intelligence, the ultimate intelligence*. Bloomsbury Publishing.

About the Contributors

Anuradha Sathiyaseelan is currently a Professor of Psychology for Christ University.

Sathiyaseelan Balasundaram is currently a Professor of Psychology for Christ University.

***

Cheena Agrawal was born in 2004 in Sendhwa, Madhya Pradesh. Cheena Agrawal is an undergrad student in the 3rd year of IPM (Integrated Programme in Management) at IIM BodhGaya. Her research interest lies in mindfulness, sustainability, HRM.

Raghu Ananthanarayanan is a behavioural scientist, yoga teacher and author. He has dedicated his life to the study and application of Yoga and Indic traditions to guide the inner transformation of individuals and shape leadership and culture building of organizations. Formally trained as an engineer with an MS in Bio-Medical Engineering from IIT, Madras, Raghu has co-founded many organizations focused on inner transformation and its application in a variety of fields. He has also authored many books and papers on Yoga, Inner transformation and Organizational Alignment. Currently, his wife Sashi and he, donning their role as Chief Mentors are working on nurturing people on a Sacred Quest at Rithambara Ashram, situated in the beautiful Nilagiris.

Elif Baykal is Assoc. Prof. at Istanbul Meidpol University. She has graduated from Bosphorus University in 2006. She has an MBA degree from Istanbul Medipol University and she has a PHD degree from Yıldız Technical University. She is teaching Management and Organisation. She has several work about Leadership, Family Firms, Positive Organizational Behavior and Workplace Spirituality.

Vijayabanu C. is currently Professor at the School of Management, SASTRA University in India. She obtained her Ph.D. in Commerce-Human Resource Management in 2000 at Bharathidasan University, India. Her current research interests focus on the areas of behavioral studies –Personality, Perception: attitudes & values . She handles courses such as Human Resource Management, organizational behaviour, and specialization courses such as Change Management, Training & Development, etc. She brings to her classes enriched knowledge of 5 years of Research & 16 years of academic experience. She has produced 5 doctoral scholars successfully and currently Guiding 2 Ph.D. scholars. She has presented papers at international and national level conferences and seminars.She has published several research articles and case studies in referred Scopus-indexed journals. She has served on the Editorial Review

Boards of several academic journals, including Business theory and practice, the Journal of Management Social Science and Humanities and the Journal of Business Economics and Management

Shreya Chawla is a Research Scholar at CHRIST (Deemed to be University). She is pursuing her research in Behavioural Intervention Technology.Her research comprises of Positive Psychology . She qualified for UGC NET in 2022 .She has earlier worked in Vallbhbhai Patel Chest Institute, Delhi University as a counselor for a project under MoH&Fw.

Noa Feuerstein is a practicing clinical psychologist and a Jungian analyst, with 30 years of experience. Studied M.A. in clinical Psychology in Bar Ilan University, and M.A. studies in Comparative religions and Indian studies at the Hebrew University, Israel. She is teaching and supervising in several schools and institute: at the 'Israeli Institute for Jungian Psychology', 'The School for Psychotherapy' in the Hebrew University counselling services, 'The school for Jungian advanced studies' at Bar Ilan University, and the 'Bi-National (Israeli-Palestinian) School for Psychotherapy', Hadassah Hospital, Jerusalem. An upcoming project is a book titled: "On Horror and Beyond: C.G. Jung's Relation to India and Upanishadic Wisdom" in which she relives the disrupted dialogue Jung had with the East, by rereading the Upanishadic literature in light of Jung's insights, answering his reservations, and opening a dialogue between the Upaniṣadic sage Yājñavalkya and Jung. In the last 4 years, she is involved with the Ritambhara Ashram, practicing inner work through intense Yoga Sutra study, and immersing in Indian itihasa (mythology). Co-moderating with Raghu Ananthanarayanan's process of Mytho-Drama, exploring the power of myth in the process of healing traumatic wounds and fostering inner transformation and enabling the process of individuation.

Madhu Giri is a licensed Clinical Psychologist, and she earned her M.phi lin Clinical Psychology from Gautam Buddha University. Driven by an unwavering commitment to make a lasting impact, Madhu Giri embarked on her doctoral journey at the Department of Psychology, Christ University, India. Under the guidance of esteemed mentors, she delved into the uncharted territories of positive psychology, exploring the profound effects of gratitude and mindfulness on mental well-being. As a JRF at the Department of Psychology, Christ University, Madhu plays a pivotal role in fostering a culture of academic excellence. Her multifaceted responsibilities include conducting independent research, assisting in teaching undergraduate and postgraduate courses, and providing counseling to help students to strive through their academic journey. She is widely regarded as a compassionate mentor, offering guidance and support to students eager to embark on their own journeys of discovery.

Ayush Gupta was born in 2002 in Kanpur, Uttar Pradesh. Ayush Gupta is an undergrad student in the 3rd year of IPM (Integrated Programme in Management) at IIM Bodhgaya. His research interests lie in hrm, ob, well-being, mental health, and mindfulness.

Sreenath. K has a Ph.D. from Bharathiar University, Coimbatore. His doctoral thesis focused on 'Enhancing Resilience through Mindfulness Intervention Program' and addressed various psychosocial issues associated with HIV-infected-adults. He has completed an introductory course in Yoga. He has also completed an online course on 'Mindfulness in Integrative Healthcare' authorized by University of Minnesota through Coursera. He was part of the extension service provided by Christ University for HIV-infected adolescents at Snehagram Vocational and Rehabilitation Centre, Krishnagiri, Tamil

Nadu. As part of the project, he has facilitated sessions on mindfulness meditation for adolescents living with HIV. He has attended the Training of Trainers workshop on Life Skills Education at Kristu Jayanti College, Bangalore. He is the coordinator of the Ph. D. program in the Dept. of Psychology at Christ University. He has published various articles in national and international journals and recently published on 'Development and Psychometric Validation of three dimensional Grit scale.' Areas of Expertise: Resilience, Yoga, Grit, Community Interventions, Review of Literature.

Bishal Patangia is a Post Graduate Student of Psychology, specialised in Human Resource Development Management at Christ University. Aspiring Public Health Practitioner, focusing on Maternal and Child Health Epidemiology.

Shashwat Ranjan is currently associated with the Indian Institute of Management Raipur as a research scholar in HRM/OB. He has his research interest in mindfulness, spirituality and value-based workplace. Shashwat has presented his work at reputed Indian conferences like the Indian Academy of Management. He is also keenly interested in the psychological aspects of work-life and the workplace.

Soumya R.R. is an Assistant Professor of Psychology.

Damini Saini is associated with IIM Raipur as an Assistant Professor in OB/HRM. She is also a key editorial member for the Journal of Applied Research in Higher Education. Dr Saini received her PhD from the prestigious Faculty of Management Studies, University of Delhi. Her research is in ethical leadership, the spiritual climate of business, and positive psychology. Recognition of her research comes from the best paper awards conferred to her work thrice. Apart from this, her scholarly interests are leadership, business ethics, the significance of ethical education in management, value-based management etc. She has contributed to various internationally acclaimed journals and book chapters. She has also actively taken part in various conferences and seminars.

Sandhya Shankar holds a doctorate from the Jawaharlal Nehru University for research with UGC-JRF in the field of Psycholinguistics. It concentrated on the cognition of time in children. Her graduation was in Elementary Education from Delhi University. The course was an integrative study of human development, subject knowledge and communication skills. She pursued her M.A. in Linguistics, with courses including semantics and developmental psycholinguistics. She has published various articles in journals and books apart from presenting papers in both national and international conferences. Her expertise lies in Language Acquisition and Pedagogy, Wellness and Language and Culture and language.

Ranjit Singha is a Doctorate Research Fellow at Christ (Deemed to be University) and a distinguished American Psychological Association (APA) member. His expertise lies in research and development across various domains, including Mindfulness, Addiction Psychology, Women Empowerment, UN Sustainable Development Goals, and Data Science. He has earned certifications from renowned institutions, including IBM and The University of Oxford Mindfulness Centre, UK, in Mindfulness. Additionally, he holds certifications as a Microsoft Innovative Educator, Licensed Yoga Professional, Certified Mindfulness Teacher, and CBCT Teachers Training from Emory University, USA. Mr Ranjit's educational qualifications include PGDBA (GM), MBA (IB), MSc in Counseling Psychology, and completion of a Senior Diploma in Tabla (Musical Instrumentation). His dedication to continuous learning is evident through his involvement in the SEE Learning® (Social, Emotional, and Ethical) Learning program. As a committed researcher and educator, Mr Ranjit focuses on mindfulness and compassion-based interventions. He has an impressive publication record, having authored twenty-three research papers, ten chapters, four books, and five edited books. His research interests encompass various aspects of mindfulness, such as assessment, benefits of mindfulness-based programs, change mechanisms, professional training, mindfulness ethics, cognitive and neuropsychology, and studies related to high-risk behaviours. Apart from his research endeavours, Mr Ranjit has extensive teaching experience, instructing courses in diverse subjects like Forensic Psychology, Positive Psychology, Organizational Planning, Strategic Management, Psycho Metric Tests, Counseling Skills, Disaster Management, Basic Computer Science, Business Planning, Business Law, and Auditing. He has mentored numerous Postgraduate and undergraduate research projects, demonstrating his commitment to nurturing young minds in psychology. Ad Hoc Reviewer at International Journal of Cyber Behavior, Psychology and Learning (IJCBPL), Reviewer and author at IGI Global, and Editor and Reviewer at TNT Publication. Furthermore, Mr Ranjit actively provides personal counselling services, showcasing his genuine concern for his students' well-being and academic success. His unwavering dedication to research and education has solidified his position as a valuable contributor to psychology.

Surjit Singha is an academician with a broad spectrum of interests, including UN Sustainable Development Goals, Organizational Climate, Workforce Diversity, Organizational Culture, HRM, Marketing, Finance, IB, Global Business, Business, AI, Women Studies, and Cultural Studies. Currently a faculty member at Kristu Jayanti College, Dr. Surjit also serves as an Editor, reviewer, and author for prominent global publications and journals, including being on the Editorial review board of Information Resources Management Journal and a contributor to IGI Global. With over 13 years of experience in Administration, Teaching, and Research, Dr. Surjit is dedicated to imparting knowledge and guiding students in their research pursuits. As a research mentor, Dr. Surjit has nurtured young minds and fostered academic growth. Dr. Surjit has an impressive track record of over 75 publications, including articles, book chapters, and textbooks, holds two US Copyrights, and has successfully completed and published two fully funded minor research projects from Kristu Jayanti College.

Vishaka Venkat has a Ph.D. from National Institute of Technology, Trichy, for her research on 'Theorising the Language of Humour in Indian Political Cartoons'. She has also specifically researched the concept of hāsya and the Indian traditions of humour. Her primary research interests include humour, Indian aesthetics, Shaktic traditions and mythology. Currently, she is researching about the Shaktic traditions in Kerala Devi temples.

Index

P

R

S

T

W

Y

www.ingramcontent.com/pod-product-compliance
Lightning Source LLC
LaVergne TN
LVHW060420300926
849162LV00006B/1480